SBAs and EMQs for MRCOG II

Chinmayee Ratha · Janesh Gupta

SBAs and EMQs for MRCOG II

Addressing the New Exam Format

🐎 Springer

Chinmayee Ratha
Fetal Medicine
Rainbow Hospitals
Hyderabad, Telangana, India

Janesh Gupta
University of Birmingham
Birmingham Women's Hospital
Birmingham, UK

ISBN 978-81-322-2687-1   ISBN 978-81-322-2689-5   (eBook)
DOI 10.1007/978-81-322-2689-5

Library of Congress Control Number: 2016931419

Springer New Delhi Heidelberg New York Dordrecht London

Printed on acid-free paper

Springer (India) Pvt. Ltd. is part of Springer Science+Business Media (www.springer.com)

Foreword

The MRCOG Part II exam is a clinical exam consisting of two parts. The first part is a written assessment of two papers each consisting of single best answer (SBA) questions and extended matching questions (EMQ), each with 50 SBAs and 50 EMQs in a 3 h paper. SBAs are worth 40 % and EMQs are worth 60 % of the total mark. The reason for this spread is that EMQs contain a wide coverage and test *clinical* judgement. Evidence supports that it is the fairest format for testing and is based on standard practice in the UK. It is a requirement to pass the written paper before proceeding to the second OSCE assessment phase. This format is going to change in September 2016 when the written paper will be separated as a Part II exam, and if successful the candidate will be allowed to keep this pass and only have to repeat the Part III OSCE exam as required. The level of the MRCOG exam is equivalent to the UK ST5 level. At this level a ST5 specialist registrar should have the degree of knowledge to be able to effectively have good clinical management skills based on the best evidence available for managing patients, both in obstetrics and gynaecology. The MRCOG Part II written and OSCE exams are blueprinted against a comprehensive syllabus which is available on the RCOG website (https://www.rcog.org.uk/en/careers-training/mrcog-exams/part-2-mrcog/syllabus/).

In preparation for the Part II exam, it is important to go through the specified syllabus, but the candidate should acquire knowledge of UK practice by reading all Green Top RCOG Guidelines, National Institute of Clinical Excellence (NICE) Guidelines, Scottish Intercollegiate Guidelines Network (SIGN) Guidelines, Good Practice Series and Scientific Statements from the Royal College. Further broad reading should be specifically *The Obstetrician & Gynaecologist* (TOG) journal, Progress Series by Studd, *Recent Advances in Obstetrics and Gynaecology* by Bonnar and *Obstetrics, Gynaecology and Reproductive Medicine* journal, which is a monthly publication providing a great revision guide for MRCOG candidates which includes sample SBA and EMQ questions. All previous reports from MBRRACE-UK ('Mothers and Babies: Reducing Risk through Audits and Confidential Enquiries across the UK') should be read. Past exam papers from the Royal College should also be practiced.

In essence the MRCOG Part II exam incorporates what a standard ST5 level specialist registrar would do on a 'day-to-day' basis of managing patients in UK hospitals. The disadvantage for non-UK graduates is that they do not have the level of exposure that the UK candidate would have in 'living and breathing' the way that patients are clinically managed. In this context non-UK candidates find 'difficult' areas such as clinical governance, risk management, clinical audit and research which are almost certain to be included in the written and OSCE exams.

As the MRCOG Part II exam is a heavily clinical biased exam, all aspects of management plans in line with clinical guidelines should be discussed with senior colleagues on a regular basis. Further, an additional good source of information can be useful from making 'hot dates' with neonatologists, bereavement counsellors, birthing centre midwives who deal with low-risk pregnancies, patient liaison services (PALS) managers who deal with patient complaints, oncology register office staff to understand how follow-up of oncology patients are organised, and attending multidisciplinary team (MDT) meetings and clinical audit meetings.

We hope that our book, which is blueprinted against the MRCOG syllabus, and written by authors who have recently been successful candidates, will help you understand how the Part II written paper is set and allow you to practice the wide range of possible questions that are derived from specific sources to which we have given the reference. There is a short explanation for the correct answer, and we have done this as far as possible throughout the book. We hope the book will also show you the wide breath of information you need to acquire to be successful in the exam. This book should also help in preparation for the OSCE exam, which is however not specifically covered in this book. We wish you all the very best in being successful, but ultimately the aim in preparing and doing the exam is that you will put into practice all the knowledge you accumulate in preparation for the MRCOG Part II exam to better the outcomes for your patients. That is in effect the ultimate aim. Good luck!

31 July 2015

Chinmayee Ratha
Janesh Gupta

Acknowledgements

This book is a result of a passion and effort put in towards preparing a comprehensive resource for candidates taking the part 2 MRCOG exam. The attempt has been to cover almost all general and subspecialty areas in obstetrics and gynaecology. The authors wish to specially acknowledge the contributions of some colleagues who provided extremely valuable inputs and helped framing questions in subspecialties. The contributions are from Dr Akanksha Sood, Sushma Hospital and Women Care Centre, Palampur, HP, India; Dr Anbu Subbian, Gynaecologic Oncology, Shankara Cancer Hospital and Research Centre & Sakra World Hospital, Bengaluru, KA, India; Dr Baljinder Kaur Chohan, ST5 O&G, Wexham Park Hospital, Slough, UK; Dr.Cecilia McKee, Northern Deanery, Royal Victoria Infirmary, Newcastle Upon Tyne, UK; Dr. Lauren Cowley University of Birmingham, Birmingham, UK; Dr Rohan Chodankar, SPR Obstetrics and Gynaecology, Frimley Park NHS Foundation Trust, Camberley, UK; and Dr Sushama Gupta, Obstetrics and Gynaecology, Birmingham Women's Hospital, Birmingham, UK, are particularly acknowledged. Their inputs provided multidimensionality in thought processes, and it is due to their contribution that the book appears to meaningfully cover most of the syllabus for the part 2 exam.

Contents

About the Authors

Dr. Chinmayee Ratha is the Lead Consultant of Fetal Medicine at Rainbow Hospitals, Hyderabad, India. She is the academic coordinator of the Department of Obstetrics and Gynecology in Rainbow Hospitals. She is an FMF (UK) approved trainer for Fetal Medicine and runs a clinical fellowship programme for subspecialty trainees in India. She has published papers in peer-reviewed, indexed journals and has received the FOGSI young author award in 2008 for the best publication in the *Journal of Obstetrics and Gynecology of India*. Her thesis paper on preeclampsia was awarded the CS Dawn Gold medal in 2003. She has received several prizes for presentations of research projects and audits at various state, national and international seminars.

Dr. Janesh Gupta is a Professor of Obstetrics and Gynaecology in the Institute of Metabolism and Systems Research, University of Birmingham Medical School and a Honorary Clinical Consultant at Birmingham Women's Hospital. He is a Consultant Obstetrician and Gynaecologist since 1995, at 31 years of age. Prior to this, he was the Consultant Obstetrician and Gynaecologist in the Department of Obstetrics and Gynaecology, Ninewells Hospital and Medical School, Dundee, Scotland, for 3 years (from 1995–1998). He has published over 150 research papers in scientific journals as well as reviews and book chapters in the fields of fetal medicine, benign gynaecology (including abnormal uterine bleeding, fibroids, endometriosis, endometrial hyperplasia) and minimal access surgery. He is an Editor-in-Chief for the *European Journal of Obstetrics and Gynecology and Reproductive Biology* (EJOG).

Abbreviations

ACE	Angiotensin-converting enzyme
ARBs	Angiotensin receptor blockers
CRL	Crown rump length
DHEAS	Dehydroepiandrostenedione
DSR	Daily symptom report
EOCs	Epithelial ovarian cancers
FGM	Female genital mutilation
FHR	Fetal heart rate
GBS	Group B streptococcus
GGT	Gamma glutamyl transferase
GS	Gestational sac
IAP	Intrapartum antibiotic prophylaxis
Ig	Immunoglobulin
LMWH	Low molecular weight heparin
MBRRACE-UK	Mothers and babies: reducing risk through audits and confidential enquiries across the UK
PEG-IFN	Pegylated interferon
TBG	Thyroxine binding globulin
THL	Transvaginal hydrolaparoscopy

Introduction

The MRCOG Part II exam is primarily designed along clinical care scenarios that test factual knowledge of the candidate as well as its practical application. The exam is based on fundamental principles of striving to provide exemplary patient care that incorporate safe practice on the basis of sound evidence. This means that success in the examination will depend on understanding the latest clinical guidelines, high-quality research articles and systematic reviews on the various subject areas. The implementation of such evidence should be evaluated through clinical audit and ensuring that best practice is done safely which is assessed through clinical governance.

This *MRCOG Part II* book is an elaborate collection of single best answer (SBA)-type questions and extended matching questions (EMQs) along with descriptive answers explaining the reasons supporting the correct alternative and excluding the distractors. Our aim is to familiarise the readers to this new pattern of questioning introduced in the membership exam from March 2015.

The exam is designed to revise your factual knowledge as well as clinical appli-cation. While reading the text you must take a moment and transpose a given fact into a clinically relevant situation and comprehend the exact answer to a given question.

Each question is designed such that it gets some important facts strongly ingrained in your mind. The distractors will help generate more inquisitiveness about the whole topic and drive you towards deeper learning.

The most productive way of using this book while preparing for the MRCOG II theory would be to practice the SBAs in this book on any one topic and then read up the given relevant reference documents. This will help you grasp the subtopics addressed in the question and will also orient you to other potential subtopics which can be presented as questions in your exam. Many questions are based on clinical case scenarios. Try and relate these situations to problems that you face in day-to-day clinical practice.

We have made an effort to cover as many varied topics as possible mapped against the MRCOG curriculum so as to provide an insight to the readers regarding potential questions.

These examinations aim at developing safe and sensitive doctors well equipped with evidence-based contemporary clinical practices and guidelines. The ultimate test of competence of any doctor is a combination of theoretical knowledge and practical application to everyday scenarios in a sensitive manner keeping the patient at the centre of the situation. This book will help you take few steps in preparing for such an assessment but more importantly allow you to put into practice what you have learned for this exam.

We wish you the best of luck for the future success in your career, remembering that this small step for being successful in the MRCOG exam will be a lifelong change in how you provide the best evidence-based clinical care for many patients in the future.

Chinmayee Ratha
Janesh Gupta

Part I

SBA: Type Questions

Antenatal Care: SBA Questions

1

ANC1

You are reviewing the notes of a 32-year-old woman in the antenatal clinic. She is 10 weeks pregnant based on her last period date and this is her third pregnancy. Her sons, aged 4 and 2 years, respectively, are fit and healthy. You are looking for risk factors to offer her screening for gestational diabetes. Which of the following conditions will you NOT offer her such screening:

A. Body mass index above 30 kg/m²
B. Family history of diabetes
C. Family origin with a high prevalence of diabetes
D. Previous macrosomic baby weighing 4.5 kg or above
E. Previous type 2 diabetes

ANC2

Q2. Commercial flights of more than 4 h duration are known to be associated with a small increase in the relative risk of:

A. Abruptio placentae
B. Antepartum depression
C. Deep vein thrombosis
D. Prelabour rupture of membranes
E. Preterm labour

© Springer India 2016
C. Ratha, J. Gupta, *SBAs and EMQs for MRCOG II*,
DOI 10.1007/978-81-322-2689-5_1

ANC3

Which antibiotics should be given to prevent early onset neonatal GBS disease to women who have accepted intrapartum antibiotic prophylaxis (IAP) and are allergic to benzylpenicillin?

A. Ampicillin
B. Clindamycin
C. Erythromycin
D. Gentamicin
E. Trimethoprim/sulfamethoxazole

ANC4

Placental abruption is seen more often in all of the following conditions except:

A. Chorioamnionitis
B. Multiple pregnancies
C. Pre-eclampsia
D. Primigravidae
E. Trauma

ANC5

The incidence of low-lying placenta in second trimester ultrasound scan is as high as:

A. 10 %
B. 15 %
C. 25 %
D. 35 %
E. 50 %

ANC6

You are preparing for the caesarean section of a multipara with central placenta previa. She is not anaemic, is haemodynamically stable and has never had any episode of vaginal bleeding. At least how many units of cross matched blood should be kept ready for use in anticipation of intraoperative blood loss?

A. 1 unit
B. 2 units
C. 3 units
D. 4 units
E. None required unless the woman has a Hb < 10 g/dL

ANC7

Women with complex social factors have been identified as those needing special provisions in their antenatal care. Which of the following pregnant women would be identified as one with a complex social factor that warrants special attention by the antenatal healthcare providers?

A. A 28-year-old primary school teacher who has recurrent migraine attacks
B. A 36-year-old housewife with previous two caesarean sections
C. A 42-year-old banker with a high paying but stressful job
D. An 18-year-old English woman who is the lead ballet dancer in a renowned troupe
E. An unmarried 38-year-old artist of Egyptian origin living legally with her partner in England for the last 12 years and running a successful boutique

ANC8

A 28-year-old woman is 22 weeks pregnant. She has long-standing type 1 diabetes mellitus. Her 20-week fetal anatomy ultrasound showed no structural fetal abnormalities. However, she is concerned about how her diabetes may cause congenital fetal anomalies in her unborn child.

Of the options listed below, which SINGLE action addresses her anxiety?

A. Amniocentesis at 22 weeks.
B. Fetal cardiac echocardiography at 24 weeks.
C. Obstetric ultrasound scan for growth and umbilical artery Doppler at 28, 32 and 36 weeks.
D. Offer reassurance as normal fetal anatomy survey at 20 weeks.
E. Quadruple maternal biochemical screening test (HCG, inhibin-A, oestriol, AFP) at 20 weeks.

ANC9

A 24-year-old woman is 12 weeks pregnant. She is attending hospital for her dating scan and routine booking serological investigations. Screening and treating for the presence of a particular pathogen during early pregnancy will reduce the risk of developing congenital fetal abnormality. Which of the pathogens listed below fulfils this criterion?

A. Hepatitis B
B. Herpes simplex virus
C. Rubella
D. Syphilis
E. Varicella zoster virus

ANC10

All pregnant women are advised to take folic acid supplements (0.4 mg, once daily) pre-pregnancy and antenatally. Nonetheless, which of the following groups of women is a dietary supplementation using a higher dose of folic acid (5 mg once daily) recommended?

A. BMI<30
B. Impaired glucose tolerance
C. Previous pre-eclampsia
D. Previous preterm delivery
E. Sickle cell disease

ANC11

All pregnant women are advised to take folic acid supplements (0.4 mg, once daily) pre-pregnancy and antenatally. Nonetheless, which of the following groups of women is a dietary supplementation using a higher dose of folic acid (5 mg once daily) recommended?

A. BMI<30
B. History of spina bifida in partner's family
C. Impaired glucose tolerance
D. Previous pre-eclampsia
E. Previous preterm delivery

ANC12

A 24-year-old woman is 22 weeks pregnant in her second pregnancy. She has had one previous caesarean delivery. Her routine 20-week obstetric ultrasound revealed a low-lying anterior placenta, partially covering the cervical os. Which SINGLE action is most appropriate?

A. Organise elective caesarean section for 39 weeks
B. Organise MRI pelvis at 32 weeks to check position of placenta.
C. Re-assess at 38 weeks and allow vaginal delivery to occur if fetal head is clinically engaged and there has been no antenatal bleeding.
D. Repeat ultrasound at 32 weeks to check position of placenta.
E. Repeat ultrasound at 38 weeks to check position of placenta.

ANC13

Which of the following is NOT a known risk factor for vasa previa:

A. Bilobed placenta
B. Placental photocoagulation
C. In vitro fertilisation
D. Multifetal pregnancy
E. Succenturiate lobes

ANC14

Drugs are prescribed in pregnancy upon the assumption that their positive effect on health outweighs the probability and severity of any harm to mother and fetus. On this basis, which of the following medications is the most likely to be contraindicated for antenatal use in pregnancy?

A. Indomethacin
B. Labetalol
C. Low-dose aspirin
D. Low molecular weight heparin
E. Metformin

ANC15

A pregnant woman is seeking advice about the effects of smoking in pregnancy. Which of the following statements is correct in relation to pregnancy risks as a consequence of her smoking during pregnancy?

A. Decreased risk of abruption
B. Increased risk of gestational diabetes
C. Increased risk of pre-eclampsia
D. Increased risk of sudden infant death syndrome (SIDS)
E. No effect on the risk of preterm delivery

ANC16

A 20-year-old woman is 33 weeks pregnant in her first pregnancy. She has a 6-h history of regular painful uterine contractions. Clinical examination confirms an appropriately sized fetus, longitudinal lie and cephalic presentation with normal fetal heart rate (155 bpm). Vaginal examination identifies a fully effaced cervix that is 5 cm dilated, with intact membranes. Which of the following is an appropriate next intervention step?

A. Administer i.m betamethasone.
B. Commence i.v. atosiban.
C. Commence oral nifedipine.
D. Insert cervical cerclage.
E. Recommend emergency caesarean section.

ANC17

A 20-year-old woman is 36 weeks pregnant in her first pregnancy and is being reviewed in the antenatal clinic. A recent obstetric growth scan confirms breech presentation of a normally grown fetus with normal liquor volume. She has no other complicating medical or obstetric disorders. She is deciding between planned vaginal or elective caesarean (LSCS) modes of delivery. Which of the following is correct in relation to the counselling she will receive?

A. External cephalic version (ECV) may be offered and has around a 50 % success rate for conversion to cephalic presentation.
B. Footling breech presentation is considered favourable for vaginal breech delivery.
C. If opting for vaginal breech delivery, induction of labour at 38 weeks is recommended to avoid excessive fetal growth.
D. Intermittent fetal heart rate monitoring is recommended for spontaneous onset vaginal breech labour.
E. LSCS and vaginal breech birth have similar rates of perinatal mortality and early neonatal morbidity.

ANC18

If the fetal crown rump length is disparate in twins at the 12 weeks scan, select the best method of dating the pregnancy.
   Gestation is age can be allotted according to:

A. Average CRL of the two foetuses.
B. CRL of the bigger fetus.
C. CRL of the smaller fetus.
D. CRL of the smaller fetus added to half the CRL of the bigger fetus.
E. Dating is best done by LMP in such cases.

ANC19

Screening for anemia in triplet pregnancy is advised at:

A. Booking, 20–24 weeks and 28 weeks
B. Booking, 20–24 weeks

C. Booking, 28 weeks and 34 weeks
D. Booking, 28 weeks
E. Booking, 26 weeks

ANC20

A 34-year-old primigravida with dichorionic twins, both fetuses in cephalic presentation, declines the offer of elective delivery at 37 weeks of gestation. You have explained to her that with uncomplicated dichorionic twin pregnancies, elective birth from 37 weeks 0 days does not appear to be associated with an increased risk of serious adverse outcomes and that continuing uncomplicated twin pregnancies beyond 38 weeks 0 days increases the risk of fetal death. What is the next step in her antenatal care?

A. Document her decision and allow pregnancy to continue for reassessment at term or when she sets into labour spontaneously, whichever is earlier.
B. Document her decision and call twice weekly for biophysical profile assessment.
C. Document her decision and call weekly for biophysical profile assessment.
D. Document her decision and take informed consent for risk of adverse outcome.
E. Refer her to another centre as the outcome is likely to be poor.

ANC21

A primigravida with twin pregnancy has booked for antenatal care at 16 weeks of gestation. Despite referral to higher centre, the chorionicity of the pregnancy could not be established by ultrasound. Fetal growth is within normal range and there are no obvious structural defects. What is the best option for further antenatal management in this case?

A. Amniocentesis to determine fetal karyotyping.
B. Chorionic villous sampling for fetal genotyping.
C. Empirically manage as dichorionic twins as this is commoner.
D. Empirically manage as monochorionic twins.
E. Offer her an MRI which will help establish chorionicity.

ANC22

With regard to advice about diet, lifestyle and nutritional supplements in multiple pregnancy, which of the following is correct?

A. Women with twins and triplets should be offered twice the dosage of supplements and asked to take an extra 220 cal per day.

B. Women with twins should take an extra 220 cal per day with twice the dosage of supplements while women with triplets 330 extra calories per day with thrice the dosage of supplements.
C. Women with twins should take an extra 220 cal per day with twice the dosage of supplements while women with triplets 330 extra calories per day with twice the dosage of supplements.
D. Women with twins and triplets should take an extra 220 cal per day with twice the dosage of supplements.
E. Women with twins and triplets should take the same diet and nutritional supplements as women with singletons.

ANC23

Ultrasound screening for structural anomalies in the second trimester of pregnancy:

A. Is optimally offered between 15 week 0 day and 20 week 0 day
B. Can be used for ruling out diagnosis of Down syndrome
C. Can be used to diagnose inborn errors of metabolism
D. Is more sensitive in women with high BMI
E. Involves echocardiography with four chamber view of heart and outflow tract routinely

ANC24

A 32-year-old second gravida at 16 weeks of gestation is about to take a long haul flight to attend a family get together. Her previous pregnancy was generally uneventful but she had a caesarean section at term due to breech presentation of the fetus. Which of the following conditions is not a contraindication for her air travel in pregnancy?

A. Haemorrhage in previous pregnancy
B. Otitis media and sinusitis
C. Recent gastrointestinal surgery
D. Recent sickling crisis
E. Severe anaemia with haemoglobin less than 7.5 g/dl

ANC25

Pregnant women with singleton pregnancies should be offered screening for anemia:

A. At booking only
B. At booking and 24 weeks

C. At booking at 26 weeks
D. At booking and 28 weeks
E. Only if there is family history of haemoglobinopathies

ANC26

The recommended dose of vitamin D supplementation for women in pregnancy and lactation is:

A. 2.5 µg/day
B. 5 µg/day
C. 7.5 µg/day
D. 10 µg/da
E. 12.5 µg/day

ANC27

In the recent "Mothers and Babies: Reducing Risk through Audits and Confidential Enquiries across the UK" (MBRRACE-UK) report, it was recommended that all women with medical disorders in pregnancy should have access to a coordinated multidisciplinary obstetric and medical clinic, thereby avoiding the need to attend multiple appointments and poor communication between senior specialists responsible for their care.

For women with pre-existing medical conditions, the ideal time for planning multidisciplinary care in pregnancy is:

A. First trimester before confirmation of fetal viability
B. First trimester after confirmation of fetal viability
C. Pre-pregnancy
D. Second trimester after screening for lethal fetal anomalies
E. Third trimester prior to confinement for delivery

ANC28

You are seeing a pregnant woman with trichorionic triplet pregnancy during her routine antenatal visit at 16 weeks. You are coordinating with a core team of midwives and sonographers for her care. You are also planning an enhanced team for referrals. You will routinely include all of the following in that team except:

A. Cardiologist
B. Dietician
C. Infant feeding specialist

D. Perinatal mental health specialist
E. Women's health physiotherapist

ANC29

Routine folic acid supplementation is advised to all pregnant women ideally starting pre-pregnancy and continuing upto 12 weeks of gestation. The advantages established with this supplementation are all of the following except:

A. Reduced risk of cardiovascular defects
B. Reduced risk of childhood asthma
C. Reduced risk of limb defects
D. Reduced risk of leukemia and pediatric brain tumors
E. Reduced risk of neural tube defects

ANC30

A pregnant woman at 26 weeks of gestation presents with minimal painless bleeding following sexual intercourse. She is haemodynamically stable and has had no such episodes in the past. Which of the following confirms the diagnosis of placenta previa?

A. Abnormal lie of the fetus with high presenting part.
B. Speculum examination showing healthy cervix and vagina and confirming bleeding through os.
C. Spongy tissue felt during per vaginal digital examination
D. Tightening of the abdomen during clinical examination
E. Ultrasound scan showing placenta inserted in the lower uterine segment

ANC31

You are about to counsel a woman with major placenta previa at 32 weeks who has just had a repeat scan for placental localisation. The ultrasound scan shows an anterior placenta covering the internal os with irregular retroplacental sonolucent zone and hypervascularity in serosa-bladder interface. Fetal parameters are appropriate for gestational age. She had her previous caesarean section for breech presentation 4 years back and has not had any episodes of bleeding in this pregnancy. What is the most appropriate course of action?

A. Immediate caesarean section.
B. Immediate MRI as it will definitively diagnose or rule out placenta accrete.
C. Plan for elective caesarean at term with appropriate precautions for placenta acreta.

D. Plan caesarean hysterectomy.
E. Rescan for placental localisation at 36 weeks as in a majority of cases; there is upward migration of placenta due to development of the lower uterine segment.

ANC32

You are seeing a 30-year-old primigravida at her booking visit. Her sister had deep vein thrombosis in her legs last year and suffered much pain and discomfort. She has heard that pregnancy increases risk for venous thrombosis and wants you to address her concern. What is the most appropriate action to take?

A. Heparin
B. Low-dose aspirin
C. Reassure
D. Test for thrombophilias
E. Warfarin

ANC33

Which of the following statements does not agree with the recommendations given by NICE for the routine antenatal care of pregnant women in the UK?

A. At the very first contact with a healthcare professional, information about folic acid supplementation, food hygiene, lifestyle advice and all antenatal screening, including screening for haemoglobinopathies, the anomaly scan and screening for Down's syndrome, as well as risks and benefits of the screening tests must be given.
B. Information about antenatal screening should not be given in group settings as it significantly hampers her privacy.
C. Information should be given in a form that is easy to understand and accessible to pregnant women with additional needs, such as physical, sensory or learning disabilities, and to pregnant women who do not speak or read English.
D. Options for management of prolonged pregnancy should be discussed at 38 weeks antenatal visit.
E. Women's decisions should be respected, even when this is contrary to the views of the healthcare professional.

ANC34

You are seeing a Somalian woman in her first pregnancy at 24 weeks of gestation. She has migrated to UK 5 years back with her husband. You are worried about the possibility of female genital mutilation.

What would be an appropriate approach to this case?

A. A preformatted sheet with pre-drawn diagrams should never be used.
B. If she volunteers the history of FGM, you should inform her sensitively that she must have an elective LSCS.
C. In case she confirms history of genital mutilation, a psychological assessment should be made.
D. If you find in her case notes a confirmation of a reversal of genital mutilation by defibulation, then it is reassuring and no further assessment in this regard is warranted.
E. You should refrain from asking about genital mutilation procedures as this is considered rude and may hurt the feelings of the woman.

ANC35

A 17-year-old college student has discovered that she is pregnant possibly because she was irregular with the COCPs she was taking for the last year. By her dates, she is expected to be 9 weeks pregnant. She plans to complete her education and settle down with her partner after few years. She is however not willing to terminate the pregnancy due to strong religious beliefs and would like to book for antenatal care.
    Which of the following will not be appropriate in your counselling?

A. Advise screening for sexually transmitted infections.
B. Explain to her that teenage pregnancy is associated with a high risk of adverse pregnancy outcome in the adolescent and has been attributed to gynaecological immaturity and the growth and nutritional status of the mother.
C. Offer her social services support to plan for delivery and child care.
D. Reassure her that with proper nutritional supplements and regular antenatal care, her pregnancy outcome can be reasonably optimised.
E. Try and convince her sensitively for a termination as you don't think the case situation has a good prognosis anyway.

ANC36

All of the following are known complications of anemia in pregnancy except:

A. Impaired psychomotor and/or mental development in infants
B. Increased childhood cardiometabolic risk factors
C. Low birth weight babies
D. Placental abruption
E. Preterm labour

ANC37

A 35-year-old rhesus-negative woman is pregnant for the third time. Her first child is 5 years old and has a rhesus-positive blood group. During her second pregnancy 2 years back, she was found to be rhesus isoimmunised and lost her baby due to hydrops fetalis at 24 weeks. She subsequently had a divorce and is now remarried and pregnant for the third time. Her pregnancy test at home was positive yesterday and she has come to seek advice for further care. Which is the most important investigation in this clinical situation that will affect the plan of antenatal care in this pregnancy?

A. Maternal anti-D antibody levels
B. Maternal blood group/rhesus typing
C. Maternal blood test for cffDNA
D. Maternal haemoglobin level
E. Paternal blood group/rhesus typing

ANC38

Based on the latest NICE recommendations for routine antenatal care of pregnant women in the UK, the number of appointments for pregnancy checkups in an uncomplicated pregnancy should be:

A. 9 for multipara and 8 for nullipara
B. 9 for nullipara and 8 for multipara
C. 10 for multipara and 7 for nullipara
D. 10 for nullipara and 7 for multipara
E. 10 for nullipara and 9 for multipara

ANC39

The commonest pathogen causing ascending genital tract infection following delivery of any type (miscarriage/abortion, termination, caesarean section, vaginal delivery) is:

A. Anaerobic bacteria
B. Amoeba
C. Chlamydia
D. Group A streptococcus
E. Group B streptococcus

ANC40

Which of the following statements regarding air travel in pregnancy is false?

A. Haemoglobin level less than 7.5 g/dl is contraindication to commercial air travel.
B. The increased cosmic radiation exposure associated with flying is not considered significant in terms of risk to mother or fetus for occasional flights.
C. The key change in environment associated with commercial air travel is cabin humidity.
D. There is 18 % increased risk of venous thromboembolism for each 2 h increase in flight duration.
E. There is no increased risk of complications in air travel in early pregnancy.

ANC41

A 30-year-old primigravida comes to the antenatal clinic at 14 weeks of gestation complaining of off and on shortness of breath such that she "needs to take a long breath". On examination she is stable with adequate air entry in both lung field and no abnormal sounds. There is no associated pallor. What will you explain to her regarding her condition?

A. About 50 % of normal pregnant women will have dyspnea before 19 weeks of gestation
B. Effects of maternal oestrogen on the respiratory centre can cause this problem.
C. Even if there is no underlying disease, this is likely to increase risk for complications during pregnancy, labour and delivery.
D. Maternal PaO2 normally decreases in pregnancy.
E. She is most likely having early stages of asthma and hence needs to see a pulmonologist urgently.

ANC42

Which of the following statements regarding physiological blood pressure changes in pregnancy is incorrect?

A. Blood pressure begins to decrease in early pregnancy and reaches a nadir at 18–20 weeks following which there is a steady rise till term.
B. Blood pressure taken in supine position during second and third trimesters of pregnancy is lower than that taken in sitting position
C. PhaseV (disappearance) rather than phase IV (muffling) of Korotkoff sounds should be taken as the diastolic reading.

D. Previously normotensive women may become transiently hypertensive following delivery.
E. Vasodilatation is the primary change in circulation in pregnancy.

ANC43

What percentage of the cardiac output is received by the gravid uterus at term pregnancy?

A. 2 %
B. 5 %
C. 10 %
D. 20 %
E. 25 %

ANC44

A 34-year-old second gravida reports to the antenatal clinic with respiratory difficulty at 28 weeks of gestation. Apart from the mechanical effects of pregnancy on her respiratory organs, her symptoms are worsened by increased oxygen consumption in the fetoplacental unit and increased respiratory drive. The substance that increases in pregnancy leading to increased respiratory drive is:

A. Aldosterone
B. Caffeine
C. Progesterone
D. Serotonin
E. Thyroxine

ANC45

A 26-year-old primigravida reports to the antenatal clinic at 32 weeks of gestation with symptoms of tingling, burning pain, numbness and a swelling sensation in her left hand. You have made a diagnosis of carpal tunnel syndrome. What is the most appropriate fact that you will you tell her about her condition?

A. Antenatal corticosteroids must be administered for fetal lung maturity.
B. Carpal tunnel syndrome is a rare condition affecting less than 4 % of pregnancies.
C. Carpal tunnel syndrome results from compression of the ulnar nerve.
D. There may be compromise of the motor function of the hand.
E. Treatment of carpal tunnel syndrome is surgical release of compressed nerve.

ANC46

You are explaining the role of vitamin supplements in pregnancy to a 30-year-old primigravida in her booking visit. Which of the following statements is true regarding the role of Vitamin B6 in pregnancy?

A. It increases homocysteine levels in pregnancy.
B. Levels increase physiologically in the third trimester of pregnancy.
C. It reduces nausea and vomiting and early pregnancy.
D. It reduces dental decay in pregnant women.
E. Routine supplementation in pregnant women is recommended in early pregnancy.

ANC47

A 26-year-old X-ray technician is pregnant and you are seeing her at her booking visit. She is 8 weeks pregnant now and has confirmed her pregnancy recently. She uses the standard safety guidelines at work but is concerned about ionising radiation exposure to her fetus. The most appropriate advice that you can give her in this regard is:

A. Her baby will receive about 1 mSv from sources of natural radiation during pregnancy. The added exposure at work should be no more than this and in practice is likely to be considerably less.
B. It is a legal requirement that she must wear an active dose meter at all times.
C. Lead aprons can be avoided as they can be uncomfortable and lead to back pain.
D. She is legally bound inform her employer about her pregnancy in writing as soon as possible.
E. X-rays affect milk production and she is at high risk of lactation failure

ANC48

For gestational age assessment of the fetus in early pregnancy, it is recommended that crown rump length be used for dating. Once the CRL exceeds 84 mm, it is recommended that dating be based on measurement of:

A. Abdominal circumference
B. Femur length
C. Head circumference
D. Humerus length
E. Transcerebellar diameter

ANC49

According to the latest maternal mortality report, "Mothers and Babies: Reducing Risk through Audits and Confidential Enquiries across the UK" (MBRRACE-UK) 2014, the rate of maternal deaths in the UK per 100,000 women giving births is:

A. 8
B. 9
C. 10
D. 11
E. 12

ANC50

You are explaining the plan of antenatal care to a woman who has come for a booking visit. Her last menstrual period was about 9 weeks back and she had a positive urine pregnancy test last week. You will offer her an ultrasound scan between 10 weeks and 13 weeks and 6 days for the following reason:

A. Detecting fetal cardiac defects
B. Detecting twin to twin transfusion in case she has MC twins
C. Reducing the incidence of induction of labour for prolonged pregnancy
D. Screening for fetal anemia
E. Screening for congenital infections

ANC51

Registrar on call receives a phone call from a GP regarding a patient, 24 weeks pregnant in her first pregnancy. She has developed chicken pox rash since one day.
    What is the most appropriate advice she should be given?

A. Antibiotics to prevent secondary bacterial infection.
B. Referred to the hospital.
C. She should receive varicella zoster immunoglobulins.
D. Start oral acyclovir.
E. Symptomatic treatment.

ANC52

A 29-year-old woman is meeting you at the antenatal clinic for her booking visit. This is her second pregnancy and she had an uneventful pregnancy 3 years back with a term delivery of a healthy boy. She has been on a diet for reducing weight off and on in the past 2 years. Her present BMI is 22 and you notice pallor during clinical examination. You have explained the risk of nutritional deficiency issues. Her haemoglobin level is 102 g/L. What is the next step in her care?

A. Blood transfusion
B. Diet modification alone
C. Iron chelation therapy
D. Oral iron supplements
E. Parenteral iron

ANC53

Ms XY is a G2P1 at 30/40 weeks with a previous vaginal delivery. She presents to the A+E with a unprovoked painless vaginal bleed (50 mls). Her 20 weeks scan suggests the presence of an anterior low-lying placenta. Examination reveals the presence of a cervical ectropion with minimal fresh bleeding. She wishes to go home, as she is reassured of the FHR on a CTG.
   Which of the following treatment options are best suited to her?

A. Admission in the maternity unit for observation until the bleeding stops.
B. Allow home as the bleeding is minimal and the APH was minor.
C. Caesarean section
D. Tocolysis and steroids
E. Ultrasound to check for persisting low-lying placenta

ANC54

Ms XY is a primigravida at 37/40 weeks. She has had low risk uncomplicated pregnancy so far. She has presented to the labour suite complaining of reduced fetal movements for 1 day. CTG is normal/reactive. She continues to perceive reduced movements despite a normal CTG. Which of the following treatment options are best suited to her?

A. Induction of labour.
B. Reassurance and kick counts at home
C. Repeat CTG in 6 h.
D. Repeat CTG in 24 h.
E. Ultrasound for fetal growth, liquor and umbilical artery doppler.

ANC55

Ms XY presents to the labour suite with a second episode of reduced fetal movements. She is 17 years old, Para 0, 39/40 weeks pregnant. She is smoker and has poor access to care. CTG is reassuring/reactive, and an ultrasound scan reveals abnormally grown fetus, with normal liquor volume and normal umbilical artery doppler. Which of the following treatment options are best suited to her?

A. Induction of labour after consultant-led counselling
B. Reassurance and kick counts at home
C. Repeat CTG in 6 h.
D. Repeat CTG in 24 h.
E. Stretch and sweep.

ANC56

Ms XY is 36/40 weeks pregnant. She is undergoing an ECV for breech presentation today. She is known to be RH-negative and non-sensitised. She had 2 anti-D injections (RAADP) at 28 and 34 weeks in keeping with the hospital policy. Which of the following treatment options are best suited to her?

A. Anti-D is not needed as she had already received it at 34/40 weeks.
B. 250 IU of anti-D.
C. 500 IU of anti-D if the test for FMH is positive.
D. 500 IU of anti-D within 72 h.
E. Postnatal anti-D administration only.

ANC57

Ms XY is a G2P0+1 at 14/40 weeks. She has had 2 previous mid-trimester spontaneous miscarriages. Transvaginal ultrasound suggests a cervical length of 28 mm with funnelling of the cervix. Which of the following treatment options are best suited to her?

A. Abdominal/laparoscopic cerclage
B. Expectant management
C. History indicated cerclage
D. Ultrasound indicated cerclage
E. Ultrasound surveillance of the cervix

ANC58

Ms XY is 30/40 weeks pregnant. Her recent MSU sample confirms the presence of significant GBS bacteriuria (>105 CFU/ml) sensitive to cephalexin. However, she is asymptomatic for a UTI. Which of the following treatment options are best suited to her?

A. Intrapartum antibiotic prophylaxis specific to GBS only.
B. Reassurance as she is asymptomatic for a UTI.

C. Repeat the MSU.
D. Treatment of the UTI and intrapartum antibiotic prophylaxis specific to GBS.
E. Treatment of the UTI only.

ANC59

Ms XY is a Para 0 and is 34/40 weeks pregnant. She has recently been diagnosed with obstetric cholestasis and commenced on ursodeoxycholic acid for the same. In view of increased obstetric surveillance, she is very concerned about fetal well being.
   Which of the following investigations would accurately predict the risk of fetal death?

A. Fetal growth scans every 2–3 weeks.
B. No such test is available.
C. Routine CTG monitoring once or twice weekly.
D. Transcervical amnioscopy for detection of meconium.
E. Weekly umbilical artery doppler.

ANC60

Ms XY is 36 weeks pregnant. She has been diagnosed with gestational diabetes, which is well controlled by diet alone. Her 36-week growth scan shows a normally grown fetus with normal liquor and Doppler. She was screened for GDM in view of her ethnicity alone. Her pregnancy has been uneventful so far.
   Up to when can Ms XY be offered elective birth if she remains undelivered?

A. 38+6
B. 39+6
C. 40+6
D. 41+6
E. Between 39 and 40 weeks

ANC61

Ms XY is primigravida, is 28 weeks pregnant and is undergoing at 75 g 2 h OGTT (oral glucose tolerance test) as her BMI is 37.
   Which of the following values is a diagnostic of gestational diabetes mellitus?

A. A fasting plasma glucose level of 5 mmol/l
B. A 1 h plasma glucose level of 5.6 mmol/l
C. A 1 h plasma glucose level of 7.8 mmol/l

D. A 2 h plasma glucose level of 7 mmol/l
E. A 2 h plasma glucose level of 7.9 mmol/l

ANC62

Ms XY is 38-year-old G5P4 with a BMI of 32. She is also a smoker but has cut down after referral to the NHS smoking cessation services. She presents to the consultant-led ANC at 6 weeks with a TV scan for threatened miscarriage, which is normal. She is 6 weeks pregnant as per the TV scan. She is otherwise fit and well. She takes routine pregnancy supplements.

Which of the following treatment options are best suited to her?

A. LMWH from 28 weeks + postpartum LMWH for 6 weeks
B. LMWH throughout the antenatal period + postpartum LMWH for 6 weeks
C. No VTE prophylaxis
D. Postpartum LMWH for 6 weeks
E. TEDS in the antenatal period

ANC63

A 42-year-old primigravida has come to discuss her antenatal care at 10 weeks of gestation. She is concerned about the chances of her baby's growth being suboptimal. Which of the following interventions will you offer her in this regard?

A. Serum PAPP-A levels at 16–18 weeks of gestation.
B. She should be offered routine abdominal palpation for detecting SGA at 28 weeks.
C. She should be offered umbilical artery Doppler from 26 to 28 weeks of gestation.
D. She should be offered uterine artery Doppler at 16 weeks of gestation.
E. She should start taking aspirin after 16 weeks of gestation.

ANC64

Which of the following is a *major* risk factor for developing an SGA fetus?

A. Daily vigorous exercise
B. Maternal age more than or equal to 35 years
C. Low maternal BMI (less than 20)
D. Low fruit intake pre-pregnancy
E. Pregnancy interval more than 5 years

ANC65

A 28-year-old woman with beta thalassemia major is planning her pregnancy. Of the following preconceptional tests that should be offered, which one need not be done routinely?

A. Bone mineral density
B. Cardiac echo, ECG and MRI (T2*)
C. Peripheral venous Doppler
D. Serum fructosamine level
E. Thyroid function tests

Maternal Medical Disorders: SBA Questions

2

MMD1

Clinical signs suggestive of sepsis include all of the following except:

A. Hypothermia
B. Polyuria
C. Pyrexia
D. Tachycardia
E. Tachypnoea

MMD2

What is false about immunisation and antibiotic prophylaxis in women at risk of transfusion related infections?

A. All women who have undergone a splenectomy should take penicillin prophylaxis or equivalent.
B. All women who have undergone a splenectomy should be vaccinated for pneumococcus and Haemophilus influenzae type B if this has not been done before.
C. Hepatitis B vaccination is recommended in HBsAg-positive women who are transfused or may be transfused.
D. Hepatitis C status should be determined.
E. The pneumococcal vaccine should be given every 5 years.

© Springer India 2016
C. Ratha, J. Gupta, *SBAs and EMQs for MRCOG II*,
DOI 10.1007/978-81-322-2689-5_2

MMD3

Which of the following features are not a hallmark of acute fatty liver of pregnancy?

A. Disseminated intravascular coagulation
B. Elevated liver enzymes
C. Hypoglycaemia
D. Hyperuricaemia
E. Proteinuria

MMD4

Of the following symptoms, mark the one 'not' included in the classical symptom-atology of Wernicke's encephalopathy:

A. Ataxia
B. Blindness
C. Confusion
D. Convulsions
E. Nystagmus

MMD5

The following are known complications of obstetric cholestasis in pregnancy except:

A. Intrauterine deaths
B. Maternal pruritus
C. Meconium staining of liquor
D. Neonatal jaundice
E. Preterm birth

MMD6

All the following are category C drugs in pregnancy except:

A. Aspirin
B. Cyclophosphamide
C. Hydroxychloroquine
D. Sulphasalazine
E. Tacrolimus

MMD7

All of the following statements about the thyroid hormones in pregnancy are true except:

A. Free T3 level is unchanged.
B. Increased thyroid binding globulin in blood.
C. Total T3 and T4 levels are increased.
D. TSH rises in the third trimester.
E. T3 crosses the placental barrier.

MMD8

Of the following statements about hyperthyroidism in pregnancy, select the correct one:

A. During pregnancy, treatment should be aimed at keeping the thyroid hormones at the lower limit of normal range.
B. Fetal hypothyroidism is a common complication in these patients.
C. Pregnancy worsens thyroid status especially in the third trimester.
D. Propylthiouracil and carbimazole can be safely continued in pregnancy.
E. Propylthiouracil and carbimazole do not cross the placenta.

MMD9

Hypopituitarism presents with all of these features except:

A. Adrenocortical insufficiency
B. Amenorrhoea
C. Anosmia
D. Failure to lactate
E. Hypothyroidism

MMD10

Hyperprolactinemia can be caused by all of the following except:

A. Dopamine antagonists
B. Hyperthyroidism
C. Pituitary adenomas
D. Polycystic ovarian disease
E. Pregnancy

MMD11

All of the following are true regarding carbohydrate metabolism in pregnancy except:

A. Decrease in insulin sensitivity in early pregnancy.
B. Fasting blood sugars are 10–20 % lower.
C. Hyperplasia of islets of Langerhans.
D. Increase in free fatty acids and ketones bodies in circulation.
E. Insulin resistance increases as pregnancy advances.

MMD12

The target range for blood sugars during labour for a pregnancy complicated by pre-existing diabetes is:

A. 2–4 mmol/L
B. 4–6 mmol/L
C. 6–8 mmol/L
D. 8–10 mmol/L
E. 10–12 mmol/L

MMD13

The following statement is true regarding metformin use in pregnancy:

A. It has no reported adverse fetal outcomes.
B. It is licensed for use during pregnancy.
C. It is effective in achieving good glycaemic control in pregnancy.
D. It is classified as a category C drug.
E. Lactic acidosis is a common complication.

MMD14

In GDM, maternal hyperglycaemia is independently and significantly linked to all of the following adverse outcomes except:

A. Caesarean delivery
B. Early miscarriages
C. Fetal hyperinsulinism
D. Macrosomia
E. Neonatal hypoglycaemia

MMD15

All of the following are pre-existing risk factors for development of type 2 diabetes except:

A. Assisted reproduction
B. Increasing parity
C. Maternal age
D. Maternal BMI
E. Twin pregnancy

MMD16

Increase in the risk of pulmonary thromboembolism in women with BMI >30 is:

A. Same as women with BMI <30
B. 3–5 times increased
C. 5–10 times increased
D. 10–12 times increased
E. 15 times increased

MMD17

Which of the following statements best describes the role of serum ferritin in pregnancy?

A. An unstable glycoprotein involved in iron transport.
B. An acute phase reactant and levels rise in infection.
C. Best test parameter to assess any type of anaemia in pregnancy.
D. Ferritin levels steadily reduce as pregnancy progresses.
E. Treatment should be started when ferritin levels are below 50 µg/l.

MMD18

The risk of recurrent urinary tract Infection in pregnancy is:

A. 1–2 %
B. 4–5 %
C. 10–15 %
D. 15–18 %
E. 20%

MMD19

A 30-year-old woman, who is 36 weeks pregnant, is seen in antenatal clinic. This is her first pregnancy. She is HIV positive. She has been fully compliant with her HAART (highly active antiretroviral therapy) throughout her pregnancy. Her latest serum viral load is <50 copies/mL. Apart from HIV, her pregnancy has been uncomplicated, and she has an appropriately grown cephalic presentation fetus. She is concerned about vertical transmission of HIV and is keen to avoid surgery if possible. Which one of the following is recommended management and advice?

A. Elective caesarean at 38 weeks gestation.
B. Elective caesarean at 39 weeks station.
C. Induce vaginal birth at 38 weeks gestation.
D. Offer spontaneous vaginal birth.
E. Postnatally, breastfeeding is considered safe as viral copy number is low.

MMD20

A 38-year-old woman is 12 weeks pregnant with a twin pregnancy. This is her second pregnancy, with her previous pregnancy complicated by gestational hypertension. Her booking blood pressure, at 12 weeks, is 135/85 mmHg. Her BMI is 34 kg/m^2. She smokes 10 cigarettes/day. Which one of the following is considered a significant (high) risk factor for the development of pre-eclampsia as her pregnancy progresses?

A. Age >35
B. BMI >30
C. Hypertensive disease during previous pregnancy
D. Multiple pregnancy
E. Smoking

MMD21

A 28-year-old woman is 12 weeks pregnant with a singleton pregnancy. This is her first pregnancy. Her booking blood pressure, at 12 weeks, is 140/90 mmHg. Her BMI is 34 kg/m^2. She smokes 10 cigarettes/day. Her mother suffered from pre-eclampsia in her pregnancies. Which one of the following is considered a significant (high) risk factor for the development of pre-eclampsia as her pregnancy progresses?

A. BMI >30
B. Elevated blood pressure at pregnancy booking
C. First pregnancy
D. Family history of pre-eclampsia
E. Smoking

MMD22

A 35-year-old woman is 33 weeks pregnant in first pregnancy. She has a one day history of headache and blurred vision. Her blood pressure is 180/110 mmHg. Urinalysis shows +++ protein. One week prior, her blood pressure was 120/70 mmHg and she had no proteinuria. Of the options listed below, select the most appropriate INITIAL drug to administer:

A. Intramuscular betamethasone
B. Intravenous magnesium sulphate
C. Intravenous furosemide
D. Intravenous diazepam
E. Oral methyldopa

MMD23

A 30-year-old woman is 16 weeks pregnant in her third pregnancy. Her blood pressure is 155/105 mmHg; 4 weeks earlier, it was 150/100 mmHg. Her urinalysis shows + protein. Her spot urinary protein/creatinine ratio is 35 mg/mmol, and a 24-h urine collection result shows 0.35 g protein. Which one of the following is considered the most likely diagnosis?

A. Chronic hypertension

B. Chronic hypertension and superimposed pre-eclampsia
C. Gestational hypertension
D. Nephrotic syndrome
E. Pre-eclampsia

MMD24

Which of the following conditions is not a known complication of maternal chicken pox in pregnancy?

A. Cholecystitis
B. Death
C. Encephalitis
D. Hepatitis
E. Pneumonitis

MMD25

Regarding pregnancy outcome after bariatric surgery in obese reproductive age women, which of the following is true?

A. Pregnancy should be delayed for at least 2 years following bariatric surgery.
B. Dumping syndrome following bariatric surgery can be provoked by 75 g GTT.
C. Ideal gestational weight gain (GWG) for pregnancies following bariatric surgery is 8–10 k.g.
D. Pregnant women need not take supplements of folic acid, vitamin B12 and iron.
E. There is increased risk of preterm deliveries and congenital anomalies.

MMD26

Which of the following statements is incorrect regarding asthma in pregnancy?

A. Asthma does not usually affect labour or delivery.
B. Asthma is a common condition that affects about 10 % of pregnant women.
C. Asthma worsens in pregnancy in 80 % of the cases.
D. Inhaled corticosteroids are the standard anti-inflammatory therapy for asthma.
E. In the postpartum period, there is not an increased risk of asthma exacerbations.

MMD27

Ms XY has is a primigravida, 29 weeks pregnant and has been diagnosed with gestational diabetes on her 2 h OGTT. Her fasting plasma glucose on the OGTT was 7.3 mmol/L. Which of the following treatment options are best suited to her?

A. Dietary modification alone
B. Diet + exercise
C. Insulin + diet + exercise
D. Metformin + diet + exercise
E. Glibenclamide + diet + exercise

MMD28

Ms XY is 38-year-old G5P4 with a BMI of 32. She presents to the consultant-led ANC at 28 weeks with a fetal growth scan, which is normal. She is otherwise fit and well. She takes routine pregnancy supplements.

In terms of VTE prophylaxis, which of the following is best suited to her?

A. LMWH from 28 weeks + postpartum LMWH for 10 days
B. LMWH from 28 weeks + postpartum LMWH for 6 weeks
C. No VTE prophylaxis
D. Postpartum LMWH for 10 days
E. TEDS in the antenatal period

MMD29

Ms XY is a primigravida, 32 weeks pregnant. She was diagnosed to have GDM on her 28-week OGTT. So far she has tried diet, exercise and metformin therapy. Her plasma glucose values are still not within target ranges for pregnancy. She declines insulin therapy, as she is needle phobic.

Which of the following treatment options are best suited to her?

A. Alpha-glucosidase inhibitors
B. Incretin-based treatments
C. SGLT-2 inhibitors
D. Sulphonylureas
E. Thiazolidinediones

MMD30

Ms XY is a Para 1 who delivered 13 weeks ago. She was diagnosed to have GDM (diet controlled). Her recent fasting plasma glucose level is 6.3 mmol/L and her HbA1C is 6 %. What is her risk of developing type 2 diabetes?

A. Current type 2 diabetes
B. High risk of developing type 2 diabetes
C. Moderate risk of developing type 2 diabetes
D. NO risk of developing type 2 diabetes
E. Low risk of developing type 2 diabetes

MMD31

Pregnant women with epilepsy have the highest risk of breakthrough seizures during:

A. First trimester
B. Intrapartum
C. Postpartum
D. Second trimester
E. Third trimester

MMD32

In cases of pheochromocytoma in pregnancy, which of the following is true?

A. Hypertension is seen in most cases.
B. Less than 1 % cases are familial.
C. More than 50 % cases are bilateral.
D. Patient should be started on alpha- and beta-adrenergic blockers immediately post diagnosis.
E. Surgery offers best cure in pregnancy.

MMD33

What percentage of pregnancies are complicated by hypertensive disorders?

A. 1–2 %
B. 1–6 %
C. 2%
D. 2–8 %
E. 10–12 %

MMD34

Ms XY is a primigravida who is 30 weeks pregnant. She presents to A + E with acute onset of shortness of breath and chest pain. She has just travelled via a long haul flight (12 h) to the UK. She has been commenced on therapeutic LMWH (dalteparin) pending investigations to rule out a PE. Her booking weight is 66 kg and she currently weighs 76 kg. What is the correct dose of dalteparin she should receive?

A. 5000 IU once daily
B. 8000 IU twice daily
C. 10,000 IU once daily
D. 12,000 IU twice daily
E. 16,000 IU once daily

MMD35

A 42-year-old primigravida at 32 weeks of gestation complains of sudden onset acute pain in her chest on the left side radiating to the shoulder and arm. She has vomiting, epigastric pain and dizziness.

Which of the following tests would be part of the first-line investigations in her case?

A. Angiography of pulmonary arteries
B. Echocardiography
C. Electrocardiography
D. Troponin T levels
E. Ultrasound of the abdomen

MMD36

In pregnant patients with prolactinomas:

A. Bromocriptine must be continued in pregnancy for all cases.
B. Cabergoline is the drug of choice during lactation.
C. MRI and prolactin levels should be done in each trimester as surveillance for patients with macroprolactinoma.
D. Patient presents with headache and visual disturbances on exacerbation.
E. Surgery can be safely performed and is the treatment of choice during pregnancy.

MMD37

Which of the following statements is false regarding hepatitis C infection in pregnancy?

A. Acute hepatitis C is a rare event in pregnancy, and the most common scenario is chronic hepatitis C virus (HCV) infection in pregnancy.
B. Coinfection with human immunodeficiency virus (HIV) increases the rate of mother-to-child transmission up to 19.4 %.
C. High viral load defined as at least 2.5×106 viral DNA copies/mL.
D. Interferon is contraindicated for treatment in pregnancy.
E. The overall rate of mother-to-child transmission for HCV is 3–5 % if the mother is known to be anti-HCV positive.

MMD38

Ms XY is a primigravida who is 30 weeks pregnant. She presents to A + E with acute onset of shortness of breath and chest pain. She has just travelled via a long haul flight (12 h) to the UK.

Which of the following investigations is not appropriate in the investigation of a suspected pulmonary embolus in pregnancy?

A. CTPA
B. CXR

C. D-Dimer
D. ECG
E. V/Q Scan

MMD39

Ms XY is a primigravida who is 32/40 weeks pregnant. She visits a friend over the weekend who informs her 5 days later that she has had shingles during their visit. Ms XY is unclear about her history of chickenpox and has recently travelled to the UK from the tropics. Which of the following treatment options are best suited to her?

A. Acyclovir.
B. Administration of varicella vaccine (live attenuated).
C. Blood test for varicella zoster immunity.
D. Immediate administration of VZIG.
E. Reassurance as shingles is rather non-infective.

MMD40

In case of maternal death due to sepsis, the postmortem protocol includes blood culture obtained from a blood sample immediately after death before opening the body. Which of the following should not be used for such sampling?

A. Brachial vein
B. Direct cardiac blood sampling
C. Femoral vein
D. Jugular vein
E. Spleen parenchyma

MMD41

Which of the following statements is true regarding pituitary insufficiency?

A. Average delay from onset to diagnosis is 7 months.
B. Failure to lactate occurs in almost all cases.
C. It is prudent to replace glucocorticoid and thyroxine in these patients during pregnancy.
D. Patients post Sheehan's syndrome/pituitary apoplexy rarely get pregnant.
E. The occurrence of Sheehan's syndrome is proportional to the amount of PPH.

MMD42

You are attending to Mrs X in the antenatal clinic. She is a 24-year-old primigravida in her ninth week of pregnancy. She is concerned about an increase in the nausea and vomiting tendency over the last week and has come to seek advice from you in this regard. You would be wrong if you told her:

A. About 30 % of pregnant women may be affected by severe nausea and vomiting, and it can cause significant morbidity.
B. In some women, the condition is so intolerable that they actually elect to have a termination of the current pregnancy
C. It is appropriately called 'morning sickness' as symptoms are severe in the morning and subside by midday.
D. Over 25,000 admissions occur per year for hyperemesis gravidarum in England.
E. Safe, effective treatments for severe nausea and vomiting of pregnancy are available.

MMD43

A 26-year-old primigravida, 26 weeks gestation has chronic hepatitis B infection. She is on Tenofovir for treatment of the HBV infection. She is HbeAg negative and the viral load is 104 IU/ml.
   Which of the following statements is true regarding her medical condition?

A. Both passive and active immunisation are warranted to prevent perinatal transmission.
B. Interferon therapy if possible is the treatment of choice in pregnancy.
C. Tenofovir should be immediately stopped.
D. The risk of perinatal transmission in her case is more than 20 %.
E. There is high chance of immunisation failure due to her viral load.

MMD44

Which of the following is true regarding Cushing's syndrome in pregnancy?

A. Distal myopathy is a distinguishing feature from signs and symptoms of pregnancy.
B. Diurnal variation of cortisol is lost in all cases.
C. More commonly due to pituitary adenomas than adrenal adenomas.
D. MRI of adrenals should always be done to rule out carcinoma.
E. Preferred screening test is imaging of adrenals, i.e., USG/MRI.

MMD45

Ms XY is a Para 1, 6 weeks postpartum. She was delivered at 27 weeks as she developed severe pre-eclampsia and HELLP syndrome. She is doing well and so is her son in special care. She is seeing a consultant today for a postnatal debrief. She is very anxious that she may develop pre-eclampsia again in the subsequent pregnancy. What is the risk of recurrence of pre-eclampsia in her subsequent pregnancy?

A. 15 %
B. 25 %
C. 35 %
D. 45 %
E. 55 %

MMD46

Ms XY is 38 + 3/40 weeks pregnant. She has a booked induction for GDM at 39/40 weeks. She has a confirmed diagnosis of chickenpox and is presently on acyclovir. Which of the following treatment options are best suited to her?

A. Caesarean section on the planned date
B. Delay delivery at least by 7 days
C. Immediate delivery by caesarean section to prevent neonatal transmission
D. Immediate induction to prevent worsening infection
E. Induction of labour on the planned date

MMD47

A 20-year-old primigravida with 30 weeks gestation has presented in the casualty with preterm labour pains. She has history of productive cough and fever since 15 days. She has a BMI of 19 and was diagnosed with gestational diabetes at 20 weeks. She has had a poor gestational weight gain. It is true to say that in this condition:

A. About 5 % of women have pre-existing or gestational diabetes.
B. FEV1 < 80 % is an absolute contraindication to pregnancy.
C. If the partner does not carry the mutation, then risk of having affected child is around 1:250.
D. Premature delivery is seen in more than half of pregnancies.
E. Women are usually infertile.

MMD48

Ms XY (para 1) is 8/52 postnatal. She was diagnosed with obstetric cholestasis in her pregnancy. Her recent LFTS are within normal limits. She is concerned about this risk of recurrence of this condition as she required an induction this time and would like a spontaneous birth in her subsequent pregnancy.

A. 1–5 %
B. 5–10 %
C. 10–20 %
D. 20–40 %
E. 45–90 %

MMD49

It is important to optimise pre-pregnancy health in a woman with sickle cell disease. You have advised many blood tests and systemic evaluations to a 29-year-old woman with sickle cell disease to help determine her pre-pregnancy health status. She is asking you for a clarification regarding the exact 'eye test' you have advised. It is most likely to be:

A. Cataract screening
B. Corneal opacity screening
C. Glaucoma screening
D. Retinal screening
E. Visual acuity screening

MMD50

All of the following statements about thalassemia syndromes are true except:

A. Are a common variety of inherited disorders.
B. The basic defect is reduced globin chain synthesis.
C. Beta-thalassemia leads to a mineral deficiency anaemia.
D. Beta-thalassemia in heterozygous state can cause mild to moderate anaemia with no significant detrimental effect on overall health
E. Thalassemia intermedia is a group of patients with beta-thalassemia whose disease severity varies.

MMD51

Ms XY is a primigravida who is 30 weeks pregnant. She presents to A + E with acute onset of shortness of breath and chest pain. She has just travelled via a long haul flight (12 h) to the UK. She has been commenced on therapeutic LMWH (Enoxaparin) pending investigations to rule out a PE. Her booking weight is 66 kg and she currently weighs 76 kg.

What is the correct dose of Enoxaparin she should receive?

A. 40 mg once daily
B. 60 mg once daily
C. 90 mg once daily
D. 40 mg twice daily
E. 80 mg twice daily

MMD52

Ms XY is a primigravida who is 38 weeks pregnant. She presents to A + E with acute onset of shortness of breath and chest pain. She has just travelled via a long haul flight (12 h) to the UK. She has been commenced on unfractionated heparin-pending investigations to rule out a PE. She has received the bolus dose of unfractionated heparin and is currently on 18 units/kg/h. Her APTT ratio 6 h after the bolus dose is 1.3. What is the most appropriate step to correctly titrate her heparin dose prior to her next APTT measurement?

A. No change in dose
B. Re-bolus 40 units/kg + 18 units/kg/h infusion
C. Re-bolus 80 units/kg + 18 units/kg/h infusion
D. Re-bolus 40 units/kg + 20 units/kg/h infusion
E. Re-bolus 80 units/kg + 20 units/kg/h infusion

MMD53

Ms XY is a primigravida, 32 weeks pregnant. Her BP on 2 occasions today (at the GP surgery) is 140/92 and 142/95 mm of Hg with ++ protein in the urine. She is asymptomatic for pre-eclampsia. Her FBC, U + Es, LFTS and uric acid are normal. Her reflexes are normal. What is the most appropriate management for her?

A. Admission to the hospital
B. Admission to the hospital + commence labetelol
C. BP and urine check with GP/CMW in 24 h

D. BP check twice weekly with GP/CMW till delivery
E. Reassurance and home

MMD54

All of the following are advantages of unfractionated heparin (UH) except:

A. The required interval between UFH and regional analgesia or anaesthesia is less (4 h) than with LMWH (12 h).
B. There is less concern regarding neuraxial haematomas with UFH.
C. Unfractionated heparin has a shorter half life compared to low molecular weight heparin (LMWH).
D. Unfractionated heparin has a complete reversal of its activity with protamine sulphate.
E. Unfractionated heparin is associated with a lower risk of thrombocytopenia as compared to LMWH.

MMD55

A 26-year-old primigravida is discussing her fears of pregnancy complications with you at the booking visit. She has heard that pregnancy and childbirth increase the risk of thromboembolism. You will be correct to tell her that the incidence of VTE in pregnancy and puerperium is:

A. 1–2/100
B. 1–2/1000
C. 1–2/10,000
D. 5–10/10,000
E. 10–15/10,000

MMD56

Which of the following statements regarding contemporary management of patients with beta-thalassemia major is true?

A. Cardiac failure is a rare cause of death.
B. Developments in MRI (magnetic resonance imaging) have helped reduce mortality.
C. Puberty is often precocious.
D. Repeated blood transfusions and iron chelation therapy is no longer the cornerstone of modern therapy.
E. Splenectomy is the mainstay of modern treatment.

Fetal Medicine: SBA Questions

3

FM1

Approximately what percentage of pregnant women are offered a choice of invasive prenatal testing?

A. 0.2 %
B. 2 %
C. 5 %
D. 10 %
E. 15 %

FM2

Third-trimester amniocentesis is associated with all of the following except:

A. Blood-stained amniotic fluid.
B. Need for multiple attempts.
C. Higher rates of culture failure for karyotyping.
D. Serious complications are rare.
E. Significant risk of emergency delivery.

FM3

Which of the following statements about prenatal invasive testing is true?

A. Decontamination of ultrasound probes can be potentially damaging.
B. In Rhesus-negative women, additional anti-D after prenatal invasive testing is not recommended if she has been on RAADP.

© Springer India 2016
C. Ratha, J. Gupta, *SBAs and EMQs for MRCOG II*,
DOI 10.1007/978-81-322-2689-5_3

C. Invasive prenatal testing cannot be carried out on women infected with HIV.
D. Severe sepsis, including maternal death, can be a complication.
E. Sterilisation of ultrasound gel is an unnecessary practice and hence not recommended.

FM4

All of the following ultrasound features suggest that the twins are dichorionic except:

A. Bicornuate uterus
B. Discordant gender
C. The 'lambda' sign
D. Twin-peak sign
E. Two separate placental masses

FM5

Chorionicity in multifetal pregnancy is best assessed at what gestation:

A. 5–6 weeks
B. 11–14 weeks
C. 16–18 weeks
D. 20–24 weeks
E. 30–34 weeks

FM6

All of the following are ultrasound criteria to diagnose twin to twin transfusion syndrome except:

A. Discordant bladder appearances
B. Discordant fluid volumes—polyhydramnios/oligoamnios
C. Discordant gender
D. Haemodynamic and cardiac compromise
E. Presence of a single placental mass

FM7

Which of the following statements regarding twin to twin transfusion syndrome (TTTS) is true?

A. Screening for TTTS should start after 24 weeks of gestation.
B. Screening for TTTS should start in the first trimester of pregnancy.
C. Severe twin–twin transfusion syndrome presenting before 26 weeks of gestation should be treated by laser ablation rather than by amnioreduction or septostomy.
D. TTTS complicates about 50 % of monochorionic twin pregnancies.
E. TTTS may sometimes complicate dichorionic pregnancies.

FM8

Possible sources of error in noninvasive prenatal testing for fetal aneuploidies include:

A. Late gestational age
B. Low maternal BMI
C. Maternal heart disease
D. Maternal malignancies
E. Placenta previa

FM9

Which of the following twin pregnancies is not possible physiologically?

A. Dichorionic monoamniotic
B. Dichorionic quadriamniotic
C. Dichorionic triamniotic
D. Monochorionic diamniotic
E. Monochorionic monoamniotic

FM10

Which of the following statements about standard Pedigree drawing is false?

A. Circles represent females.
B. Consanguineous mating is represented by a single horizontal line.
C. Diamonds represent unspecified gender.
D. Square represents males.
E. Usually three generations are drawn.

FM11

When using two measurements of AC or EFW to estimate growth velocity, to minimise false-positive rates for diagnosing FGR, the measurements should be:

A. 1 week apart
B. 2 weeks apart
C. 3 weeks apart
D. 4 weeks apart
E. 6 weeks apart

FM12

The following conditions have a 25 % recurrence risk except:

A. Achondroplasia
B. Beta-thalassemia
C. Cystic fibrosis
D. Propionic academia
E. Spinal muscular atrophy

FM13

All of the following ultrasound signs help in the diagnosis of chorionicity in twin pregnancies except

A. Concordant fetal sex
B. Lambda sign
C. Presence of separate placental masses
D. 'T' sign
E. Thickness of the intertwin membrane

FM14

In a couple with a previous child with congenital adrenal hyperplasia, the risk of having a subsequent virilised female is:

A. 1:2
B. 1:4
C. 1:8
D. 1:16
E. 1:32

FM15

All of the following statements are true about the management of a woman with a previous child with congenital adrenal hyperplasia except:

A. Dexamethasone should be started prior to 7 weeks' gestation.
B. Dexamethasone regimen reduces the need for corrective surgery for virilisation.
C. Dexamethasone is successful in preventing virilisation in all cases of affected female fetuses.
D. Dexamethasone should be stopped if the fetus is male or an unaffected female.
E. Dexamethasone has significant maternal side effects.

FM16

The commonest enzyme deficiency seen in congenital adrenal hyperplasia

A. 11 β-hydroxylase
B. 17 α-hydroxylase
C. 17 hydroxysteroid dehydrogenase
D. 18 hydroxylase
E. 21 hydroxylase

FM17

Incidence of chromosomal abnormalities in sporadic first trimester miscarriage is:

A. 10–22 %
B. 20–30 %
C. 40–50 %
D. 50–60 %
E. 70 %

FM18

A 40-year-old woman is 12 weeks pregnant. She is attending hospital antenatal clinic for her dating scan. She is concerned about her risk of having a child affected by Down syndrome. Which SINGLE action is the most appropriate management action given her anxiety and consistent with current routine antenatal screening advice for the UK?

A. Measure nuchal translucency and check for presence/absence of fetal nasal bone at 12 weeks.
B. Measure nuchal translucency and maternal serum PAPP-A and HCG at 12 weeks.
C. Offer amniocentesis at 15 weeks.
D. Offer detailed fetal anatomy ultrasound to check for fetal congenital malformation at 20 weeks.
E. Offer maternal biochemical quadruple screening test at 16 weeks.

FM19

Normally fetal blood volume is about:

A. 30–50 ml/kg
B. 50–60 ml/kg
C. 80–100 ml/kg
D. 100–150 ml/kg
E. 150–170 ml/kg

FM20

A 24-year-old woman is 12 weeks pregnant. She is attending hospital for her dating scan and routine booking serological investigations. Screening and treating for the presence of a particular pathogen during early pregnancy will reduce the risk of developing congenital fetal abnormality. Which ONE of the pathogens listed below fulfils this criteria?

A. Hepatitis B
B. Herpes simplex virus
C. Rubella
D. Syphilis
E. Varicella zoster virus

FM21

A 28-year-old woman is 22 weeks pregnant. She has long standing type 1 diabetes mellitus. Her blood sugars have remained well controlled in pregnancy. However, she is concerned about how her diabetes may cause congenital fetal anomalies in her unborn child.

Of the options listed below, which SINGLE action best addresses her anxiety?

A. Amniocentesis at 22 weeks
B. Anomaly scan and fetal cardiac echocardiography at 20 weeks
C. Obstetric ultrasound scan for growth and umbilical artery Doppler at 28w, 32w and 36w
D. Offer reassurance as HbA1C is normal
E. Quadruple maternal biochemical screening test (HCG, Inhibin-A, oestriol, AFP) at 20 weeks

FM22

Severe twin to twin transfusion syndrome (TTTS) diagnosed before 26 weeks is best treated by:

A. Amnioreduction
B. Laser ablation of vessels
C. Selective fetal reduction
D. Septostomy
E. Termination of pregnancy

FM23

A 24-year-old woman experiences an antepartum stillbirth at 34 weeks gestation. Which one of the following maternal serological investigations may be helpful in identifying a cause for the stillbirth?

A. Group A streptococcus
B. Hepatitis B
C. Human parvovirus B19
D. Influenza
E. Varicella zoster virus

FM24

The following are statements relating to intrauterine fetal growth restriction (IUGR) and small for gestational age (SGA). Which ONE of the following statements is correct?

A. All fetuses that are IUGR are in less than the 10th percentile for estimated gestational age-specific fetal weight (EFW).
B. All fetuses that are SGA are IUGR.
C. Constitutionally small SGA fetuses are at increased risk of antepartum stillbirth.
D. SGA is defined as growth at the 10th or less percentile for weight of all fetuses at that gestational age.
E. The most common cause for SGA is fetal chromosomal abnormality.

FM25

A 20-year-old woman is 33 weeks and 4 days weeks pregnant in her first pregnancy. She has a 6-h history of regular painful uterine contractions with intact membranes. Obstetric ultrasound confirms appropriate for gestational age fetus and cephalic presentation. A diagnosis of early-stage preterm labour is made. Which ONE of the following is most appropriate in relation to the counselling she will receive?

A. Administering prophylactic antibiotics improves neonatal outcome.
B. Antenatal corticosteroids are not indicated as tocolysis may successfully prevent preterm birth.
C. Antenatal corticosteroids will reduce the risk of neonatal respiratory distress syndrome and neonatal mortality if preterm birth occurs.
D. Fetal fibronectin testing is necessary to predict the time interval for preterm delivery.
E. Tocolysis (such as oral nifedipine or i.v. atosiban) is strongly recommended.

FM26

Listed below are paired environmental factor and corresponding characteristic fetal abnormality.
  Select the SINGLE correctly matched pair:

A. Carbon monoxide poisoning—congenital cyanotic heart disease
B. Excessive vitamin A—fetal cranial–neural–crest abnormalities
C. Folic acid deficiency—choroid plexus cysts
D. Human parvovirus B19—deafness
E. Smoking—macrosomia

FM27

In a case of twin pregnancy, splitting at the two-cell stage results in:

A. Conjoint twins
B. Craniopagus
C. Dichorionic diamniotic
D. Monochorionic monoamniotic
E. Monochorionic diamniotic

FM28

Rate of transplacental transmission of human parvovirus B19 infection in pregnancy is:

A. About 15 % in first trimester, 20 % in second trimester and 70 % in third trimester
B. About 90 % in first trimester,40 % in second trimester and negligible at term
C. More than 80 % in first trimester, 60 % in second trimester and 15 % in third trimester
D. Negligible in first trimester, 10 % in second trimester and 40 % in third trimester
E. Uniformly about 10–20 % at any stage in pregnancy

FM29

The most common fetal infection with an incidence of 0.5–2 % in pregnant population is:

A. Cytomegalovirus
B. Human parvovirus B19
C. Rubella
D. Toxoplasma
E. Varicella

FM30

Ms XY is 38-year-old primigravida who is 15 +2 days pregnant. Her recent bloods suggest a high risk for Down's syndrome (1 in 100). She opts to have amniocentesis as a diagnostic test.
   What additional risk of miscarriage does amniocentesis carry?

A. 0 %
B. 0.5 %
C. 1 %
D. 2 %
E. 10 %

FM31

Ms XY is 22 weeks pregnant with anti-D antibodies. She presents to the consultant-led clinic for follow-up.
   What titres of anti-D antibodies are associated with severe HDFN (haemolytic disease of the fetus and newborn)?

A. 4iu/ml
B. 6iu/ml

C. 12iu/ml
D. 16iu/ml
E. 32iu/ml

FM32

Mrs. X has come to see you in her booking visit at 9 weeks gestation. This is her second pregnancy, and her previous pregnancy was terminated at 10 weeks due to confirmed primary Rubella infection.

This time she has been told that she is immune to Rubella, but she is still very concerned about reinfection in this pregnancy.

What fact can you tell her regarding reinfection of Rubella?

A. Antibiotic prophylaxis can effectively reduce the risk of reinfection.
B. If reinfection occurs, then the risk of fetal infection is 90 % before 12 weeks of gestation, about 55 % at 12–16 weeks, and it declines to 45 % after 16 weeks.
C. Reinfection cannot occur in Rubella; hence, she need not worry further in this regard.
D. Reinfection can occur but is less likely in natural immunity than with vaccine-induced immunity.
E. Reinfection is clinically more severe than the primary infection.

FM33

Incidence of conjoined twinning is:

A. 900–1000 pregnancies
B. 9000–10,000 pregnancies
C. 90,000–100,000 pregnancies
D. 900,000–1,000,000 pregnancies
E. 0.9 % of all twin pregnancies

FM34

All of the following statements regarding surveillance methods for small fro gestational age fetuses are true except:

A. CTG should not be used as the only form of fetal surveillance.
B. Interpretation of the amniotic fluid volume on ultrasound should be based on the single deepest vertical pocket.
C. The BPP is time consuming, and the incidence of an equivocal result is high in severely SGA fetuses.

D. MCA Doppler should be used to time delivery in preterm SGA fetuses with normal umbilical artery Doppler.

E. DV Doppler has moderate predictive value for academia and adverse outcome.

FM35

During a 20 weeks anomaly scan on a 26-year-old pregnant woman, the fetus is found to have an occipital encephalocele, polydactyly and bilateral polycystic kidneys. The most likely diagnosis is:

A. Arnold–Chiari malformation
B. Beckwith–Wiedemann syndrome
C. Meckel–Gruber syndrome
D. Noonan syndrome
E. Seckel syndrome

FM36

Twin to twin transfusion occurs in about 15 % of monochorionic pregnancies. When the Doppler studies are critically abnormal in either twin and are characterised as abnormal or reversed end-diastolic velocities in the umbilical artery, reverse flow in the ductus venosus or pulsatile umbilical venous flow, this corresponds to the following stage in Quintero's system:

A. Stage 1
B. Stage 2
C. Stage 3
D. Stage 4
E. Stage 5

FM37

Which of the following fetal anomalies can be diagnosed with certainty by antenatal ultrasound?

A. Down syndrome
B. Edwards syndrome
C. Gangliosidosis
D. Hydrops fetalis
E. Tay–Sachs disease

FM38

Which of the following statements about intrauterine fetal deaths is false?

A. In most cases of stillbirths, the cause remains unexplained.
B. Over one-third of stillbirths are small-for-gestational-age fetuses.
C. Stillbirth is a common occurrence.
D. The stillbirth rate has remained generally constant since 2000.
E. Whenever a late IUFD is suspected, urgent CTG should be arranged.

FM39

A 28-year-old woman in her first pregnancy was diagnosed to have a chicken pox infection at 14 weeks gestation. She was referred for a detailed fetal anomaly scan at 19 weeks gestation which revealed no obvious fetal structural defects, and she was reassured by the doctor. She is very anxious about the risk of fetal varicella syndrome (FVS) and is considering an amniocentesis. Which of the following statements best describe the role of amniocentesis in this situation:

A. If the amniotic fluid is negative for varicella DNA, it definitely rules out FVS.
B. If the amniotic fluid is positive for varicella DNA, it definitely confirms FVS.
C. It is late to do an amniocentesis now as it should have been done during the acute phase.
D. Negative predictive value of amniocentesis is better than positive predictive value in detecting FVS.
E. The presence of VZV DNA has a high specificity but a low sensitivity for the development of FVS.

FM40

A 27-year-old primigravida has monochorionic diamniotic twin pregnancy with severe twin to twin transfusion at 25 weeks of gestation. She has undergone LASER ablation of the anastomotic vessels.
    She is concerned about the recurrence of the problem. What will you tell her about the risk of recurrence of twin to twin transfusion post LASER?

A. 1 %
B. 5 %
C. 10 %
D. 15 %
E. 20 %

FM41

Which of the following is an indication for immediate delivery by LSCS of an SGA fetus:

A. EFW 480 g, gestational age 28 weeks, steroid covered and AREDV
B. EFW 1220 g, gestational age 35 weeks, steroid covered and UA Doppler normal
C. EFW 1350 g, gestational age 35 weeks, steroid covered and static growth for 3 weeks
D. EFW 1800 g, gestational age 37 weeks, steroid not covered and UA Doppler normal
E. EFW 1800 g, gestational age 37 weeks, steroid covered and UA Doppler normal

FM42

Which of the following statements regarding managing antenatal care and delivery of a woman whose fetus is diagnosed with a lethal anomaly is true?

A. Early induction of labour where the fetus has a lethal anomaly is not an option in the UK.
B. Epidural analgesia should be avoided due to increased risks.
C. Labour should ideally be induced at 37 weeks of gestation in these cases.
D. Women will not need more frequent visits than the usual antenatal care schedule.
E. Women should not be allowed to labour in private or in a single room.

FM43

A. Abdominal palpation or symphysio-fundal height measurement.
B. Ultrasound biometry such that more than 15 % discordance between the fetuses is an indicator of IUGR.
C. Ultrasound biometry should be done at intervals less than 28 days.
D. Ultrasound biometry should be based on fetal abdominal circumference measurements.
E. Umbilical artery Doppler should be used to monitor IUGR in twin pregnancies.

FM44

The most suitable method of selective feticide in a monochorionic twin pair with structural discordance endangering the viability of one fetus is by:

A. Bipolar cautery
B. Intra-abdominal potassium chloride
C. Intracardiac potassium chloride
D. Mifepristone
E. Oxytocin

FM45

A 38-year-old pregnant woman meets you in the antenatal clinic with the report of her 20 weeks anomaly scan. The report states that there is excessive amniotic fluid and a 'double bubble' sign in the fetal abdomen. The 'double bubble' sign seen in fetal ultrasound is suggestive of:

A. Anorectal malformation
B. Arteriovenous fistula in the fetal liver
C. Colonic perforation
D. Duodenal atresia
E. Tracheoesophageal fistula

FM46

Which of the following statements is true about the fetal risks due to maternal infection with chicken pox in pregnancy:

A. Combination of ultrasound scan and amniocentesis is diagnostic for FVS.
B. FVS does not occur at the time of initial fetal infection.
C. If maternal serological conversion occurs in the first 28 weeks of pregnancy, she has a high risk of FVS.
D. Risk of FVS is highest in the first trimester.
E. Risk of spontaneous miscarriage is increased if chickenpox occurs in the first trimester.

FM47

The most sensitive, noninvasive method to diagnose fetal anaemia is:

A. Amniotic fluid spectrophotometry
B. Fetal Doppler of middle cerebral artery

C. Fetal hepatic vein Doppler indices
D. Maternal uterine artery Doppler
E. Maternal hepatic artery Doppler

FM48

MS XY is 8 weeks pregnant. She is being screened for risk factors for an SGA baby. Which of the following is not a major risk factor for development of an SGA fetus?

A. Cocaine use
B. Daily vigorous exercise
C. PAPP-A <0.4MoM
D. Paternal SGA
E. Smokes 10 cigarettes/day

FM49

Ms XY is a primigravida who is 34 weeks pregnant. Her last two serial scans have shown an SGA fetus growing on the 9th centile. Her last scan shows positive EDF with a normal PI. She reports having good fetal movements. How should further fetal surveillance be undertaken?

A. Fortnightly umbilical artery Doppler
B. Twice weekly CTG
C. Twice weekly umbilical artery Doppler
D. Weekly CTG
E. Weekly umbilical artery Doppler + CTG

FM50

Ms XY is 22 weeks pregnant with anti-C antibodies. She presents to the consultant-led clinic for follow-up. At what minimum titres of anti-C antibodies would you consider referral to the fetal medicine centre?

A. 4 iu/ml
B. 5 iu/ml
C. 6 iu/ml
D. 15 iu/ml
E. 20 iu/ml

Labour and Delivery: SBA Questions

4

LD1

Q1. Mrs X, primigravida at term is in second stage of labour. After delivery of the fatal head, shoulder dystocia was diagnosed and the McRoberts manoeuvre has nor effected the delivery of the shoulders, which is the next method to be used:

A. All-fours position
B. Delivery of posterior arm
C. Suprapubic pressure
D. Internal rotation manoeuvres
E. Zavanelli manoeuvre

LD2

Elective caesarean section is best recommended to prevent morbidity from shoulder dystocia in which of the following clinical situations:

A. All women at term with suspected macrosomia
B. Diabetic women with suspected macrosomia
C. Prelabour rupture of membranes at term
D. Previous shoulder dystocia
E. Women with previous two caesarean births

LD3

Q.3 Which of the following statements about timing of delivery in multiple pregnancy is true?

© Springer India 2016
C. Ratha, J. Gupta, *SBAs and EMQs for MRCOG II*,
DOI 10.1007/978-81-322-2689-5_4

A. All monochorionic twin pregnancies should be delivered by elective caesarean section.
B. Monochorionic monoamniotic twins should be monitored by weekly biophysical profiles till 36 weeks of gestation.
C. Women with triplets should be offered delivery after 35 completed weeks of pregnancy after a course of antenatal corticosteroids.
D. Women with uncomplicated dichorionic twin pregnancies should not be offered elective delivery prior to 40 weeks of gestation.
E. Women with uncomplicated monochorionic twin pregnancies should be offered delivery after 35 completed weeks of pregnancy after a course of antenatal corticosteroids.

LD4

Regarding shoulder dystocia, which of the following statements is true?

A. A large majority of infants with a birth weight of $\geq$4500 g do not develop shoulder dystocia.
B. All women with history of shoulder dystocia should be offered elective caesarean section in their subsequent pregnancies.
C. Conventional risk factors predicted about 96 % of shoulder dystocia that resulted in infant morbidity.
D. Induction of labour prevents shoulder dystocia in nondiabetic women with a suspected macrosomic fetus.
E. While managing shoulder dystocia, suprapubic pressure should not be used.

LD5

All of the following are known factors for anal sphincter injury during delivery except:

A. Expected fetal weight more than 4 kg
B. Induction of labour
C. Mediolateral episiotomy
D. Primiparous
E. Second stage more than 1 h

LD6

Massive blood loss is defined as loss of:

A. 1 blood volume in 12 h
B. 1 blood volume in 24 h

C. 50 % of blood volume loss in 2 h
D. 50 % of blood volume loss in 4 h
E. 50 % of blood volume loss in 24 h

LD7

Of the following, the most consistent finding in uterine rupture is:

A. Abnormal CTG
B. Acute scar tenderness
C. Haematuria
D. Maternal tachycardia
E. Severe abdominal pain referred to the shoulder tip

LD8

History of previous vaginal birth in a woman with a caesarean section attempting to deliver vaginally is associated with the planned VBAC success rate of:

A. 50 %
B. 60–67 %
C. 72–76 %
D. D.85–90 %
E. 99 %

LD9

Ms XY is a primigravida, gestational diabetic, 38 weeks in spontaneous labour. She was assessed at 13:00 h and had progressed to 5 cms cervical dilatation. She was examined at 17:00 h and was found to be 6 cms dilated, 0.5 long, with intact membranes, vertex at spines.
    What is the next appropriate step in managing her labour?

A. Adequate progress of labour. VE in 4 h
B. ARM + oxytocin + VE in 2 h
C. ARM + oxytocin + VE in 4 h
D. ARM + VE in 2 h
E. ARM + VE in 4 h

LD10

A 20-year-old woman is 36 weeks pregnant in her second pregnancy and is being reviewed in the antenatal clinic. She has had a previous caesarean delivery. A recent obstetric growth scan confirms cephalic presentation of a normally grown fetus. She has no other complicating medical or obstetric disorders. She is deciding between planned vaginal birth after caesarean (VBAC) and elective repeat caesarean section (ERCS) modes of delivery. Which ONE of the following is correct in relation to the counselling she will receive?

A. ERCS is usually performed at commencement of 38th week of gestation.
B. ERCS is recommended as chances of successful VBAC are less than 50 %.
C. Future pregnancy, after two caesarean deliveries, is not recommended due to increased surgical risks of a third caesarean delivery.
D. If planning VBAC, induction of labour is safer than spontaneous onset of labour.
E. The risk of uterine scar rupture in spontaneous onset of labour and planned VBAC is 0.2–0.5 %.

LD11

A 32-year-old woman is 36 weeks pregnant in first pregnancy with DCDA (dichorionic diamniotic) twins and is being reviewed in the antenatal clinic. A recent obstetric growth scan confirms both fetuses are normally grown. Both twins are longitudinal lie and cephalic presentation. She has no other complicating medical or obstetric disorders. She is deciding between planned vaginal or elective caesarean modes of delivery. Which ONE of the following is correct in relation to the counselling she will receive?

A. About 10 % of twin pregnancies result in spontaneous birth before 37 weeks, 0 days.
B. Continuing twin pregnancies beyond 38 weeks, 0 days increases the risk of fetal death.
C. Maternal antenatal corticosteroids are routinely recommended for all twin pregnancies.
D. Offer elective birth from 37 weeks, 0 days after a course of maternal corticosteroids has been administered.
E. There is strong evidence to show caesarean delivery is safer for mother and fetuses than vaginal mode of delivery.

LD12

Which one of the following statements is correct in relation to the third stage of labour?

A. Active management reduces the risk of haemorrhage and shortens the third stage compared to physiological management.

B. Early cord clamping achieves better infant haematological outcomes than delayed cord clamping.

C. If actively managed, the mean duration is 30 min.

D. If the placenta is retained, then its manual removal should only be conducted under general anaesthesia.

E. Physiological management involves cord clamping, and the placenta is delivered by controlled cord traction, but no use of oxytocin.

LD13

Hypoxic-ischaemic encephalopathy (HIE) is a rare neonatal condition that is a consequence of intrapartum fetal oxygen deprivation. Which ONE of the following statements is characteristic of neonates diagnosed with HIE?

A. Apart from CNS, there is no evidence of any other organ dysfunction (e.g. kidney, lungs, liver, heart, intestines).

B. Five-minute Apgar score is >9.

C. Mild hypothermia via selective head cooling is neuroprotective in term neonates with HIE.

D. In most cases, there are no identifiable preconception, antenatal or intrapartum risk factors that increase susceptibility for HIE.

E. Umbilical cord artery pH at birth is between 7.25 and 7.30.

LD14

Which ONE of the following statements represents the correct sequence of events in relation to the mechanism of labour for a vertex presentation?

A. Descent, flexion, engagement, internal rotation, restitution and external rotation, extension, expulsion

B. Descent, engagement, flexion, extension, restitution and external rotation, internal rotation, expulsion

C. Engagement, descent, flexion, extension, restitution and external rotation, internal rotation, expulsion

D. Engagement, descent, flexion, internal rotation, restitution and external rotation, extension, expulsion

E. Engagement, descent, flexion, internal rotation, extension, restitution and external rotation, expulsion

LD15

A 38-year-old woman has breech presentation at 39 weeks and is opting for elective caesarean section (LSCS) for mode of delivery. Her BMI is 28. She has no other medical or obstetric disorders and has not had any previous surgery. When counselling about elective LSCS, which one of the following statements is valid?

A. All women should receive antibiotic prophylaxis just prior to skin incision.
B. All women should receive thromboprophylaxis with low molecular weight heparin just prior to skin incision.
C. Elective LSCS should be performed at 40 weeks +0 days gestation to maximise fetal growth.
D. General anaesthesia is safer than regional anaesthesia.
E. On average, women need 5 days to recover in hospital following LSCS.

LD16

A 25 year old, who is 40 weeks pregnant in her first pregnancy, is in the second stage of labour. She has been actively pushing for 2 h and is exhausted. CTG shows a baseline of 150 bpm, normal baseline variability, occasional accelerations and infrequent typical variable decelerations. She is contracting 3–4 every 10 min. Vaginal examination reveals a fully dilated cervix with the fetal head in a direct occipito-anterior position and at station +1 below spines. Which of the following is the most appropriate next management step?

A. Caesarean section delivery
B. Episiotomy
C. Fetal blood sampling
D. Instrumental delivery
E. Start IV oxytocin augmentation

LD17

A 25 year old, who is 40 weeks pregnant in her first pregnancy, is in the second stage of labour. She has been actively pushing for 1 h. CTG shows a baseline of 180 bpm, reduced baseline variability, no accelerations and frequent atypical variable decelerations. She is contracting 3–4 every 10 min. Vaginal examination reveals a fully dilated cervix with the fetal head in a direct occipito-anterior position and at station +1 below spines. Which of the following is the most appropriate next management step?

A. Caesarean section delivery
B. Episiotomy
C. Fetal blood sampling

D. Instrumental delivery

E. Start IV oxytocin augmentation

LD18

Mrs. X, 32-year-old second gravida, previous vaginal birth, suffered a spinal cord injury at the level of T8 at 32 weeks of gestation. She had a singleton fetus with an anterior high placenta, and her fetal scan after the accident revealed an AGA fetus with normal amniotic fluid, fetal activity, Dopplers and no signs of internal bleeding in the placenta.

She was managed as an inpatient with multidisciplinary care at the obstetric unit. Which of the following statements is appropriate for her care?

A. At caesarean section, regional anaesthesia should not be offered.

B. First choice of muscle relaxant at GA is rocuronium as suxamethonium is avoided.

C. She must be counselled about the chances of lactation failure due to spinal injury.

D. Thromboprophylaxis is avoided as it can lead to spinal hematomas.

E. Vaginal delivery is contraindicated.

LD19

You are counselling a 28-year-old primigravida with a singleton pregnancy at the antenatal clinic at 38 weeks regarding her options for delivery. Her clinical history has been normal so far and is perceiving good fetal movements, and she has a fetus in cephalic presentation. Which of the following statements is incorrect?

A. Membrane sweeping can be offered as it reduces the need for induction of labour.

B. If she does not set into spontaneous labour, she will be offered induction of labour at 40 weeks.

C. The choice of induction agent will be intravaginal PGE2.

D. If one attempt of induction fails, another attempt may be made.

E. If one attempt of induction fails, a caesarean section will be offered.

LD20

Induction of labour should not be offered if:

A. Multipara,39 weeks, breech presentation, ECV failed, wanting a vaginal birth

B. Primigravida,34 weeks, PPROM for 1 week, clinically stable on oral erythromycin—no signs of chorioamnionitis

C. Primigravida,37 weeks, severe FGR with reduced amniotic fluid and suspicious CTG

D. Primigravida,40 weeks, uneventful pregnancy so far, requests induction of labour as her partner is moving abroad
E. Primigravida,41 weeks AGA fetus, maternal perception of reduced fetal movements but normal amniotic fluid, normal CTG

LD21

Ms XY is 30/40 weeks pregnant in her first pregnancy. She is in established preterm labour, although not in advanced labour. The cause of preterm labour appears to be an untreated E. coli UTI.

Ms XY is haemodynamically stable and apyrexial. Her lactate levels are 0.5. Which treatment is most likely to improve neonatal outcome?

A. Atosiban to suppress preterm labour
B. Betamethasone IM with tocolysis
C. Cephalexin to treat UTI
D. Erythromycin to treat preterm labour
E. Oral dexamethasone with tocolysis

LD22

What is the risk of neonatal transmission with vaginal births and recurrent genital herpes?

A. 0 %
B. 0–3 %
C. 5–10 %
D. 10–20 %
E. 50 %

LD23

While counselling a low-risk primigravida about planning her delivery, the following information should be given to her:

A. A home birth or midwifery-led unit (freestanding or alongside) is not particularly suitable for her.
B. A small increase in risk of adverse outcomes to her baby exists if she plans to deliver at home.
C. An admission CTG will be performed if she is admitted to the labour ward with suspected but not established labour.
D. She must not ask for the cord to be cut later than 5 min after delivery.
E. The success rate of vaginal deliveries in midwifery-led units is due to timely and higher rate of interventions.

LD24

Ms XY is a G3P2 at 30 weeks with a previous CS done 3 years ago for presumed fetal distress. She would like to attempt a VBAC this time. What success rate would you quote for VBAC?

A. 72–75 %
B. 75–80 %
C. 80–85 %
D. 87–90 %
E. >90 %

LD25

Ms XY is 38/40 weeks pregnant with one previous CS. She presents in spontaneous labour and has an agreed plan for a VBAC. She now complains of pain in the site of the CS scar. Which of the following is most consistently associated with a uterine rupture?

A. Abnormal CTG
B. Acute onset scar tenderness
C. Hematuria
D. Severe abdominal pain, persisting in between contractions
E. Vaginal bleeding

LD26

Ms XY is 32/40 weeks pregnant with a cervical cerclage inserted at 14/40. She presents to the labour suite with a confirmed diagnosis of PPROM.

Inflammatory markers are normal. Ms XY is clinically well and demonstrates no uterine activity. Which of the following treatment options are best suited to her?

A. Delayed removal of the cerclage only if signs of infection appears
B. Delayed removal of the cerclage till labour ensues
C. Immediate removal of the cerclage
D. Removal of cerclage at 34/40
E. Removal of the cerclage in 48 h for steroid administration

LD27

Which of the following women should be offered intrapartum antibiotic prophylaxis for prevention of early-onset GBS disease in the neonate?

A. 28 year old, nullipara, established preterm labour at 29 weeks gestation

B. 28 year old, second gravida with previous caesarean section for breech, now planning for a vaginal birth after caesarean section (VBAC).

C. 29 year old, second gravida, previous child had congenital diaphragmatic hernia, now has PROM at 38 weeks gestation

D. 30 year old, nullipara, no antenatal risk factors, in established labour at 38 weeks gestation having temperature of 38.2°

E. 30 year old, second gravida, previous preterm birth, now with PPROM at 32 weeks gestation

LD28

You are evaluating Mrs X who has been in first stage of labour for the past 10 h. Which of the following information is least relevant to your further clinical management?

A. Cervical dilatation and rate of change
B. Ethnicity
C. Parity
D. The woman's emotional state
E. Uterine contractions

LD29

A 23-year-old primigravida is in threatened preterm labour at 32 weeks of gestation. As there is a possibility of imminent preterm birth, a decision to administer antenatal corticosteroids is taken. While explaining the rationale of this treatment to her, all of the following statements are correct except that antenatal corticosteroids:

A. Are known to be safe to the mother
B. Reduce the risk of intraventricular haemorrhage
C. Reduce the risk of maternal inflammation
D. Reduce the risk of neonatal death
E. Reduce the risk of respiratory distress syndrome

LD30

A 32-year-old primigravida presents at 38 weeks with history of leaking of clear fluid per vaginam for the last 2 h. On clinical examination, fundal height is about 36 weeks, uterus is relaxed, cephalic presentation (3/5 palpable) and fetal heart rate is normal. Per speculum examination confirms clear fluid leaking.

What would you tell her about her condition?

A. About 40 % of pregnancies may be affected by term PROM.
B. Cesarean section will be offered after 24 h if she does not set into spontaneous labour.

C. Immediate induction of labour may be offered.
D. Intravaginal PGE2 cannot be used as there is leaking per vaginam.
E. Oxytocin has definite advantages and should be preferred over PGE2 (oral/vaginal).

LD31

The recommended gestational age to offer delivery to an uncomplicated triplet pregnancy is:

A. 34 weeks after a course of antenatal steroids
B. 35 weeks after a course of antenatal steroids
C. 34 weeks without steroids as the role of steroids in triplets is not established
D. 35 weeks without steroids as the role of steroids in triplets is not established
E. 37 weeks to avoid risks of prematurity

LD32

Mrs X, a 28-year-old primigravida has leaking of fluid per vaginam for the past 3 h at 32 weeks of gestation. Per speculum examination confirms leakage of clear amniotic fluid per vaginam. She is clinically stable with no signs of infection. Ultrasound shows a singleton fetus in cephalic presentation, appropriate for gestation with normal liquor and Dopplers.

You are explaining her clinical situation to her. You would be correct to say that:

A. Almost 10 % of pregnancies have PPROM.
B. Digital vaginal examination is recommended to help to assess her Bishop score.
C. Erythromycin should be given orally for 10 days following diagnosis of PPROM.
D. If NICU beds are available, it is better to deliver her immediately after steroid cover.
E. Vaginal PGE2 can be used for inducing her labour now.

LD33

Which of the following is correct regarding the use of misoprostol for induction of labour:

A. It is licenced for induction of labour in the UK.
B. Oral dose should not exceed 25 micrograms.
C. Risk of hyperstimulation is dose dependent.
D. Vaginal misoprostol 25 micrograms is superior to vaginal PGE2 for induction of labour.
E. When the cervix is unfavourable, doses above 25 micrograms are associated with higher rates of successful induction of labour.

LD34

The overall risk of obstetric anal sphincter injury during vaginal deliveries is:

A. 1 %
B. 1.5 %
C. 2 %
D. 2.5 %
E. 3.5 %

LD35

A primigravida at term, in first stage of labour had uterine hyperstimulation following oxytocin augmentation. The oxytocin drip was stopped, but after a few minutes, she had hypotension, tachycardia and a feeble pulse showing signs of collapse. Resuscitative efforts could not restore any cardiac output for 4 min, and a decision for perimortem caesarean section was taken. Which of the following is the correct approach in conducting the perimortem caesarean section?

A. If an epidural is not sited earlier, a general anaesthesia can be used.
B. The patient must be immediately shifted to the nearest emergency operating theatre.
C. The procedure must be done within 5 min of collapse after confirming fetal viability.
D. There is no need for checking fetal viability.
E. When resuscitation is ongoing, the procedure should be deferred.

LD36

Ms XY is 38/40 weeks pregnant in her first pregnancy. She has been treated for a GBS UTI at 32 weeks. She presents with a history of PROM with clear liquor. CTG is reassuring. Which of the following treatment options are best suited to her?

A. Antibiotics for the baby only, immediate postpartum
B. Antibiotics for the baby only, postpartum based in culture reports
C. Induction of labour in 24 h + IV benzylpenicillin immediately
D. Induction of labour + IV benzylpenicillin in active labour
E. Induction of labour + IV benzylpenicillin immediately

LD37

Ms XY is a G3P2 and term undergoing an emergency caesarean section under GA, as she presents in labour with previous 2 caesarean sections with an APH. During the CS, an anterior low-lying placenta fails to separate after delivery of the baby. A clear cleavage plane cannot be identified. The bleeding is minimal. She has consented to a sterilisation, as her family is now complete. Which of the following treatment options are best suited to her?

A. Attempt to separate placenta and caesarean hysterectomy if bleeding occurs
B. Elective caesarean hysterectomy
C. Leaving the placenta in situ with postoperative methotrexate
D. Removal of the bulk of the placenta and cord and closure
E. Removal of the placenta piecemeal and closure of bleeding points

LD38

Ms XY is primigravida at 41/40 weeks in spontaneous labour. She is Indian (Asian ethnicity) and has a baby in direct OP position. She has been pushing for 2 h and using epidural analgesia. The total duration of her second stage has been 3 h. She has been consented for a trial of instrumental delivery in theatre as birth is not imminent. Which of the following risk factors has the strongest association with obstetric anal sphincter injury?

A. Ethnicity
B. Occipito posterior position
C. Prolonged 2nd stage
D. Shoulder dystocia
E. Ventouse delivery with episiotomy

LD39

Which type of female pelvis favours direct occipito-posterior position?

A. Android pelvis
B. Anthropoid pelvis
C. Contracted pelvis
D. Gynaecoid pelvis
E. Platypelloid pelvis

LD40

Ms XY is 39/40 weeks pregnant. She presents to the labour suite in active labour with intact membranes. Her recent vaginal swabs were negative for GBS. Her previous baby has been affected by early-onset neonatal GBS disease. Which of the following treatment options are best suited to her?

A. Intrapartum antibiotic prophylaxis specific to GBS
B. No maternal antibiotic prophylaxis in labour
C. Neonatal antibiotic prophylaxis specific for GBS at birth

D. Routine neonatal cultures and antibiotic prophylaxis accordingly
E. Reassurance only as recent swabs negative for GBS

LD41

Ms XY is a primigravida who is 38 weeks pregnant. She presents with a history of PROM for a few hours. Examination reveals clear liquor. Maternal observations are normal.

What is the percentage of women that will spontaneously labour in 24 h of PROM at term?

A. 30 %
B. 40 %
C. 50 %
D. 60 %
E. 70 %

LD42

Which of the following is recommended as a method of induction of labour?

A. Extra-amniotic PGE2
B. Intracervical PGE2
C. Intravaginal PGE2
D. Intracervical PGE2
E. Oral PGE2

LD43

Ms XY is 35/40 weeks pregnant in her first pregnancy. Her USS today reveals a baby with extended breech presentation.

What is the incidence of breech presentation at term?

A. <1 %
B. 1–2 %
C. 3–4 %
D. 4–8 %
E. 8–10 %

LD44

Ms XY is 35/40 weeks pregnant in her first pregnancy and presented to her GP with white vaginal itchy discharge. Her vaginal swab collected 2 days ago revealed the presence of Group B streptococcus. She is very concerned and would like antibiotics for the same. Which of the following treatment options are best suited to her?

A. Antibiotics for the baby only, immediate postpartum
B. Antibiotics for the baby only, postpartum based in culture reports
C. IV benzylpenicillin as prophylaxis during an ELECTIVE caesarean section
D. IV benzylpenicillin in active labour
E. Oral penicillin V for 5 days

LD45

Ms XY is primigravida at 41/40 weeks in spontaneous labour. She is Indian (Asian ethnicity) and has a baby in direct OA position. She has been pushing for 1 h and using epidural analgesia. Birth is imminent. Perineum appears overstretched and distended. What angle of a mediolateral episiotomy is most likely to prevent an OASI?

A. 30° from the midline
B. 40° from the midline
C. 45° from the midline
D. 60° from the midline
E. 90° from the midline

LD46

Ms XY is a primigravida who is 38 weeks pregnant. She presents with a history of PROM for a few hours. Examination reveals clear liquor. Maternal observations are normal. What is the risk of serious neonatal infection with ruptured membranes at term?

A. 0.1 %
B. 0.5 %
C. 1 %
D. 5 %
E. 10 %

LD47

Ms XY is a primigravida who is 39 weeks pregnant in spontaneous active labour. She also has diet-controlled GDM. She is theatre as the FHR/CTG showed a fetal bradycardia for 8 mins. At 9 mins in theatre, the FHR has recovered. Examination reveals she is 7 cms dilated with clear liquor in direct OA position. Ms XY is very keen on a vaginal birth only if it safe for her labour to continue. She is currently using Entonox for analgesia.

What should be the next appropriate management plan?

A. Allow labour to continue
B. FBS
C. Proceed with CS under spinal anaesthesia
D. Proceed with CS under GA
E. Recommend epidural analgesia

LD48

Ms XY is 38/40 weeks pregnant. She has developed confirmed primary genital herpes. She is presently being treated with acyclovir. She has confirmed SROM since 2 h. Which of the following treatment options are best suited to her?

A. Caesarean section after adequately nil per oral (6 h later)
B. Caesarean section after corticosteroid cover (24–48 h later)
C. Immediate caesarean section
D. Immediate induction of labour with IV acyclovir
E. Induction of labour after 24 h with IV acyclovir

LD49

A 32-year-old second gravida came in preterm labour at 29 weeks of gestation. She was administered the first dose of antenatal corticosteroids, but she delivered just after 6 h of the first dose. It will be correct to tell her that the effect of the antenatal corticosteroids in her case:
A. Is not likely to be of any benefit
B. Is likely to reduce the risk of intraventricular haemorrhage
C. Is likely to reduce the risk of maternal inflammation
D. Is likely to reduce the risk of neonatal death
E. Is likely to reduce the risk of respiratory distress syndrome

LD50

You are conducting a lower segment caesarean section on a full-term primigravida with a free-floating fetal head. Peroperatively, there is difficulty is delivering the fetal head. Choose the single best option from the alternatives given below:

A. Ask for fundal pressure
B. Avoid any attempts of pushing from below
C. Breech extraction is an unacceptable option
D. Try gently to put your hand into the pelvis
E. Use of forceps is best avoided

Postpartum Issues: SBA Questions

5

PP1

You have just examined Mrs X in the postpartum clinic. She is complaining of breast pain and discomfort. You have established a diagnosis of postpartum mastitis.

All of the following are treatment options for her except:

A. Analgesics
B. Antibiotics if infective mastitis
C. Gentle hand expression to promote drainage
D. Local measures like hot and cold compress
E. Stopping breastfeeding

PP2

The commonest urinary problem occurring in the postpartum period is:

A. Detrusor instability
B. Mixed incontinence
C. Stress incontinence
D. Urinary tract infection
E. Vesicovaginal fistula

PP3

A 24-year-old woman presents to delivery suite with a 12 h history of right-sided chest pain and shortness of breath. She is at 7 days' postnatal having delivered her baby by emergency caesarean section at 34 weeks. Her pregnancy was complicated by severe hypertension and postpartum haemorrhage of 1 L. She has a BMI of 32. Her BP is 130/80 mmHg, pulse is 108 bpm, temperature is 37.2 and oxygen saturations are 94 % in air. What is the SINGLE most likely diagnosis?

A. Anaemia
B. Myocardial infarction
C. Pneumonia
D. Pulmonary embolism
E. Subphrenic abscess

PP4

A 40-year-old woman, who has had a previous caesarean delivery, experiences brisk vaginal bleeding immediately following vaginal delivery of a 36-week gestation baby (birth weight 3.8 kg). 10 min prior to the delivery, there was acute onset fetal bradycardia and cessation of uterine contractile activity. The urinary catheter shows haematuria. The placenta was delivered without complication.

Bimanual compression of the uterus is extremely painful for the woman. Despite an estimated blood loss of 500 ml, she appears pale and clammy with BP 90/30 and pulse 120 bpm. Which one of the following is the most likely cause for the excessive genital tract bleeding?

A. Excessive epidural analgesia
B. Retained placenta
C. Uterine atony
D. Uterine inversion
E. Uterine rupture

PP5

A 40-year-old woman, who has had three previous vaginal deliveries, experiences brisk vaginal bleeding immediately following vaginal delivery of 36-week gestation twins (birth weights 2.0 and 1.9 kg). An episiotomy was not required. The placenta was delivered without complication. She received an epidural top-up 30 min before delivery. The estimated blood loss is 700 ml. Which one of the following is the most likely cause for the excessive genital tract bleeding?

A. Excessive epidural analgesia
B. Retained placenta
C. Uterine atony
D. Uterine inversion
E. Uterine rupture

PP6

A 32-year-old woman presents to delivery suite with a 3-day history of worsening pelvic pain and vaginal bleeding with clots. She is at 5 days postnatal having delivered her baby by kiwi cup vacuum delivery at 41 weeks' gestation. She has a BMI of 32. Her BP is 130/80 mmHg, pulse is 108 bpm, temperature is 37.9 and oxygen saturations are 95 % in air. She has pelvic tenderness on examination.

What is the SINGLE most likely diagnosis?

A. Cervical carcinoma
B. Bacterial vaginosis
C. Endometritis
D. Urinary tract infection
E. Uterine rupture

PP7

Which one of the following statements is correct in relation to postpartum depression?

A. Antidepressants (paroxetine, sertraline, tricyclic group) are contraindicated if breastfeeding.
B. Postpartum blues occur in around 5 % of new mothers.
C. Postpartum depression affects around 10 % of women,
D. Postpartum psychosis has a low risk of recurrence.
E. Women with postpartum blues commonly think about committing infanticide.

PP8

Which one of the following best defines secondary postpartum haemorrhage?

A. Abnormal genital tract bleeding that occurs 24 h after delivery to 7 days' post partum
B. Abnormal genital tract bleeding that occurs between delivery to 7 days
C. Abnormal genital tract bleeding that occurs between delivery to 6 weeks' postpartum
D. Abnormal genital tract bleeding that occurs 24 h after delivery to 6 weeks' postpartum
E. Abnormal genital tract bleeding that occurs 48 h after delivery to 6 weeks' postpartum

PP9

Which one of the following correctly states how much energy is provided by human milk through breastfeeding?

A. 5 kcal per dL
B. 20 kcal per dL
C. 70 kcal per dL
D. 200 kcal per dL
E. 500 kcal per dL

PP10

Which one of the following correctly states the calorific energy requirements for a newborn infant born at term gestation?

A. 15 Kcal/kg/day
B. 30 Kcal/kg/day
C. 60 Kcal/kg/day
D. 120 Kcal/kg/day
E. 240 Kcal/kg/day

PP11

Postpartum anaemia is defined as a haemoglobin less than:

A. 100 g/l
B. 102 g/l
C. 105 g/l
D. 108 g/l
E. 110 g/l

PP12

A 34-year-old woman attends the postpartum clinic with complaints of superficial dyspareunia. She delivered a 4.5 kg baby with the help of outlet forceps 2 months back. She is currently breastfeeding. On local examination the perineum is healthy, no signs of atrophic vaginitis. On palpation, there is definite tenderness in the episiotomy scar. What will be your advice to her:

A. Antibiotics to reduce local infection.
B. Avoid sexual intercourse till the pain subsides.
C. Local anaesthetic application 30 min prior to intercourse.

D. Local corticosteroids for a week.

E. Surgical refashioning of the perineum will be a permanent solution.

PP13

A 25-year-old low-risk woman delivered a healthy baby at term by an emergency caesarean section for massive APH. Estimated blood loss was 1.5 L, uneventful recovery.

What is the risk of abruption in her next pregnancy?

A. 1.5 %

B. 2.5 %

C. 3.5 %

D. 4.5 %

E. 5.5 %

PP14

Ms. XY is brought to the A + E department, unwell. She is a para 1, post-SVD 3 days ago with ragged membranes noted at delivery. Her observations include pulse 128 bpm, BP 80 systolic, RR 24 breaths/min and temp 39° C and she feels cold and clammy. She reports heavy offensive lochia.

She has been fluid resuscitated now and commenced on oxygen by mask.

What is the next immediate step in her management?

A. Broad spectrum IV antibiotics

B. Blood cultures, HVS, MSU

C. EUA in theatre with removal of retained tissue

D. Imaging—pelvic USS

E. Measurement of serum lactate

PP15

Ms. XY is a para 1 who delivered 1 week ago. She was diagnosed to have GDM (diet controlled), and her plasma glucose levels have now returned to normal.

What follow-up should she have postpartum?

A. 75 g 2 h OGTT 6 weeks' postpartum

B. 75 g 1 h OGTT 6 weeks' postpartum

C. Fasting plasma glucose at 4 weeks' postpartum

D. Fasting plasma glucose at 12 weeks' postpartum

E. Random plasma glucose at 6 weeks' postpartum

PP16

Ms. XY is a para 1, day 1 postpartum and known to have essential hypertension and asthma. She was not medicated throughout her pregnancy. Her blood pressures postpartum have been 150–160 (S) and 95–100 (D). Her urine PCR is 20. She is breastfeeding.

Which of the following treatment options are best suited to her ?

A. Amlodipine
B. Enalapril
C. Labetelol
D. Methyldopa
E. Thiazide diuretics

PP17

Ms. XY is brought to the A + E department, unwell. She is a para 1, post-SVD 3 days ago with ragged membranes noted at delivery. Her observations include pulse 128 bpm, BP 80 systolic, RR 24 breaths/min and temp 39° C and she feels cold and clammy. She reports heavy offensive lochia. She has been fluid resuscitated now and commenced on oxygen by mask. Which of the following blood results reflect severe sepsis?

A. CRP 160 mg/L
B. D dimer—1600 ng/mL
C. ESR 90 mm/h
D. Serum lactate (arterial)—6 mmol/L
E. WCC—16×109/L

PP18

Ms. XY is brought to the A + E department, unwell. She is a para 1, post-SVD 3 days ago with ragged membranes noted at delivery. Her observations include pulse 128 bpm, BP 80 systolic, RR 24 breaths/min and temp 39° C and she feels cold and clammy. She reports heavy offensive lochia. Which of the following antibiotics are best suited to her?

A. Co-amoxiclav
B. Co-amoxiclav + gentamicin
C. Co-amoxiclav + metronidazole
D. Piperacillin—tazobactam
E. Piperacillin—tazobactam + clindamycin

PP19

Ms. XY is now a para 1, with A negative blood group. She has just delivered in the midwifery-led unit and has had to theatre for a manual removal of a retained placenta. Her baby at 0+ve. Kleihauer test suggests a fetomaternal haemorrhage of 6 mLs. How much anti-D should she receive?

A. 500 IU
B. 625IU
C. 750IU
D. 1000 IU
E. 1500IU

PP20

Drugs are prescribed in pregnancy upon the assumption that their positive effect on health outweighs the probability and severity of any harm to the mother and fetus. On this basis, which SINGLE drug is most likely to be contraindicated for maternal use when breastfeeding?

A. Cabergoline
B. Low-molecular-weight heparin
C. Nifedipine
D. Progestogen-only pill
E. Warfarin

PP21

Ms. XY was diagnosed to have an acute DVT at 34 weeks of gestation. She received antenatal LMWH. She has delivered this morning (38 weeks). She would like to discuss warfarin for postpartum thromboprophylaxis as she would rather avoid needles. She would like to breastfeed.
   Which of the following treatment options are best suited to her ?

A. Warfarin commenced at 48 h postpartum.
B. Warfarin commenced at 72 h postpartum.
C. Warfarin commenced at 96 h postpartum.
D. Warfarin commenced at 120 h postpartum.
E. Warfarin contraindicated, as she is breastfeeding.

PP22

Ms. XY is on day 1 postpartum following a vaginal delivery at home. She presents to the A + E department in septic shock. She gives history of a fever and sore throat leading up to the delivery.

What is the most likely organism responsible for her condition?

A. *E. Coli*
B. *C. difficile*
C. *H. Influenzae*
D. *S. aureus*
E. *S. pyogenes*

PP23

Ms. XY is in theatre recovery after repair of a 3B perineal tear. You come to debrief her about the procedure.

What percentage of women are asymptomatic after EAS repair at 12 months ?

A. 20–30 %
B. 40–50 %
C. 50–60 %
D. 60–80 %
E. >90 %

Early Pregnancy Care: Questions

6

EP1

The incidence of clinically recognised miscarriage in pregnancy is about:

A. Less than1 %
B. 1–2 %
C. 5–10 %
D. 10–20 %
E. 20–30 %

EP2

The most common indication for women attending gynaecology emergency in the UK is:

A. Bleeding in early pregnancy
B. Missing IUCD
C. Pain in the lower abdomen
D. Pelvic organ prolapse
E. Urinary incontinence

EP3

Which of the following routes of administration is inappropriate for the drug misoprostol:

A. Oral
B. Subdermal

© Springer India 2016
C. Ratha, J. Gupta, *SBAs and EMQs for MRCOG II*,
DOI 10.1007/978-81-322-2689-5_6

C. Sublingual
D. Rectal
E. Vaginal

EP4

Which one of the following ultrasound descriptions is diagnostic of miscarriage (GS, gestational sac; CRL, crown-rump length; FHR, fetal heart rate)?

A. Mean GS diameter 25 mm, with no obvious yolk sac or fetal pole
B. Mean GS diameter 25 mm containing a fetal pole with CRL = 3 mm without evidence of FHR
C. Mean GS diameter 40 mm containing a fetal pole with CRL = 7 mm with evidence of FHR
D. No identifiable intrauterine or extrauterine GS with serum βhCG 200 IU/L
E. No identifiable intrauterine or extrauterine GS with serum βhCG 1500 IU/L

EP5

A 20-year-old, who is at 12 weeks' gestation, has a 2-day history of vaginal bleeding and lower abdominal pain. Ultrasound shows a 25 mm fetal pole with absent fetal heart rate. Pelvic examination reveals her cervix to be 4 cm dilated with bulging intact membranes. Which one of the following is the most likely diagnosis?

A. Cervical incompetence
B. Incomplete miscarriage
C. Inevitable miscarriage
D. Pregnancy of uncertain viability
E. Threatened miscarriage

EP6

A 29-year-old, who is at 6 weeks' gestation, is diagnosed to have a right tubal ectopic pregnancy by transvaginal pelvic ultrasound. Which one of the following factors would enable systematic methotrexate to be offered as a medical treatment option for the ectopic pregnancy?

A. Ectopic adnexal mass is 5×4 cm in size.
B. Initial serum hCG 1000 IU/L.
C. Presence of fetal heart beat in ectopic pregnancy.
D. Ultrasound evidence of haemoperitoneum >50 mL.
E. The woman has had previous salpingectomy so further salpingectomy surgery is contraindicated.

EP7

A 29-year-old, who is at 6 weeks' gestation, presents with slight vaginal spotting. Transvaginal pelvic ultrasound shows no evidence of any intrauterine or extrauterine pregnancy. A serum βhCG is measured at initial presentation and repeated 48 h later. Which one of the following βhCG results is suspicious for a clinically significant ectopic pregnancy?

A. 500, 1200
B. 800, 200
C. 1000, 400
D. 1000, 3000
E. 2000, 2500

EP8

A patient with a positive pregnancy test, small amount of PV bleeding and no abdominal pain present has a single transvaginal ultrasound scan, showing an intrauterine gestational sac, with a crown-rump length (CRL) of 5 mm, with no fetal heart beat. Which of the following would be the most appropriate management plan?

A. Advise a to carry out a pregnancy test in 3 weeks.
B. Offer medical management of miscarriage.
C. Offer rescan after a minimum of 7–10 days.
D. Offer rescan in 48 h.
E. Offer surgical management of miscarriage.

EP9

A 25-year-old woman presents to the A+E department with left iliac fossa pain, vaginal bleeding and a positive pregnancy test. Which symptoms may be associated with an ectopic pregnancy?

A. Passage of tissue
B. Urinary symptoms
C. Rectal pressure and/or pain on defecation
D. Breast tenderness
E. All of the above

EP10

A 25-year-old woman presents to the A+E department with abdominal pain and a positive pregnancy test (8/40). USS is performed to rule out a miscarriage. USS shows an intrauterine gestational sac with the ratio of transverse to anteroposterior dimension, greater than 1.5 with cystic spaces in the placenta. What is the likely ultrasonographic diagnosis?

A. Complete molar pregnancy
B. Incomplete miscarriage
C. Missed miscarriage
D. Partial molar pregnancy
E. Pseudosac of an ectopic pregnancy

EP11

Ms. XY is a primigravida who presents to the A + E department with dark-brown discharge PV for 1 day and mild lower abdominal discomfort. She is 7/40 pregnant as per her LMP. Her TV scan shows the presence of a gestational sac and yolk sac with a fetal pole of 7.5 mm and no fetal heart activity.

Which of the following treatment options are best suited to her?

A. Discuss management options for miscarriage
B. Rescan in 1 week
C. Serum βhCG now and in 48 h
D. Serum hCG and progesterone
E. Serum progesterone to assess viability

EP12

Ms. XY is a primigravida who is 9/40 weeks' pregnant and has confirmed diagnosis of missed miscarriage (she had 2 transvaginal scans a week apart). After discussion of the various options, she opts for medical management for missed miscarriage. She is extremely anxious about the discomfort associated with the procedure and has a low pain threshold.

Which of the following is appropriate for medical management of missed miscarriage?

A. Mifepristone 200 mg PO + misoprostol 400 mcg PV
B. Misoprostol 800 mcg + NSAIDS for analgesia
C. Misoprostol 800 mcg
D. Oral Misoprostol 600 mcg
E. Vaginal Misoprostol 600 mcg

EP13

Ms. XY is a primigravida who presents to the A + E department with dark-brown discharge PV for 1 day and mild lower abdominal discomfort. She is 7/40 pregnant as per her LMP. Her transvaginal scan shows the presence of a gestational sac measuring 26 mm with no fetal pole. Which of the following treatment options are best suited to her?

A. Discuss management options for miscarriage.
B. Rescan in 1 week.
C. Serum βhCG now and in 48 h.
D. Serum hCG and progesterone.
E. Serum progesterone to assess viability.

EP14

Ms. XY is 9/40 weeks' pregnant. She presents to the early pregnancy clinic with a history of a painful vaginal heavy bleed 96 h ago. Ultrasound reveals a live fetus at 9/40 weeks with a 5×5 cm subchorionic haematoma. Booking bloods reveal she is A negative with no atypical antibodies.

Which of the following treatment options are best suited to her with regard to administration of anti-D?

A. Anti-D is not necessary (<12/40 weeks).
B. Anti-D is unlikely to be effective (>72 h).
C. Anti-D should be given in a dose of 250 IU.
D. Anti-D should be given in a dose of 500 IU.
E. Anti-D should be given after an appropriate test for FMH.

EP15

A 25-year-old woman diagnosed with a complete mole (16/40) is scheduled to undergo surgical evacuation in theatre. Which is the only acceptable management plan in her case?

A. Cervical priming using prostaglandins
B. Routine oxytocin infusion prior to commencement of evacuation
C. Oxytocin infusion in cases of life-threatening haemorrhage
D. Routine oxytocin infusion at the end of evacuation
E. IUCD for long-term contraception immediately post-procedure

EP16

Which of the following statements is appropriate in women presenting with early pregnancy with bleeding:

A. hCG measurement can determine the location of pregnancy.
B. If on expectant management pain and bleeding are resolved in 7–14 days, the UPT should be repeated after 3 weeks.

C. Mifepristone can be used in missed abortion and incomplete abortion.
D. Post-salpingotomy, 1 in 10 patients may need further treatment in the form of methotrexate or salpingectomy.
E. Serum progesterone measurements can be used as an adjunct to diagnose viable intrauterine/ ectopic pregnancy.

EP17

Medical management for an ectopic pregnancy can be considered if:

A. Unruptured ectopic pregnancy of <45 mm.
B. Cardiac activity is demonstrable.
C. hCG is <3500 IU/ml.
D. There is abdominal pain.
E. There is no evidence of intrauterine pregnancy.

EP18

The incidence of gestational trophoblastic disease in the UK is calculated as:

A. 1in 287 live births
B. 1 in 346 live births
C. 1 in 563 live births
D. 1in 714 live births
E. 1in 976 live births

EP19

Which of the following is not an example of gestational trophoblastic disease:

A. Chorioangioma
B. Choriocarcinoma
C. Complete mole
D. Partial mole
E. Placental site trophoblastic tumour

EP20

Which of the following statements is correct about molar pregnancy:

A. Complete moles usually (75–80 %) arise as a consequence of dispermic fertilisation of an 'empty ovum'.

B. Complete moles show evidence of mature fetal red blood cells.
C. Partial moles occur rarely due to dispermic fertilisation of an ovum.
D. Some complete moles (20–25 %) arise after duplication of a single sperm following fertilisation of an 'empty ovum'.
E. 10 % of partial moles represent tetraploid or mosaic conceptions.

Gynaecological Problems: SBA Questions

7

GYN1

Which of the following is a selective progesterone receptor modulator?

A. Dinoprostone
B. Misoprostol
C. Ormeloxifene
D. Raloxifene
E. Ulipristal

GYN2

Medical management of fibroids is best indicated when:

A. Fibroid is less than 3 cm, not distorting the cavity and asymptomatic.
B. Fibroid is less than 3 cm, distorting the cavity and asymptomatic.
C. Fibroid is less than 3 cm, not distorting the cavity and causing heavy bleeding.
D. Fibroid is more than 3 cm, distorting the cavity and asymptomatic.
E. Fibroid is more than 3 cm, not distorting the cavity and asymptomatic.

GYN3

The incidence of chronic pelvic pain in women of reproductive age group is:

A. 2–5 %
B. 5–10 %
C. 10–15 %

© Springer India 2016
C. Ratha, J. Gupta, *SBAs and EMQs for MRCOG II*,
DOI 10.1007/978-81-322-2689-5_7

D. 15–25 %
E. 40–50 %

GYN4

The commonest pathology identified at diagnostic laparoscopy in patients with chronic pelvic pain is:

A. Adhesions
B. Endometriosis
C. Fibroids
D. No pathology detected
E. Pelvic inflammatory disease

GYN5

The incidence of adnexal pathology detected for the first time in pregnancy is:

A. 0.5 %
B. 2–5 %
C. 5–6 %
D. 10 %
E. 15–20 %

GYN6

The preferred period for intervention for an ovarian mass in pregnancy is:

A. 8 weeks
B. 10 weeks
C. 12 weeks
D. 14 weeks
E. 20 weeks

GYN7

Pick the correct statement regarding management of ovarian cysts in pregnancy.

A. All suspected dermoid cysts need to be excised due to risk of torsion.
B. Following cyst aspiration, recurrence occurs in <5 % of women.

C. Persistent simple cysts larger than 10 cm can be offered cyst aspiration.
D. Simple cysts smaller than 5 cm persist in 20 % of women.
E. Torsion commonly occurs in the third trimester.

GYN8

A 45-year-old woman presents with right-sided nipple discharge. Clinical examination and mammography showed no abnormalities. Which one of the following is the next most appropriate action?

A. Cytology.
B. Microdochectomy.
C. MRI scan.
D. Ultrasound of the breast.
E. Underlying cancer is a common finding; therefore, organise surgery for mastectomy.

GYN9

Which one of the following is correct in relation to polycystic ovarian syndrome, PCOS?

A. Increased risk of type II diabetes or gestational diabetes.
B. Increased risk of uterine polyps.
C. No induction of uterine bleeding following 5 days of oral progestogen therapy.
D. Resistant to clomiphene citrate ovulation induction in 50 % of cases.
E. Virilisation is common.

GYN10

Obstetric outcomes in pregnancy after uterine artery embolisation—which of the following is not true?

A. The caesarean section rate is about 50 %.
B. Miscarriage rates are increased.
C. PPH is increased due to abnormal placentation.
D. Rate of preterm delivery is increased up to 16 %.
E. There is higher rate of malpresentation.

GYN11

A 14-year-old girl presents in the gynaecology OPD with a history of irregular bleeding per vaginam for the last 4–5 months. She has been rather stressed out with her school and theatre group activities which is adversely affecting her routine life and cannot recollect her dates or menstrual pattern well.

She was on the pill for the past year. Of late she has loss of appetite with nausea and vomiting and fullness of the lower abdomen. She has lost weight in the last 3 months due to poor food intake. On examination vesicles are seen in the vagina close to the external cervical os.

What is the most likely clinical diagnosis?

A. Contact dermatitis
B. Genital herpes
C. Molar pregnancy
D. Sarcoma botryoides
E. Vaginal carcinoma

GYN12

Ms. XY is 64 years old and is postmenopausal. She has recently been diagnosed with a 4 cm ovarian cyst on a transabdominal scan. The scan could not identify the other ovary as the bowel obscured it.

The scan was being undertaken for suspected gallstones with the cyst being an incidental finding. Ms. XY is very anxious that this may represent ovarian cancer. Which of the following investigations are best suited to her to further investigate the ovarian cyst?

A. CA-125
B. CT Abdomen and pelvis
C. MRI
D. Transvaginal ultrasound with Doppler studies
E. Transvaginal ultrasound + CA-125

GYN13

Ms. XY is 32 years old, otherwise fit and well and using the progesterone-only pill for contraception. She has recently been diagnosed (incidentally) with a 55 mm simple right ovarian cyst with anechoic fluid.

Her CA-125 results are 5 u/ml. She is very anxious about the prospect of surgery. She has been risk assessed for VTE and is at low risk for using the COCP.

Which of the following treatment options are best suited to her?

A. Offer COCP for three cycles and repeat the USS.
B. Offer laparoscopic ovarian cystectomy.

C. Repeat USS in 12 months, unless symptomatic.
D. Reassure and discharge from care.
E. Stop the POP as it is associated with ovarian cysts.

GYN14

Ms. XY, 22 years old, has recently been diagnosed with PCOS. Her BMI is 23. Her modified GTT was normal. She has very irregular oligomenorrheic cycles. She is extremely anxious about her general health and the risk of cancer. She is not planning a pregnancy in the near future. She suffers from migraines. Which of the following treatment options are best suited to her?

A. Annual screening for breast cancer
B. Annual screening for ovarian cancer
C. Annual modified GTT
D. COCPs
E. Three monthly withdrawal bleeds with gestagens

GYN15

Ms. XY is 35 years old with a Mirena IUD in situ. She presents to the colposcopy clinic with her latest smear showing *Actinomyces*-like organisms (ALO). She complains of pelvic pain, deep dyspareunia and vaginal discharge for a week. She is not sexually active presently.

Which of the following treatment options are best suited to her?

A. PID outpatient antibiotics (ceftriaxone IM followed by doxycycline and metronidazole).
B. Remove Mirena and send for culture + PID outpatient antibiotics.
C. Remove Mirena and send for culture + amoxicillin PO.
D. Triple swabs (STI) and treat after culture results.
E. Triple swabs (STI) + PID outpatient antibiotics.

GYN16

Which of the following statements is true about endometrial polyps?

A. Endometrial polyps are common among women under the age of 20 years.
B. Endometrial polyps are usually symptomatic and cause heavy menstrual bleeding.
C. In both pre- and postmenopausal women, endometrial polyps lose their apoptotic regulation and overexpress oestrogen and progesterone receptors.

D. The malignant potential of endometrial polyps is high.

E. There is no role of conservative management for endometrial polyps.

GYN17

A 45-year-old woman with a BMI of 48 is requesting for a hysterectomy in order to have a permanent solution to her menorrhagia. She has been having heavy bleeding since the last 5–6 months and her haemoglobin is 100 g/L. Her colleague at work had a hysterectomy 6 months back for long-standing menorrhagia, and she is relieved after the surgery, so she also wants to have the operation as soon as possible. You are reluctant to plan a surgery right away as there are serious risks associated with surgery in obese women.

Which of the following approach is not recommended?

A. Explain to her that both laparoscopic and open surgery would carry serious risks in her case.

B. If she is insistent, then plan for the hysterectomy as soon as possible with adequate precautions.

C. Offer advice regarding weight loss (food intake, exercise, support, medication, bariatric surgery).

D. Offer alternative treatment like a levonorgestrel intrauterine system.

E. Tell her that she should seriously consider alternate therapy options if it can help her avoid surgery.

GYN18

A 26-year-old woman presents to her OPD with complaints of dyspareunia. She has been having a painful period for the past 1 year, and the pain has increased lately. She has some vaginal discharge which is not foul smelling or associated with pruritus. She also complains of becoming irritable during her periods in the past few months. Speculum examination reveals the presence of blue nodules in the vagina.

What is the most likely diagnosis?

A. Bacterial vaginosis

B. Cervicitis

C. Endometriosis

D. Pelvic inflammatory disease

E. Vulvovaginitis

GYN19

During embryological development of the normal female reproductive system in humans, which of the following does not occur?

A. Both male and female fetuses initially have both a Wolffian (mesonephric) duct that lies medially and a Müllerian (paramesonephric) duct that lies laterally.
B. Primordial germ cells form by week 8, subsequently migrating into the developing ovary at week 11 and differentiating into oogonia.
C. The paramesonephric duct develops into the uterus and fallopian tubes, while the vagina develops from the vaginal plate.
D. The two Müllerian ducts fuse at the caudal end to form the body of the developing uterus, and the unfused lateral arms form the fallopian tubes.
E. The urogenital system develops from the intermediate mesothelium of the peritoneal cavity and the endoderm of the urogenital sinus.

GYN20

Some procedures are recommended while conducting a routine gynaecological examination. Which of the following is not appropriate?

A. Presence of a chaperone is considered essential.
B. Should the patient decline the presence of a chaperone, the doctor should send the chaperon out of the room.
C. The consent for the examination should be recorded in the notes.
D. Verbal consent should be obtained in the presence of the chaperone.
E. Whenever there is an indication for breast examination, verbal consent should be obtained, again in the presence of a chaperone.

GYN21

The reported incidence of psychosexual disorders in women attending gynaecology clinics is around:

A. 2–3 %
B. 5–7 %
C. 7–10 %
D. 20–30 %
E. 50–60 %

GYN22

Women with premature ovarian insufficiency are not at increased risk of:

A. Atherosclerosis
B. Breast cancer
C. Cerebrovascular accidents

D. Osteoporosis
E. Vulvovaginitis

GYN23

A 26-year-old woman presents to her GP complaining of new onset vaginal discharge. She is sexually active and uses condoms for protection against STIs although she has been regularly using the pill for the last 6 months. She has had 2 partners in the last 6 months. She is particularly worried because she has had spotting per vaginam after sexual intercourse in the last few weeks. Her Pap smear done last year was normal. Speculum examination reveals the presence of an erythematous raw-looking cervix.

What is the most likely diagnosis?

A. Aphthous ulcer
B. Bacterial vaginosis
C. Cervical polyp
D. Chlamydia
E. Ectropion

GYN24

From an outflow tract perspective, the only uterine anomaly that may cause a problem is:

A. Arcuate uterus
B. Bicornuate uterus
C. Complete septate uterus
D. Noncommunicating rudimentary horn
E. Unicornuate uterus

GYN25

A worried mother gets her 16-year-old girl to her GP. She is concerned that her daughter has not as yet commenced her periods. On examination there is poor development of secondary sexual characters, cubitus valgus, evidence of webbed neck and short stature. Which of the following investigations will help you confirm the diagnosis?

(a) Estimation of serum FSH:LH
(b) Karyotyping
(c) MRI of the pelvis
(d) Ultrasound of the pelvis
(e) X ray of the limbs

GYN26

In the use of SSRI/SNRIs for treatment of severe PMS, all of the following statements are true except:

A. Possible side effects of SSRIs include nausea, insomnia and reduction of libido.
B. SSRI/SNRI should be considered as first-line pharmacological intervention for severe PMS.
C. SSRIs should be withdrawn gradually when given full cycle to avoid withdrawal symptoms.
D. There is good evidence that it can be combined with hormonal contraceptives for better control of symptoms.
E. Total premenstrual daily symptom report (DSR) scores were better with luteal phase dosing than full-cycle dosing.

GYN27

A 43-year-old woman is having a diagnostic hysterolaparoscopy as part of the investigations for abnormal uterine bleeding. During laparoscopy, you see an ovarian cyst in the left ovary which is possible for an endometrioma.

You have taken consent only for diagnostic hysterolaparoscopy. What is the most appropriate course of action?

A. Complete the diagnostic procedure now and discuss with her treatment for the ovarian cyst later.
B. Do an ovarian cystectomy as you have anyway put her under anaesthesia, and technically you can complete the process right away.
C. Proceed for an exploratory laparotomy as the surgery may present unexpected complications if done laparoscopically.
D. Proceed for a hysterectomy as she was considering this as an option when you discussed the treatment plan for abnormal uterine bleeding with her last month in the OPD.
E. Take consent from her relatives for the ovarian cyst/ovary removal, go ahead with the procedure and debrief her later.

GYN28

Of the following complementary therapy options, choose the one with evidence of effect in the treatment of premenstrual syndrome:

A. Evening primrose oil
B. *Ginkgo biloba*
C. Magnesium

D. St John's wort
E. Vitamin A

GYN29

A 34-year-old nullipara is undergoing treatment for primary infertility. She has irregular periods with a cycle length varying from 45 to 60 days. Her last menstrual period was about 7 weeks back. She was posted for diagnostic hysterolaparoscopy, and during laparoscopy you find an unexpected ectopic pregnancy in the left fallopian tube. She is hemodynamically stable and the right fallopian tube appears healthy.

You have taken consent only for diagnostic hysterolaparoscopy. What is the most appropriate course of action?

A. Abandon the procedure now and discuss with her treatment for ectopic pregnancy later.
B. Do bilateral salpingectomy to prevent further ectopic pregnancies and plan fertility treatment later.
C. Proceed for an exploratory laparotomy.
D. Remove the ectopic pregnancy at the same sitting and debrief her later.
E. Report your junior staff for negligence for not ruling out pregnancy prior to procedure.

GYN30

A 53-year-old woman who is amenorrheic for the past 1 year complains of vaginal dryness, superficial dyspareunia and urinary urgency. She has been treated for urinary infection 2 months back, and there is no active urinary infection now although symptoms persist. She has been on HRT for the past 6 months due to severe palpitations, hot flushes and night sweats, and she is relieved of those symptoms.

Which of the following statements is appropriate for her?

A. Low-dose local corticosteroids are the most effective treatment in this case.
B. Reassure her as she is already on HRT that these symptoms will also subside gradually.
C. Start treatment with vaginal oestrogen for relief of symptoms.
D. These symptoms cannot be due to oestrogen deficiency as she is already on HRT.
E. Urodynamic study should be advised.

Subfertility and Endocrinology: SBA Questions

8

SFE1

All of the following are causes of premature ovarian failure except:

A. Fragile X syndrome
B. Kallmans syndrome
C. Mumps oophoritis
D. Pelvic irradiation
E. Turner's syndrome

SFE2

Among the following, select the strongest prognostic factor associated with recurrent miscarriages:

A. Fibroids
B. Increasing maternal age
C. Polycystic ovarian disease
D. Positive anticardiolipin antibodies
E. Smoking

SFE3

All of the following may adversely affect male fertility except:

A. Anabolic steroids
B. Cannabis addiction
C. Moderate alcohol consumption

© Springer India 2016
C. Ratha, J. Gupta, *SBAs and EMQs for MRCOG II*,
DOI 10.1007/978-81-322-2689-5_8

D. Tobacco consumption
E. Varicoceles

SFE4

Post testicular causes account for the following percentage of male infertility:

A. 10 %
B. 20 %
C. 30 %
D. 40 %
E. 50 %

SFE5

Choose the first option of management for mild male factor infertility:

A. In vitro fertilisation
B. Six cycles of IUI along with clomiphene citrate
C. Six cycles of IUI alone
D. Three cycles of IUI with clomiphene citrate
E. Three cycles of IUI alone

SFE6

Average pregnancy rated with ICSI (intracytoplasmic sperm injection)

A. 10–15 %
B. 15–25 %
C. 30–40 %
D. 50–60 %
E. 60–70 %

SFE7

The growth factor implicated in mediating the effects of ovarian hyperstimulation is:

A. Insulin-like growth factor
B. Placental growth factor
C. Transforming growth factor α

D. Transforming growth factor β
E. Vascular endothelial growth factor

SFE8

Which one of the following statements is correct regarding recurrent miscarriage?

A. Antiphospholipid syndrome, if found to be the cause of recurrent miscarriage, is untreatable.
B. Antiphospholipid antibodies are present in 15 % of women with recurrent miscarriage.
C. Cervical weakness (incompetence) is a recognised cause of first-trimester recurrent miscarriage.
D. One of the partners carries a chromosomal abnormality in at least 25 % of couples with recurrent miscarriage.
E. Recurrent miscarriage is defined as the loss of two or more consecutive pregnancies before 24 weeks gestation.

SFE9

Which ONE of the following is correct in relation to the prevalence of the main causes of infertility in the UK?

A. Factors in the male causing infertility (10 %)
B. Fibroids (30 %)
C. Ovulatory disorders (10 %)
D. Tubal damage (50 %)
E. Unexplained infertility (no identified male or female cause) (25 %)

SFE10

Which ONE of the following clinical scenarios is considered diagnostic of polycystic ovarian syndrome?

A. Infrequent periods, elevated testosterone
B. Infrequent periods, infertility, low day 21 serum progesterone
C. Infrequent periods, impaired glucose tolerance, obesity
D. Polycystic ovaries, obesity, low day 21 serum progesterone
E. Polycystic ovaries, elevated LH:FSH ratio, obesity

SFE11

A 34-year-old woman, who has been trying to conceive for 3 years, is referred to the infertility clinic for further management. Which ONE of the following is an appropriate discussion issue during her clinic counselling?

A. Altering smoking, alcohol or caffeine intake has no impact on spontaneous or IVF pregnancy success.
B. Despite having regular monthly menstrual cycles, a mid-luteal serum progesterone test is recommended in order to confirm ovulation.
C. Laparoscopy is the only reliable method to screen for tubal abnormalities.
D. Low serum progesterone in the mid-luteal phase of their cycle confirms ovulation.
E. There is a need for an endometrial biopsy to exclude luteal phase defect.

SFE12

A 40-year-old woman, who has been trying to conceive for 3 years, is offered IVF (in vitro fertilisation) as a treatment option by her fertility specialist. Which ONE of the following is an appropriate discussion issue during her clinic counselling?

A. Ovarian volume, ovarian blood flow and inhibin B usefully predict IVF success rate.
B. Preimplantation genetic diagnosis (PGD) of the embryo is required prior to its uterine transfer.
C. Progesterone administration is not required following embryo transfer.
D. Salpingectomy prior to IVF is beneficial in women with hydrosalpinges.
E. The chance of a live birth following IVF treatment increases with rising female age.

SFE13

Which ONE of the following clinical scenarios is considered diagnostic of polycystic ovarian syndrome?

A. Hirsutism, obesity, elevated testosterone
B. Hirsutism, elevated LH:FSH ratio, impaired glucose tolerance
C. Infertility, infrequent periods, obesity
D. Infrequent periods, elevated LH:FSH ratio, obesity
E. Infrequent periods, elevated testosterone

SFE14

Which ONE of the following is likely to predict a favourable ovarian response to gonadotrophin stimulation in IVF (in vitro fertilisation)?

A. Anti-Mullerian hormone ≤5.4 pmol/l
B. Follicle-stimulating hormone <4 IU/l
C. Increased ovarian blood flow on pelvic ultrasound
D. Oestradiol (E2) >500 pmol/L
E. Total antral follicle count ≤4 on pelvic ultrasound

SFE15

A 30-year-old woman has been trying to conceive for 3 years. She has infrequent menstrual cycles. Ultrasound confirms a normal uterus and polycystic ovaries. X-ray hysterosalpingogram has confirmed bilateral patent fallopian tubes. Her partner's semen analysis is reported as within normal limits. Her BMI is 25 kg/m². She has normal prolactin, FSH, oestradiol and testosterone. Of the options listed, which one of the following therapies is considered the most appropriate initial therapy?

A. Bromocriptine
B. Clomiphene citrate
C. Gonadotrophin
D. Laparoscopic ovarian drilling
E. Metformin

SFE16

The WHO classification of ovulation disorders describes three classes. Which one of the following is characteristically associated with low FSH and low oestrogen (WHO Class I)?

A. Hyperprolactinaemia
B. Ovarian endometriosis
C. Ovarian failure
D. Polycystic ovarian syndrome
E. Weight loss (low BMI)

SFE17

The WHO classification of ovulation disorders describes three classes. Which one of the following is characteristically associated with high FSH and low oestrogen (WHO Class III)?

A. Hyperprolactinaemia
B. Ovarian endometriosis
C. Ovarian failure
D. Polycystic ovarian syndrome
E. Weight loss (low BMI)

SFE18

In cases of infertility:

A. All mild to moderate endometriosis patients with infertility should have laparoscopy+adhesiolysis with an expert before IVF.
B. Gonadotrophins can be offered as second-line treatment in cases of clomiphene resistant PCOS patients.
C. In cases of mild male factor infertility, it is recommended that sperm concentration and IUI should be done for three cycles.
D. In cases of unexplained infertility, stimulated IUI is better than no treatment.
E. NICE recommends IVF as the treatment of choice in cases of unexplained infertility if not conceived after 1 year of unprotected intercourse.

SFE19

The mother of a 10-year-old girl with beta-thalassemia major seeks consultation in order to enquire about how the fertility prospects of her daughter may be affected due to her medical condition.
   Which of the following statements would be incorrect to tell her?

A. Her daughter's fertility may be reduced due to iron overload.
B. Hormonal contraceptives are contraindicated in these women.
C. Ovulation induction with injectable gonadotrophins may be needed.
D. Prolonged period of iron chelation therapy may be required prior to induction of ovulation and pregnancy.
E. Puberty is often delayed and incomplete in girls with beta-thalassemia major.

SFE20

A 40-year-old man undergoes a semen analysis test. Which one of the following components listed in his test result is considered to be ABNORMAL according to WHO 2010 semen analysis criteria?

A. Progressive motility 25 %
B. Sperm concentration 50×106 per ml

C. Total (progressive and nonprogressive motility) 75 %
D. Total sperm number 200×106 spermatozoa per ejaculate
E. Volume 4.0 ml

SFE21

The single largest cause of acquired tubal pathology is:

A. Acinetobacter
B. Bacterial vaginosis
C. Chlamydia trachomatis
D. Group A streptococcus
E. Mycobacterium tuberculosis

SFE22

Ms XY is 38 years old and suffers from primary infertility and endometriosis. Her recent TV scan suggests the presence of a 2.5 cm endometrioma. Her pain is well controlled using simple analgesics.

She is due to undergo IVF. Which treatment is best suited to deal with her endometrioma?

A. Expectant management
B. Laparoscopic ovarian cystectomy
C. Laparoscopic ovarian cyst aspiration
D. Laparoscopic ovarian cyst fenestration and drainage
E. Laparoscopic salpingoophorectomy

SFE23

Ms XY (30 years) and her male partner (26 years) have been trying to conceive naturally for the last 3 years. They have had infertility investigations over the last year. These include a normal semen analysis, normal USS pelvis, normal HSG, normal TSH, prolactin, D3 FSH, LH and normal AMH.

Her day 21 progesterone suggest ovulation. Ms XY is rubella immune and has negative swabs for an STI. Her recent cervical smear is normal. Which of the following treatment options are best suited to her?

A. Clomiphene citrate
B. IUI
C. IVF-ICSI
D. IVF
E. Letrozole

SFE24

Which of the following statements correctly describes salpingitis isthmica nodosa?

A. It involves endosalpingeal but not myosalpingeal compartments of the fallopian tube.
B. It is the most common cause of distal tubal disease.
C. Is associated with perihepatic adhesions.
D. Leads commonly to hydrosalpinx.
E. Results of tubal resection and anastomosis for SIN have poor success rates.

SFE25

Women with OHSS are specially prone to:

(a) Thrombosis of vessels in calf
(b) Thrombosis of vessels in upper body
(c) Thrombosis of vessels in the spleen
(d) Thrombosis of vessels in the kidney
(e) Thrombosis of vessels in the liver

SFE26

Measures to predict ovarian response to gonadotrophin stimulation in IVF are all except:

(a) Antral follicle count less than four
(b) Antral follicle count more than 16
(c) Anti-Mullerian hormone
(d) FSH levels
(e) Ovarian volume

SFE27

Fertiloscopy is an outpatient technique that includes (THL = transvaginal hydrolaparoscopy):

A. Hysteroscopy, falloposcopy and salpingoscopy
B. Hysteroscopy, falloposcopy and THL
C. Hysteroscopy, THL and salpingoscopy
D. Hysterolaparoscopy and salpingoscopy
E. Hysterolaparoscopy, THL, falloposcopy and salpingoscopy

SFE28

Risk of transmission of HIV from HIV-positive male to female partner is negligible when all the following criteria are met except:

(a) Man is compliant with HAART.
(b) The plasma viral load is <50 copies/ml for 3 months.
(c) There are no other infections present.
(d) Unprotected intercourse is limited to the time of ovulation.
(e) Male/female condoms are regularly used.

SFE29

Hypogonadotropic hypogonadism as a cause for male subfertility is seen in:

(a) <1 %
(b) 5 %
(c) 10 %
(d) 15 %
(e) 20 %

SFE30

Which of the following statements regarding androgen metabolism in women is not true?

A. In healthy women, 80 % of circulating testosterone is bound to sex hormone-binding globulin (SHBG), 19 % is bound to albumin and 1 % circulates freely in the blood stream.
B. Most of the circulating testosterone is metabolised in the liver into androsterone and etiocholanolone.
C. Of the circulating androgens, only testosterone and DHEA-S are able to activate androgen receptors.
D. Some androgen production occurs in all healthy women and is required for the synthesis of estrogens.
E. Urinary 17-ketosteroids are end products of androgen metabolism.

SFE31

In counselling women planning for fertility treatment about the risk of malignancy associated with use of fertility drugs, which of the following statements is true?

A. Aetiology of malignant melanoma, and to a lesser extent that of thyroid cancer, is known to involve endogenous and exogenous hormones; hence, there is a significant association of IVF cycles to non-gynaecological cancers.
B. Most fertility medications are associated with significantly increased risk of breast cancer.
C. There is strong evidence linking infertility treatment with childhood cancers.
D. There is strong evidence to link multiple IVF cycles to development of uterine cancer.
E. When counselling, patients in general should be reassured about the current data: that there is no significant increase in risk of cancer with IVF treatment for them or their offspring.

SFE32

Surgical reversal of tubal sterilisation:

A. Is as successful as IVF.
B. NHS funds surgical reversal of tubal sterilisation.
C. NHS funds IVF in this patient group.
D. Results are independent of woman's age.
E. Residual tubal length less than 4 cm is a good prognostic factor.

SFE33

The primary metabolic problem in congenital adrenal hyperplasia is a deficiency in production of:

A. Adrenocorticotrophic hormone (ACTH)
B. Aldosterone
C. Cortisol
D. Corticotrophin-releasing hormone (CRH)
E. Dehydroepiandrostenedione

SFE34

Ms XY is 7 weeks pregnant. She has been diagnosed with her 3 consecutive first-trimester miscarriages before this pregnancy. She is 28 years old and with the same partner. She is presently on folic acid supplementation. Her miscarriages remain unexplained. Which of the following treatment options are best suited to her?

A. Aspirin
B. Aspirin and LMWH

C. HCG injections
D. Progesterone supplementation
E. Reassurance and expectant management

SFE35

The direct biochemical evidence of hyperandrogenism is obtained by measurement of serum:

A. Androstenedione
B. Anti-Mullerian hormone
C. DHEAS (dehydroepiandrostenedione)
D. Levonorgestrel
E. Testosterone

Sexual and Reproductive Health: SBA Questions

9

SRH 1

The incidence of hot flushes in surgically induced menopause:

A. 25 %
B. 50 %
C. 60 %
D. 75 %
E. 90 %

SRH2

A 22-year-old woman presents to her GP for advice regarding the most appropriate postnatal contraception. She had an uncomplicated vaginal delivery 6 weeks back at 40 weeks gestation. She is intermittently breastfeeding and bottle feeding her baby. She and her partner are keen to space out child bearing by 2–3 years and requesting for the most reliable form of contraception. She admits to having difficulty in remembering to take contraceptive medication. Select the SINGLE most appropriate contraceptive option:

A. Combined contraceptive vaginal ring
B. Combined oral contraceptive pill
C. Condoms
D. Lactational amenorrhoea
E. Progestogen only implant

© Springer India 2016
C. Ratha, J. Gupta, *SBAs and EMQs for MRCOG II*,
DOI 10.1007/978-81-322-2689-5_9

SRH3

A 22-year-old woman presents to her GP for advice regarding the most appropriate postnatal contraception. She had an uncomplicated vaginal delivery at 40 weeks gestation 3 weeks prior.

She is bottle feeding her baby. She and her partner are keen to space out child bearing by 1–2 years and wishing a reliable form of contraception. She has a history of irregular menstrual cycles and polycystic ovarian syndrome. Select the SINGLE most appropriate contraceptive option:

A. Combined oral contraceptive pill
B. Copper intrauterine device
C. Levonorgestrel-releasing intrauterine system (Mirena)
D. Progestogen only pill
E. Progestogen only injectable

SRH4

Which one of the following is correct in relation to vaginal discharge?

A. Empirical treatment, based on history taking alone, is appropriate if BV or candida is clinically suspected and the risk of PID is considered very low.
B. Is more characteristic with chlamydia than trichomonas vaginalis infection.
C. The presence of Gardnerella vaginalis alone is sufficient to diagnose BV.
D. Vaginal pH measurement can help distinguish between bacterial vaginosis and trichomonas vaginalis.
E. Wet microscopy of the discharge is unreliable and unlikely to yield causative organism.

SRH5

A 26-year-old woman sought contraceptive advice, and after considering all her options, she decided to start on the combined oral contraceptive pill. As you have to advise her on the best method of using these pills, you are giving her some directions. Which of the following statements is incorrect in this regard?

A. If you start the pill on the first day of your period, you will be protected from pregnancy immediately.
B. If you start the pill at any other time in your menstrual cycle, you will need to use additional contraception, such as condoms, for the first 7 days of pill taking.

C. If you miss one pill anywhere in your pack or start the new pack 1 day late, you will need to use additional contraception, such as condoms, for the first 7 days of pill taking.
D. You can also start the pill up to, and including, the fifth day of your period and you will be protected from pregnancy immediately.
E. You can start the pill any time in your menstrual cycle if you are sure you are not pregnant.

SRH6

Which one of the following is correct in relation to syphilis?

A. Identified preferentially by culture of genital ulcer exudate in artificial media.
B. Dark field microscopy of genital ulcer (chancre) exudate is non-diagnostic.
C. Antibacterial treatment in early pregnancy does not prevent congenital syphilis.
D. Primary syphilis is associated with a mucocutaenous rash.
E. Secondary syphilis is associated with generalised lymphadenopathy.

SRH7

Which one of the following is correct in relation to neisseria gonorrhoea?

A. Culture requires anaerobic medium.
B. Is not a recognised cause for neonatal ophthalmia neonatorum (neonatal 'sticky eye').
C. Infects superficial mucosal surfaces lined with squamous epithelium.
D. Untreated, may cause a syndrome of fever, skin lesions, arthritis and endocarditis.
E. Vaccine preventing transmission exists.

SRH8

Which one of the following is correct in relation to chlamydia?

A. Chlamydial infection is the second most common bacterial sexually transmitted infection in the UK.
B. If diagnosed during pregnancy, antibiotic treatment should be deferred till after delivery.
C. May cause triad of arthritis, conjunctivitis and urethritis in young men.
D. More likely to be symptomatic than asymptomatic in women.
E. Previous chlamydia does not increase the risk of ectopic pregnancy.

SRH9

Which one of the following is correct in relation to diagnosing and treating acute pelvic inflammatory disease (PID)?

A. All cases diagnosed with PID require transvaginal ultrasound scanning.
B. Long-term sequelae are unrelated to the severity of PID at presentation.
C. Outpatient antibiotic treatment should not be commenced prior to identification of organisms on swabs or knowing their sensitivities.
D. Over the long term, a copper IUD is associated with a lower rate of PID compared to Mirena LNGIUS.
E. The absence of endocervical or vaginal pus cells on a wet-mount vaginal smear reliably excludes PID.

SRH10

Which one of the following drugs, if given in combination with the combined oral contraceptive (COC), will reduce the contraceptive efficacy of COC?

A. Ampicillin
B. Doxycycline
C. Erythromycin
D. Rifampicin
E. Sodium valproate

SRH11

The contraceptive injection, which lasts for 3 months, contains which one of the following:

A. Depot medroxyprogesterone acetate
B. Ethinyl estradiol
C. Etonogestrel
D. Levonorgestrel
E. Norethindrone

SRH12

Which one of the following is characteristically associated with the use of combined oral contraceptive pill?

A. 'Contraceptive failure is more likely if miss 2 pills mid-packet than beginning or end of a packet'.
B. Contraindicated if previous personal history of hydatidiform mole.
C. Decreases the risk of ovarian and endometrial cancer.
D. Reduces the risk of breast and cervical cancer.
E. Routine thrombophilia testing is required prior to commencing COC because of it increasing the risk of thromboembolism.

SRH13

Which one of the following is characteristically associated with the use of progestogen-only pill contraceptive?

A. Causes reduced bone mineral density.
B. Decreases the risk of breast cancer.
C. Decreases the risk of functional ovarian cysts.
D. Inhibits lactation.
E. Menstrual irregularities tend to resolve on long-term treatment.

SRH14

Which one of the following is appropriate when counselling a woman who is requesting emergency contraception following unprotected sexual intercourse (UPSI)?

A. Copper IUCD insertion is effective provided it is inserted no more than 5 days after known ovulation.
B. No oral medication exists if >72 h elapsed from unprotected intercourse.
C. No emergency contraception is available over the counter without a prescription.
D. Tablet methods are more effective than copper-IUCD at preventing pregnancy.
E. Ulipristal is a prostaglandin that is effective if taken within 120 h of UPSI.

SRH15

Which one of the following is appropriate when counselling a woman who is requesting postnatal contraception?

A. COC can be used from 3 weeks postpartum in breast feeding mothers.
B. Cu-IUCD or Mirena IUS may be fitted 4 weeks after a vaginal or caesarean birth.
C. Lactational amenorrhoea (requires fully breastfeeding and amenorrhoea) has around 0.5 % failure rate, even if menses occur.

D. No contraception is needed till 42 days postpartum as this is the earliest ovulation can recommence.
E. POP inhibit lactation and are contraindicated if breastfeeding.

SRH16

In relation to the law on young people, confidentiality and consent, which one of the
following statements is correct?

A. A doctor is unable to give contraceptive treatment or advice to a person under
   the age of 16 year.
B. Gillick competency and Fraser guidelines are interchangeable.
C. There is a legal obligation to report underage sex.
D. The Sexual Offences Act specifically prohibits teachers, nurses, youth workers
   from providing sexual healthcare advice to minors.
E. Under the Sexual Offences Act 2003, it is an offence for a person aged 18 or
   over to have sexual intercourse/any form of sexual touching with a person under
   16.

SRH17

A 36-year-old woman is diagnosed with mild-stage pelvic endometriosis at diagnostic laparoscopy. She has regular menstrual cycles. Her partner has normal semen
analysis. The couple have been trying to conceive for 2 years. Which one of the
following management options is the preferred initial treatment choice?

A. Clomiphene citrate ovulation induction
B. Gonadotrophin-releasing hormone agonist (GnRHa)
C. Gonadotrophin-releasing hormone antagonist
D. Laparoscopic excision/ablation of peritoneal endometriosis
E. Selective progesterone receptor modulator

SRH18

When explaining surgical termination of pregnancy, which ONE of the following is
appropriate to discuss during counselling for the procedure?

A. Antibiotic prophylaxis is not necessary.
B. Genital tract infection occurs in less than 1 % of cases.
C. Suction termination done at <7 weeks gestation has inferior results than that
   done between 7 and 12 weeks gestation.

D. The risk of damage to the external cervical os at the time of surgical abortion is minimised by using pre-procedure intravaginal oestrogen gel.
E. The risk of uterine perforation is 5 %.

SRH19

Which of the following is a recommended protocol for antibiotic prophylaxis for women requesting an induced abortion?

A. Azithromycin 1 g orally on the day of abortion, **plus** metronidazole 1 g orally prior to or at the time of abortion
B. Azithromycin 1 g orally on the day of abortion, **plus** metronidazole 800 mg rectally prior to or at the time of abortion
C. Doxycycline 200 mg orally twice daily for 7 days, starting on the day of the abortion, **plus** metronidazole 1 g rectally prior to or at the time of the abortion
D. Doxycycline 200 mg orally twice daily for 7 days, starting on the day of the abortion, **plus** metronidazole 800 mg orally prior to or at the time of the abortion
E. Metronidazole 1 g rectally or 800 mg orally prior to or at the time of abortion for women who have tested negative for *C. trachomatis* infection

SRH20

Ms XY has an ERPC/SMM 1 week ago for a missed miscarriage following an unplanned pregnancy at 10/40 weeks. The histology results suggest a molar pregnancy. Ms XY is keen on contraception to avoid a further unplanned pregnancy. Her beta hCG levels are 960 mIU/l today.
    Which of the following contraceptives are best suited to her?

A. Barrier contraception
B. Combined oral contraception
C. Copper IUCD
D. Minipill
E. Mirena IUS

SRH21

Ms XY is 10 weeks pregnant. She has been diagnosed with her third consecutive missed miscarriage. She is 28 years old and with the same partner. She opts for surgical management of miscarriage.
    Which of the following investigations are appropriate?

A. Karyotyping of the products of conception
B. Karyotyping of the products of conception and karyotyping of both partners
C. Maternal karyotyping
D. Paternal karyotyping
E. Prenatal diagnostic testing in the subsequent pregnancy

SRH22

Ms XY presents to the GUM clinic seeking emergency contraception. She recalls her last unprotected sexual intercourse was 4 days ago. She has erratic cycles otherwise, and exact time of ovulation cannot be confidently determined. She consents to STI screening. Which of the following treatment options are best suited to her?

A. Copper IUCD
B. Levonorgestrel
C. Mirena IUS
D. Medroxyprogesterone acetate
E. Ulipristal acetate

SRH23

Which of the following is true regarding Qlaira?

A. Qlaira contains estradiol valerate and desogestrel.
B. Qlaira has continuous 28 days cycle with 26 active pills with decreasing oestrogen and increasing progesterone dose followed by 2 placebos.
C. There are clinically significant benefits over the pills containing synthetic oestrogen.
D. This is a triphasic pill.
E. While taking Qlaira if the pills are missed, the same pills rules apply as other combined oral contraceptive pills.

SRH24

You have to counsel a 28-year-old woman for an appropriate method of contraception. She had a complete molar pregnancy which was evacuated last week. What is the correct advise you can give her:

A. Barrier contraceptives have a low failure rate.
B. Barrier methods provide the added advantage of preventing sexually transmitted infections.
C. Combined oral contraceptive pills are absolutely contraindicated for her.

D. Combined oral contraceptive pills can be started if hCG levels show a decreasing trend.
E. Intrauterine devices should not be used till hCG levels are normal.

SRH25

Which of the following is not true about Neisseria gonorrhoea infection?

A. Almost half of the cases with gonorrhoea may be asymptomatic.
B. Heavy menstrual bleeding is a known symptom.
C. Neisseria gonorrhoea are Gram-negative bacilli.
D. Pharyngitis, meningitis and endocarditis are known presentations.
E. Postcoital or intermenstrual bleeding can be seen in cases with cervicitis.

SRH26

In evaluation and management of women with vaginal discharge, which of the following statements is incorrect?

A. Allergic reactions can cause excessive vaginal discharge.
B. Douching the vagina as part of daily hygiene helps reduce vaginal discharge.
C. Exclusion of infective and other causes can help confirm that a vaginal discharge is physiological.
D. There is some association between methods of contraception and vaginal discharge.
E. Women with cervical ectopy may complain of increased physiological discharge.

SRH27

Mrs XY is a 35-year-old woman who is a known case of congenital heart disease with a single ventricular physiology and on regular follow-up with the cardiologist. She is stable in regard to her cardiac condition and wants an intrauterine contraceptive device (IUCD) inserted. Her cardiologist has given his consent for the same after reviewing her case.

Which of the following is appropriate regarding the arrangements for the IUCD insertion in this case?

A. Her own GP can do it in his clinic.
B. It does not matter where the IUCD is inserted as long as someone experienced does it.
C. It should be done in the hospital setting with involvement of the cardiologist.

D. The main concern here is to prevent any infection.

E. Women with cardiac disease should not be encourage to use the IUCD.

SRH28

Which of the following statements is appropriate for contraceptive advice to women with inflammatory bowel disease?

A. Condoms are the preferred method in women who are on medication for IBD as its efficacy cannot be affected by them.

B. Laparoscopic sterilisation is an appropriate method of contraception for women with IBD who have had previous pelvic or abdominal surgery.

C. Women can be informed that there is a causal association between combined oral contraception (COC) use and onset or exacerbation of IBD so it is best avoided.

D. Women should be advised that the efficacy of oral contraception is unlikely to be reduced by large bowel disease but may be reduced in women with Crohn's disease who have small bowel disease and malabsorption.

E. Women using combined hormonal contraception do not need any additional contraception while taking antibiotic courses.

SRH29

Which of the following is a recommended regimen for medical abortion less than 49 days of gestation?

A. Mifepristone 200 mg orally followed 12–24 h later by misoprostol 800 µg given by the vaginal, buccal or sublingual route

B. Mifepristone 200 mg orally followed 24–48 h later by misoprostol 800 µg given by the vaginal, buccal or sublingual route

C. Mifepristone 400 mg orally followed 12–24 h later by misoprostol 800 µg given by the vaginal, buccal or sublingual route

D. Mifepristone 400 mg orally followed 24–48 h later by misoprostol 800 µg given by the vaginal, buccal or sublingual route

E. Mifepristone 600 mg orally followed 24–48 h later by misoprostol 800 µg given by the vaginal, buccal or sublingual route

SRH30

High vaginal swabs (HVS) may be used to aid the diagnosis of BV, VVC, TV or other genital tract infections (e.g. streptococcal organisms) which may be the cause of vaginal discharge, but their use should generally be reserved for some specific situations.

In the following list, HVS is of very limited value in which of the following situation:

A. Failed treatment
B. Pregnancy, postpartum, postabortion or post-instrumentation
C. Presence of thick, curdy white discharge with itching in vulva with vaginal pH <4.5
D. Recurrent symptoms
E. When symptoms, signs and/or pH are inconsistent with a specific diagnosis

Gynaecologic Oncology: SBA Questions

10

GYNONCO1

The most common cause of death from gynaecological malignancy in the developed world:

A. Cervical cancer
B. Endometrial cancer
C. Ovarian cancer
D. Vaginal cancer
E. Vulval cancer

GYNONCO2

The risk of endometrial cancer is increased in the following condition:

A. Asherman syndrome
B. Behcet's syndrome
C. Ehlers–Danlos syndrome
D. Lynch syndrome
E. Marfan's syndrome

GYNONCO3

Oral contraceptive pills reduce the risk of endometrial cancer by:

A. 2–5 %
B. 5–10 %
C. 10–15 %

© Springer India 2016
C. Ratha, J. Gupta, *SBAs and EMQs for MRCOG II*,
DOI 10.1007/978-81-322-2689-5_10

D. 40–50 %
E. 75 %

GYNONCO4

The incidence of occult ovarian cancers detected in women with BRCA mutation who undergo risk reducing salpingo-oophorectomy is:

A. 1–2 %
B. 5–7 %
C. 10–12 %
D. 25–30 %
E. 40–50 %

GYNONCO5

The following statements are true regarding borderline ovarian tumours except:

A. Laparoscopic management is associated with possibilities of cyst rupture, development of port-site metastases and understaging of disease.
B. No role for chemotherapy has been demonstrated for borderline ovarian tumours.
C. Risk is not increased in BRCA mutations.
D. The incidence of invasive disease at recurrence varies from 8 % to 73 %.
E. The risk of recurrence varies between 0 % and 58 %.

GYNONCO6

Borderline tumours of the ovary are commonly associated with the following genetic mutation:

A. Braf/Kras pathway
B. BRCA
C. MSH2
D. PMS1/PMS2
E. p53

GYNONCO7

The recommended first line of treatment in Lichen sclerosus is:

A. Antifungals
B. Local antibiotics

C. Local anaesthetic creams
D. Tacrolimus
E. Ultrapotent corticosteroids

GYNONCO8

Lichen sclerosus commonly presents in the following age group:

A. Adolescent
B. Postmenopausal
C. Premenarchal
D. Premenopausal
E. Reproductive age group

GYNONCO9

Flat-topped violaceous purpuric plaques on the vulva are characteristic of:

A. Eccrine hamartoma
B. Lichen planus
C. Lichen sclerosus
D. Lichen simplex
E. Vulval intraepithelial neoplasia

GYNONCO10

A 50-year-old woman presented with 20 mm mass in the left breast associated with skin indentation. Which one of the following is the next most appropriate action?

A. Breast conserving surgery.
B. Chemotherapy is strongly recommended.
C. Ductal carcinoma in situ is the underlying histological type.
D. MRI.
E. The clinical picture is that of locally advanced breast cancer; therefore, offer radiotherapy.

GYNONCO11

A 72-year-old woman was diagnosed with 10 mm, grade II, oestrogen receptor negative invasive left breast cancer. She had a palpable left axillary lymph node. Which one of the following is the next most appropriate action?

A. Adjuvant tamoxifen should be given for 5 years.
B. Axillary lymph node clearance.
C. Chemotherapy is strongly recommended.
D. Needle biopsy of the axillary node.
E. Sentinel node biopsy and primary axillary surgery.

GYNONCO12

Which one of the following correctly describes the NHS breast cancer screening programme?

A. Those aged 25–50 years, screen every 3 years, and those aged 50–64 years, screen every 5 years.
B. Those aged 40–70 years, screen every 3 years.
C. Those aged 45–65 years, screen every 3 years.
D. Those aged 50–70 years, screen every 3 years.
E. Those aged 60–80 years, screen every 2 years.

GYNONCO13

A 34-year-old woman presents with 6 weeks' history of a lump in the upper outer quadrant of the right breast. She has a family history of breast cancer. Clinical examination of the breast suggests a benign lump (E2 grading on examination). Which one of the following is the next most appropriate action?

A. Breast cancer is a likely diagnosis.
B. Fibroadenoma is the likely diagnosis.
C. Mammogram should be a part of her triple assessment.
D. The patient should be reassured and discharged.
E. Ultrasound scan of the breast.

GYNONCO14

What percentage of patients in dedicated vulval cancers present with Lichen sclerosus?

A. 5 %
B. 10 %
C. 25 %
D. 40 %
E. 60 %

GYNONCO15

Untreated VIN (vulva intraepithelial neoplasia) may progress to carcinoma of vulva in:

A. 1–2 %
B. 5 %
C. 10 %
D. 15 %
E. 25 %

GYNONCO16

The commonest HPV type to be associated with vulval carcinoma and vulval intraepithelial carcinoma is:

A. HPV 6
B. HPV 11
C. HPV 16
D. HPV 18
E. HPV 31

GYNONCO17

In management of invasive vulval cancer, inguinofemoral lymphadenectomy can be avoided in all except:

A. Basal cell carcinoma
B. Melanoma with clinically uninvolved nodes
C. Squamous cell carcinoma with depth of invasion <1 mm
D. Squamous cell carcinoma with depth of invasion >1 mm
E. Verrucous carcinoma

GYNONCO18

All the following are true about endometrial cancers except:

A. 80 % of endometrial cancers are type 1.
B. Type 1 cancers arise on a background of atypical hyperplasia.
C. Type 1 cancers are causally related to hyperoestrogenic risk factors.
D. Type 1 cancers occur in older women.
E. Type 1 cancers are frequently related to obesity, infertility and nulliparity.

GYNONCO19

What percentage of endometrial cancers are inherited?

A. <5 %
B. 7–8 %
C. 10 %
D. 10–15 %
E. 20 %

GYNONCO20

In staging of vulvar carcinoma, a tumour of any size, with or without extension to adjacent perineal structures, and with more than three positive inguinofemoral nodes is:

A. Stage II
B. Stage IIIA
C. Stage IIIB
D. Stage IIIC
E. Stage IVA

GYNONCO21

The first malignancy that was recognised to be linked to obesity is:

A. Cervical adenocarcinomas
B. Endometrial cancers
C. Epithelial ovarian tumours
D. Germ cell tumours
E. Gestational trophoblastic tumours

GYNONCO22

The most prevalent cancer affecting pregnancy and puerperium is:

A. Breast cancer
B. Choriocarcinoma
C. Leukaemias
D. Ovarian cancer
E. Thyroid cancer

GYNONCO23

The following are recommended by FIGO for staging of cervical cancer except:

A. Chest X-ray
B. Cystoscopy
C. Examination under anaesthesia
D. Intravenous pyelogram
E. Ultrasonography of the abdomen and pelvis

GYNONCO24

All of the following about adenocarcinomas of the cervix are true except:

A. Adenocarcinomas account for 20 % of cervical cancers.
B. They are likely to be diagnosed in younger women.
C. They are associated with delay in diagnosis compared to their squamous counterparts.
D. They are associated with a poorer prognosis in comparison with squamous carcinomas of the cervix.
E. HPV 16 is commonly related to adenocarcinomas.

GYNONCO25

Detection rates of endometrial cancer with the Pipelle in postmenopausal women are:

A. 50 %
B. 60 %
C. 70 %
D. 90 %
E. 99 %

GYNONCO26

Regarding peritoneal cytology in endometrial cancer, the following is true:

A. In patients with stage I and II endometrial cancer, positive peritoneal cytology adversely affects survival.
B. Postoperative radiotherapy is indicated in the presence of positive peritoneal cytology.

C. Positive peritoneal cytology may carry a poor prognostic significance when the disease has spread beyond the uterus.
D. Positive peritoneal cytology after the 2009 FIGO staging warrants chemotherapy.
E. Positive peritoneal cytology, when found, is termed stage IIIB.

GYNONCO27

Regarding lymphatic involvement in endometrial cancer, pick the incorrect statement.

A. Lymphadenectomy helps to individualise postoperative adjuvant treatment.
B. Lymphatic spread is related to the grade of the tumour and myometrial involvement.
C. Para-aortic nodes are commonly involved even in the absence of pelvic nodal involvement.
D. Para-aortic spread occurs directly from lymphatics draining the fundus of the uterus.
E. Spreads are common to the pelvic and para-aortic nodes.

GYNONCO28

The 5-year overall survival for endometrial cancer is:

A. 50 %
B. 60 %
C. 70 %
D. 80 %
E. 90 %

GYNONCO29

Call–Exner bodies are found in:

A. Dermoid tumours
B. Granulosa cell tumours
C. Mature teratomas
D. Serous cystadenomas
E. Theca cell tumours

GYNONCO30

Ms. XY is 64 years old, postmenopausal. Her recent TV ultrasound scan reveals the presence of a 4 cm right ovarian cyst. The cyst is multiloculated and shows the presence of a solid area. There is no free fluid. The left ovary is normal. Her CA125 is 50 u/ml. She has been explained of her RMI results. What is her RMI score based on the information provided?

A. 25
B. 100
C. 150
D. 250
E. 450

GYNONCO31

Ms. XY is 64 years old, postmenopausal. Her recent TV ultrasound scan reveals the presence of a 4 cm right ovarian cyst. The cyst is multiloculated and shows the presence of a solid area. There is no free fluid. The left ovary is normal. Her CA125 is 50 u/ml. She has been explained of her RMI results (450). Which of the following treatment options are best suited to her?

A. Laparoscopy and bilateral salpingo-oophorectomy
B. Laparoscopy and right salpingo-oophorectomy
C. Laparotomy and staging procedure (including TAH+BSO+infracolic omentectomy)
D. MRI abdomen–pelvis
E. PET scan

GYNONCO32

Ms. XY is 64 years old, postmenopausal. Her recent TV ultrasound scan reveals the presence of a 4 cm right ovarian cyst. The cyst shows anechoic fluid with no solid areas. There is no free fluid. The left ovary is normal. Her CA125 is 5 u/ml. Which of the following treatment options are best suited to her?

A. Discharge from care.
B. Laparoscopy and unilateral or bilateral salpingo-oophorectomy.
C. Repeat TVS + CA-125 at 4 months' intervals for a year.
D. Repeat TVS + CA-125 at yearly intervals for 2 years.
E. Ultrasound guided cyst aspiration.

GYNONCO33

Ms. XY is 35 years old and had a LLETZ recently. The histology results confirm the presence of CIN 2, which has been completely excised. How should she be followed up under the NHS cervical screening programme if her subsequent tests are normal?

A. Colposcopy at 6 and 12 months + annual cytology for 9 years prior to routine recall
B. Colposcopy at 6 and 12 months + annual cytology for 5 years prior to routine recall
C. Cytology at 6 and 12 months + annual cytology for 5 years prior to routine recall
D. Cytology at 6 and 12 months + annual cytology for 9 years prior to routine recall
E. Cytology at 6, 12 and 24 months prior to routine recall

GYNONCO34

Lifetime increase in risk of breast cancer with CTPA:

A. 0.1 %
B. 1 %
C. 10 %
D. 13 %
E. 25 %

GYNONCO35

All of the following statements regarding borderline ovarian tumours are true except:

A. BRCA gene mutation carriers are not at increased risk for the development of borderline ovarian tumours.
B. Complete surgical staging is the cornerstone of management.
C. Lactation is found to be protective against borderline ovarian tumours.
D. Oral contraceptive use is protective against the development of borderline ovarian tumours.
E. Stromal invasion is not seen.

GYNONCO36

Ms. XY is 8 weeks' pregnant. Her last smear result suggested mild dyskaryosis. She is due for a repeat smear. Which of the following treatment options are best suited to her?

A. Defer smear until 6 weeks' postpartum.
B. Perform colposcopy 6 weeks' postpartum.
C. Perform smear in the mid-trimester.
D. Perform smear immediate postpartum.
E. Perform smear when due.

GYNONCO37

Ms. XY is 55 years old. She underwent a TAH + BSO, 4 weeks ago. Her preoperative histology following a prior loop excision of the cervix suggested incompletely excised CIN 3. She is at a consultant-led follow-up clinic to discuss her further management. Which of the following treatment options are best suited to her?

A. Colposcopy at 6, 12 and 24 months
B. No further follow-up
C. Vault cytology at 6 and 12 months
D. Vault cytology at 6, 12 and 24 months
E. Vault cytology at 6 and 12 months, followed by 9 annual vault cytology samples

GYNONCO38

The risk of contralateral lymph node involvement in a laterally placed lesion of vulval carcinoma is:

A. <1 %
B. 1–2 %
C. 2–4 %
D. 3–5 %
E. 5 %

GYNONCO39

During surgery for ovarian tumour, if the frozen section report is a borderline ovarian tumour, which of the following is not a recommended procedure?

A. Appendicectomy in the case of mucinous tumours.
B. Conservative surgery in women wishing to retain fertility.
C. Total abdominal hysterectomy ,bilateral salpingo-oophorectomy and infracolic omentectomy in women who do not wish to preserve fertility.
D. Exploration of the entire abdominal cavity with peritoneal washings.
E. Systematic biopsies of a macroscopically normal contralateral ovary are recommended to exclude recurrent disease in women where conservative surgery is done.

GYNONCO40

The role of the sentinel lymph node mapping is most established in this gynaeco-logical malignancy:

A. Cervical cancer
B. Endometrial cancer
C. Ovarian cancer
D. Vaginal cancer
E. Vulval cancer

Urogynaecology and Pelvic Floor: SBA Questions

11

UGN1

Q1. The nerve that is susceptible to entrapment injuries during sacrospinous ligament fixation as it runs behind the lateral aspect of the sacrospinous ligament is the:

A. Genitofemoral nerve
B. Obturator nerve
C. Peroneal nerve
D. Pudendal nerve
E. Sciatic nerve

UGN2

The main complication of mesh repair in vaginal prolapse:

A. Bladder injury
B. Bowel injury
C. Mesh erosion
D. Infection
E. Recurrence of prolapse

UGN3

Painful bladder syndrome is characterised by all of the below except:

A. Increased frequency
B. Increased night-time frequency
C. Pain related to bladder filling

© Springer India 2016
C. Ratha, J. Gupta, *SBAs and EMQs for MRCOG II*,
DOI 10.1007/978-81-322-2689-5_11

D. Positive urine cultures
E. Urgency

UGN4

In the female pelvis, the ureter forms an important relation with the ovaries and lies:

A. Anterior to ovary
B. Inferior to ovary
C. Medial to ovary
D. Lateral to ovary
E. Posterior to ovary

UGN5

Which of the following is not true about postpartum voiding dysfunction?

A. It is defined as failure to pass urine spontaneously within 6 h of vaginal delivery or catheter removal after delivery.
B. It is seen in 0.7–4 % deliveries.
C. Epidural anaesthesia is a risk factor.
D. All postpartum patients' measurement of residual urine volume helps identifying women with voiding dysfunction.
E. If a patient does not void within 6 h of delivery and if the residual urine volume is >500 ml, then it is advisable to keep an indwelling catheter for 24 h.

UGN6

Vault prolapse can be prevented at the time of vaginal hysterectomy by:

A. Cruikshank's closure
B. DeLancey's procedure
C. McCall culdoplasty
D. Moschcowitz procedure
E. Simple peritoneal closure

UGN7

Ms. XY is 60 years old. She presents with a picture of mixed incontinence with stress as a predominant feature. A urinary tract infection has been ruled out. She does not smoke or consume caffeine. A grade 1 cystocele is noted on examination. Which of the following treatment options are best suited to her?

A. Anticholinergics
B. Gel horn pessary
C. Pelvic floor muscle training
D. TVT
E. Urodynamic studies

UGN8

Ms. XY is 60 years old. She presents with symptoms suggestive of an overactive bladder. Urine dip is negative for leucocytes and nitrites. She does not smoke or consume caffeine. Examination reveals no prolapse. Which of the following is the most appropriate advice?

A. Bladder diary—72 h
B. Bladder scan
C. Filling and voiding cystometry
D. Flexible cystoscopy
E. MSU for culture

UGN9

Ms. XY is 60 years old. She presents with symptoms suggestive of an overactive bladder. Urine dip is negative for leucocytes and nitrites. She does not smoke or consume caffeine. Examination reveals no prolapse. Conservative therapies and OAB drugs have failed to improve her symptoms. After an MDT discussion, a decision is reached to try botulinum toxin A. Which of the following is an appropriate starting dose of the toxin?

A. 50 units
B. 150 units
C. 200 units
D. 250 units
E. 300 units

References http://www.lasvegasurogynecology.com/POPstix%20insert_opt.pdf

UGN10

Ms. XY is 70 years old. She presents to the urogynaecology specialist nurse with the complaint to feeling a bulge per vaginum. She has had a TAH +BSO 15 years ago.

Which point corresponds to the vaginal vault/cuff scar on the POP –Q (pelvic organ prolapse quantification system)?

A. Aa
B. Ba

C. C
D. Ap
E. Bp

UGN11

Ms. XY is 70 years old. She presents to the urogynaecology specialist nurse with the complaint of feeling a bulge per vaginam. She has had a TAH+BSO 15 years ago.

Which of the following points on the POP-Q system will not be recorded as a part of her assessment?

A. Aa
B. Ba
C. C
D. D
E. Bp

UGN12

Which of the following is not true about duloxetine?

A. Duloxetine is believed to act by increasing sphincter activity in the storage phase of the micturition cycle.
B. It is a serotonin and noradrenaline (norepinephrine) reuptake inhibitor.
C. It has clinically important interactions with other drugs including warfarin and antidepressants.
D. It is approved for the treatment of urinary incontinence.
E. With the use of duloxetine, overweight women tended to have a lesser improvement in incontinence quality-of-life score than women with a BMI <28.

UGN13

Which of the following is a contraindication to suprapubic catheterisation?

A. Neurogenic bladder
B. Inability to self-catheterise
C. Intractable self injury
D. Severe incontinence
E. Very obese patients

UGN14

All of the following statements regarding anterior wall repair are true except:

A. Anterior repair is performed for symptomatic anterior vaginal wall prolapse.

B. Continuous sutures produce a more robust repair than intermittent sutures.

C. The procedure provides support along the whole length of the anterior vaginal wall, thereby supporting both the urethra and the bladder base.

D. Use of a nonabsorbable graft reduces the risk of operative failure or recurrence but is associated with a risk of graft erosion and bladder injury.

E. While troublesome urinary symptoms may be improved by anterior repair, a significant proportion of women develop new urinary symptoms following surgery, which will be particularly unwelcome if they were symptom-free before.

UGN15

Which of the following is not an example of a problem arising from pelvic floor dysfunction?

A. Faecal incontinence

B. Incompetent cervix

C. Pelvic organ prolapse

D. Sexual dysfunction

E. Urinary incontinence

UGN16

'Long-term' intraurethral catheters are kept in situ for at the most:

A. 2 weeks

B. 4 weeks

C. 8 weeks

D. 12 weeks

E. 16 weeks

UGN17

A 57-year-old, post menopausal woman complains of 'something coming out of her vagina' and difficulty in opening her bowels. She had four children uneventfully with vaginal births. Her last child birth was 18 years back. The most likely diagnosis is:

A. Anterior vaginal wall prolapsed

B. Genuine stress incontinence

C. Overflow incontinence

D. Posterior vaginal wall prolapse

E. Stress incontinence

UGN18

Which of the following statements about urethral diverticulum is true?

A. Congenital cases may occur from remnants of Gartner's duct or abnormal union of primordial folds or persisting cell rests, especially Müllerian, and are commonly found in children.
B. Most cases are acquired and result from repeated infections and obstruction of the periurethral glands.
C. The UD usually dissects within the urethral pelvic ligament with the orifice/ neck at 11 o'clock.
D. Traumatic childbirth, especially with assisted delivery, has been suggested as a cause of UD development, and they never develop in nulliparous patients.
E. Urethral diverticulum presents with the classical triad of dysuria, post-void dribbling and dyspareunia in most of the patients.

UGN19

Ms. XY is 55 years old. She suffers from symptoms of an overactive bladder. Bladder retraining has not helped her. Her recent urine analysis is negative for infection.
    What is next step in her management?

A. Botulinum A toxin
B. Mirabegron
C. Darifenacin once daily
D. Transcutaneous posterior tibial nerve stimulation
E. Urodynamic studies

UGN20

A third-degree perineal tear is defined as:

A. Complete disruption of the anal sphincter muscles, which may involve either or both the external (EAS) or/and internal anal sphincter (IAS) muscles with partial involvement of the rectal mucosa
B. Partial or complete disruption of the anal sphincter muscles, which may involve the external (EAS) but not the internal anal sphincter (IAS) muscles
C. Partial but not complete disruption of the anal sphincter muscles, which may involve either or both the external (EAS) or/and internal anal sphincter (IAS) muscles and one third of rectal mucosa
D. Partial or complete disruption of the anal sphincter muscles, which may involve either or both the external (EAS) or/and internal anal sphincter (IAS) muscles without involvement of rectal mucosa
E. Partial or complete disruption of the anal sphincter muscles, which may involve either or both the external (EAS) or/and internal anal sphincter (IAS) muscles with some involvement of rectal mucosa

Core Surgical Skills and Postoperative Care: SBA Questions

12

CSPO1

Regarding the use of adhesion prevention agents, which of the following is true?

A. Steroids must be used in fertility-conserving surgery for prevention of adhesions.
B. Dextran when used as an anti-adhesive agent can cause anaphylaxis.
C. The use of Adept in gynaecological surgeries has not shown significant reduction in de novo adhesions.
D. Seprafilm is oxidised regenerated cellulose.
E. Evidence shows definite benefit of using adhesion prevention agents in caesarean section.

CSPO2

Select the single most appropriate statement with reference to abdominal incisions and preoperative preparations in a gynaecological surgery:

A. Horizontal incisions cause minimum nerve damage.
B. Preoperative showering with antiseptics reduces the infection rate to almost half.
C. A scalpel should be changed after superficial incision for a deep incision.
D. Vertical skin incisions have better cosmetic results and greater strength.
E. Wound infection rates are less if no hair is removed as compared to depilatory preparation.

© Springer India 2016
C. Ratha, J. Gupta, *SBAs and EMQs for MRCOG II*,
DOI 10.1007/978-81-322-2689-5_12

CSPO3

A 45-year-old woman undergoes an abdominal hysterectomy for a large fibroid uterus. She is found to have a fibroid in broad ligament, and there is a concern that her ureter may have been damaged during the difficult surgery. Which of the following is the least possible site of ureteric injury in this surgery?

A. At the level of the uterosacral ligament
B. Lateral to the uterine vessels
C. Renal pelviureteric junction
D. The area of the ureterovesical junction close to the cardinal ligaments
E. The base of the infundibulopelvic ligament as the ureters cross the pelvic brim at the ovarian fossa

CSPO4

Regarding nonabsorbable suture materials, which of the following statements is correct?

A. All nonabsorbable sutures are monofilamentous and have lower incidence of wound infection.
B. Polypropylene has higher tissue reactivity than polytetrafluoroethylene.
C. Surgical silk has higher tensile strength than nylon.
D. The incidence of wound dehiscence and hernia is lower for nonabsorbable than slowly absorbable sutures.
E. The incidence of prolonged wound pain and suture sinus is significantly higher with a nonabsorbable suture.

CSPO5

A patient who underwent an abdominal hysterectomy a few days ago complains of numbness over the skin over the anterior aspect of the upper thigh. This could be attributed to neuropathy of the:

A. Femoral nerve
B. Obturator nerve
C. Peroneal nerve
D. Pudendal nerve
E. Sciatic nerve

CSPO6

Staples are used for wound closure. Which of the following statements about the use of staples in a gynaecological surgery is incorrect?

A. A nonabsorbable staple made of stainless steel has the highest tensile strength of any wound closure material.
B. Contaminated wounds closed with staples have a lower incidence of infection compared with those closed with sutures.
C. Disadvantages of staples include the potential for staple track formation, bacterial migration into the wound bed and discomfort during staple removal.
D. Prior to stapling, it is useful to grasp the wound edges with forceps to evert the tissue so as to prevent inverted skin edges.
E. Staples have a high tissue reactivity.

CSPO7

Following massive blood transfusion, what is the recommended dose of fresh frozen plasma to be administered to prevent coagulation problems?

A. 10–12 ml/kg for every 4 units of red cells
B. 12–15 ml/kg for every 4 units of red cells
C. 15–18 ml/kg for every 4 units of red cells
D. 12–15 ml/kg for every 6 units of red cells
E. 15–18 ml/kg for every 8 units of red cells

CSPO8

Axonotmesis is best described as an iatrogenic nerve injury which involves:

A. Axon transection injury related to incorrect incision sites
B. Damage occurring to the axon with preservation of the supporting Schwann cells
C. Long recovery period usually extending to few years
D. Need for restorative surgery in most cases
E. Poor chances of regeneration despite restorative surgery

CSPO9

Which of the following statements regarding laparoscopic entry in cases of previous abdominal surgery is false?

A. In patients with previous abdominal surgery with midline scar, the open-entry incision can be placed well lateral to the midline and beyond the lateral border of the rectus muscle.
B. Infraumbilical closed-entry techniques should not be used in patients with a previous abdominal surgery with midline scar.
C. Infraumbilical closed-entry techniques are very safe in patients with previous transverse suprapubic incisions as there is negligible risk of periumbilical adhesions.
D. Open-entry techniques like the Hasson method are definitely preferred for thin patients.
E. Palmer's point entry is unsafe for patients with previous splenectomy.

CSPO10

Which of the following is an example of a self-retaining retractor?

A. Balfour
B. Deaver
C. Doyen's
D. Langenbeck
E. Morris

CSPO11

Ms. XY is a Para 1 who has had an emergency caesarean section for failure to progress. Her epidural catheter was removed at 8:00 AM today, 6 h after her CS. She is written up to have prophylactic LMWH daily, commencing today for 10 days. Her postnatal check is satisfactory. Which of the following times is most appropriate for her to have the LMWH?

A. 9:00
B. 10:00
C. 11:00
D. 12:00
E. 8:00 on the subsequent day

CSPO12

Ms. XY, 48 years old, para 3, is due to undergo a NovaSure endometrial ablation in theatre for heavy menstrual bleeding. A WHO surgical safety checklist is in progress. Which of the following is not a component to the sign out?

A. Any surgical or anaesthetic delays.
B. Hat instrument, sponge and needle counts are correct (or not applicable).
C. The specimen is labelled.
D. The surgeon, anaesthesia professional and nurse review the key concerns for recovery and management of this patient.
E. Whether there are any equipment problems to be addressed.

CSPO13

A surgical position which involves the patient in supine position of the body with hips flexed at 15° as the basic angle and with a 30° head-down tilt is known as:

A. Lithotomy position
B. Lloyd–Davies position
C. Sim's position
D. Trendelenburg position
E. Ward Mayo position

CSPO14

Ms. XY is 35 years old. She is a para 3 with 2 previous caesarean sections and desires permanent contraception. She has opted to have a laparoscopic tubal occlusion/ sterilisation procedure. Her BMI is 33. She has had a successful Veress needle insufflation (first pass). What level of pressure must be obtained before passing the trocar?

A. 0–5 mm of Hg
B. 10–15 mm of Hg
C. 15–20 mm of Hg
D. 20–25mm of Hg
E. 30–35 mm of Hg

CSPO15

Intraoperative cell salvage is a strategy to reduce the use of banked blood. If IOCS is done for nonsensitised rhesus negative women at the term of a term caesarean section, which of the following statements is true regarding the minimum dose of anti-D to be administered?

A. 250 iu stat within 72 h.
B. 500 iu two doses 6 weeks apart.
C. 1000 iu stat within 72 h.
D. 3000 iu stat within 72 h.
E. Anti-D is not administered if the baby's blood group is rhesus negative.

CSPO16

All of the following are true about surgical needles except:

A. Blunt-point needle is used for patients with hepatitis B.
B. Needles with 'eye' are rarely used nowadays.
C. Surgical needles have three basic components—the attachment point, the body and the point.
D. The deeper the pane of surgery, the more curved the needle should be.
E. The diameter of the needle is generally bigger than that of the suture material.

CSPO17

Which of the following is correct regarding synthetic tissue adhesives?

A. All synthetic tissue adhesives are non-biodegradable.
B. Cyanoacrylate is associated with increased microbial infection.
C. Cyanoacrylates polymerise upon contact with blood, forming a solid film that bridges the wounds.
D. Fibrin-based glues are biological, while gelatin-based hydrogels are synthetically prepared.
E. Synthetic tissue adhesives can be used for surface applications but not for internal use.

CSPO18

A downward and inward muscle-splitting incision from the McBurney point that allows extraperitoneal drainage of abscesses is called:

A. Elliot incision
B. Gridiron incision
C. Kustner incision
D. Mouchel incision
E. Rockey–Davis incision

CSPO19

The ilioinguinal and iliohypogastric nerves can be injured during a gynaecological surgery. Which of the following describes these nerves the best?

A. Both nerves pass laterally through the head of the psoas muscle before running diagonally along quadratus lumborum.

B. The iliohypogastric nerve is both sensory and motor, while the ilioinguinal nerve has a sensory function only.

C. The ilioinguinal nerve arises from the L5–S1 nerve root, while the iliohypogastric nerve arises from the T12-L1 nerve root.

D. The ilioinguinal nerve pierces the external oblique aponeurosis above the superficial inguinal ring, while the iliohypogastric nerve emerges through it.

E. The reported incidence of ilioinguinal or iliohypogastric neuropathy following a Pfannenstiel incision is less than 1 %.

CSPO20

Which of the following is not a known risk factor for nerve injury during a gynaecological surgery?

A. Entrapment of the psoas muscle
B. Narrow pelvis
C. Operating time more than 4 h
D. Thin-body habitus
E. Well-developed abdominal wall muscles

CSPO21

The inferior epigastric artery originates from:

A. The external iliac artery anterior to the inguinal ligament
B. The external iliac artery posterior to the inguinal ligament
C. The internal iliac artery anterior to the inguinal ligament
D. The internal iliac artery inferior to the inguinal ligament
E. The internal iliac artery posterior to the inguinal ligament

CSPO22

A 34-year-old woman had a caesarean section after 24 h of labour due to secondary arrest of cervical dilatation and maternal exhaustion. Two hours post-LSCS, she complained of acute-onset left-sided chest pain radiating to the left shoulder and arm along with breathlessness. She had no previous known medical conditions or family history of cardiac disease. Which of the following statements is true regarding investigations planned to rule out acute myocardial infarction?

A. Acute MI is highly unlikely in this clinical scenario, and precious time and efforts should not be wasted on the same in this scenario.

B. Coronary angiography is useful in diagnosing and treating acute MI in postpartum patients.

C. Isoenzyme MB will be more specific and should be used in this case.

D. Normal ECG would rule out acute myocardial infarction.

E. Troponin T levels may increase in prolonged labour or caesarean section and hence cannot be used in this case.

CSPO23

While operating on a patient in lithotomy position, the padding between the lateral fibular heads and the stirrup prevents injury to:

A. Common peroneal nerve

B. Lateral cutaneous nerve of the thigh

C. Obturator nerve

D. Pudendal nerve

E. Tibial nerve

CSPO24

Ms. XY is in theatre for repair of a 3C tear. She has been given spinal anaesthetic and antibiotics. Which suturing technique is most suited for the torn IAS (internal anal sphincter)?

A. Continuous locked 3–0 PDS

B. Continuous unlocked 3–0 PDS

C. End-to-end technique (interrupted)

D. Figure-of-8 stitches

E. Overlap technique

CSPO25

Ms. XY is in theatre for repair of a 3C tear. She has been given spinal anaesthetic and antibiotics. What structures are torn in a 3C tear?

A. Both EAS+IAS

B. EAS+IAS+anal mucosa

C. IAS only

D. Less than 50 % EAS

E. More than 50 % EAS

Surgical Procedures: SBA Questions

13

SP1

Q1. Safety measures to prevent laparoscopic electrosurgical complications include all of the following except:

A. Inspect insulation carefully before use.
B. Use the highest possible effective power setting.
C. Use available technology; newer tissue response generators and active electrode monitoring technology eliminate concerns about insulation failure and capacitive coupling.
D. Use a low-voltage waveform for monopolar diathermy (cut).
E. Use bipolar electrosurgery when appropriate.

SP2

The following statements regarding energy sources in endoscopy are true except:

A. The bipolar device avoids risk of burn injury to the patient.
B. Bipolar circuits form a circuit within the instrument.
C. Both require non-electrolytic solutions when used in operative hysteroscopy.
D. Monopolar energy needs the patient to be part of the circuit.
E. A return electrode is attached to the patient in monopolar circuit.

SP3

All of the following risks can commonly occur with diagnostic hysteroscopy except:

© Springer India 2016
C. Ratha, J. Gupta, *SBAs and EMQs for MRCOG II*,
DOI 10.1007/978-81-322-2689-5_13

A. Failure to visualise the cavity
B. Injury to the bladder
C. Pelvic infection
D. Uterine perforation
E. Vaginal bleeding

SP4

Ms. XY is 35 years old. She is a Para 3 with two previous caesarean sections and desires permanent contraception. She has opted to have a laparoscopic tubal occlusion/sterilisation procedure. Her BMI is 33. She has had two failed attempts at Veress needle insertion through the umbilical route. Which of the following treatment options are best suited to her?

A. Abandon the procedure.
B. Direct trocar insertion.
C. Hysteroscopic Essure sterilisation (also permanent).
D. Palmer's point entry.
E. Third attempt by a different operator.

SP5

All of the following are safe surgical principles during placement of a primary trocar in laparoscopic surgery except:

A. Emptying the bladder
B. Maintaining an intra-abdominal pressure of 25 mmHg
C. Open laparascopy in high-risk patients
D. Saline test after Veress placement
E. Trendelenburg position

SP6

The best route to perform a hysterectomy (if technically feasible) is:

A. Abdominal
B. Laparascopically assisted vaginal hysterectomy
C. Robot-assisted hysterectomy
D. Total laparoscopic hysterectomy
E. Vaginal

SP7

Defibulation is the reversal of female genital mutilation (infibulation) and is carried out to restore the anatomy to help minimise obstetric complications. Which of the following statements is correct about defibulation?

A. Antenatal surgical correction should be planned only after 34 weeks to minimise risk of preterm birth.
B. Cutting diathermy should not be used.
C. Defibulation can restore physical and emotional normality.
D. Incision should be made along the vulval excision scar.
E. Urethral catheterisation may cause further trauma and hence should be avoided.

SP8

The most effective method of preventing enterocele formation after vaginal hysterectomy is:

A. MacDonald culdoplasty
B. Mackenrodt culdoplasty
C. Mackenzie culdoplasty
D. McCall culdoplasty
E. McRobert culdoplasty

SP9

Which of the following is least likely to be a complication of lower segment caesarean section?

A. Anal sphincter injury
B. Bladder dome injury
C. Colonic perforation
D. Intra-abdominal haemorrhage
E. Transient tachypnea of the newborn

SP10

Ms. XY, 48 years old, a Para 3, is due to undergo a NovaSure endometrial ablation in theatre for heavy menstrual bleeding. A WHO surgical safety checklist is in progress. Which of the following components of the checklist need to be completed before the surgical procedure begins?

A. Sign in and sign out
B. Sign in and time in
C. Sign in and time out
D. Time in and time out
E. Time in and sign out

Clinical Governance: SBA Questions

14

CG1

A 32-year-old is in labour for the last 8 h. She had a previous uneventful vaginal birth at term. She has just broken her waters and there is meconium staining of the liquor amnii. The CTG shows late decelerations. Per vaginam examination shows that the cervix is 6 cm dilated with presenting part at −3 station. You suggest an emergency caesarean section in view of fetal distress, but she declines the same and wants to continue trying for a vaginal birth as she believes she will be fine as it is her second delivery. What should you do?

A. Contact social services for the interest of the unborn fetus who is at risk of harm.
B. Inform her husband and get him to consent for the caesarean section.
C. Respect her choice and continue monitoring and documenting the labour.
D. Stop treating her as she is obviously determined to pursue her own wishes.
E. Transfer her care to another consultant as she is not listening to you.

CG2

Ethics is the understanding of the nature of conflicts arising from duties and obligations. The *four-principle approach* provides a way of thinking about ethical issues/ problems in a simple and accessible way that should cut across cultural differences. Which of the following is not included in these 'four principles'?

A. Beneficence
B. Maleficence
C. Obligation to avoid causing harm
D. Justice
E. Respect for autonomy

© Springer India 2016
C. Ratha, J. Gupta, *SBAs and EMQs for MRCOG II*,
DOI 10.1007/978-81-322-2689-5_14

CG3

A clinical teacher plays all roles except:

A. Assessor
B. Examiner
C. Facilitator
D. Planner
E. Role model

CG4

A 17-year-old girl attends the gynaecology outpatient with complaints of irregular periods. She migrated to the UK with her family a year back and gives history suggestive of female genital mutilation (FGM). As a doctor practising in the UK, which of the following is an appropriate action for you as a gynaecologist?

A. Inform the police about her genital mutilation issue within 1 month.
B. Confirm from her parents if the surgery was done in safe and hygienic conditions.
C. Reassure her that FGM is a known practice in many countries and it is appropriate to conduct such procedures due to cultural reasons.
D. Treat her for her irregular periods only as that is her primary complaint.
E. You are not obliged to inform the police of the FGM procedure that was done with the girl's consent.

CG5

A 30-year-old primigravida receives her 12th week booking blood test results and finds that she has hepatitis C infection. She abused psychotropic drugs in the past and relates that to her infection. After consulting the gastroenterologist, she wants to opt for interferon therapy and hence wants a termination of pregnancy. She has told you that she wants to keep the information about the infection confidential. Her husband and her mother do not understand why she wants a termination and want an answer from you. Which of the following is applicable to this situation?

A. You can tell the husband as he has a right to know the reason for termination.
B. You can tell her mother as she would act in the woman's best interest.
C. The unborn fetus is being compromised so you must inform child protection authorities and try to save the fetus.
D. You do not have to tell either the husband or the mother.
E. You should advise her to delay her treatment with interferon.

CG6

Which of the following is not an essential component of elements that fulfil the criteria of a valid consent?

A. Communicating
B. Deciding
C. Motivating
D. Retaining
E. Understanding

CG7

The mental capacity act applies to people over the age of:

A. 12 years
B. 14 years
C. 16 years
D. 18 years
E. 20 years

CG8

Which is not a component of five steps of 'the 1-min preceptor'?

A. Commitment
B. Positive reinforcement
C. Judgement
D. Application
E. Correction of mistakes

CG9

What is the most appropriate statement regarding a lawsuit on medical negligence?

A. Medical negligence is part of the tort law and is part of criminal law.
B. The plaintiff can claim a breach of moral duty by the defendant to take care resulting in damage to claimant.
C. The plaintiff has to establish that the defendant owed him/her a duty of care.
D. A breach of duty need not be established in all cases.
E. Once a breach of care is established, the onus is on the defendant to disprove the causal link on a balance of probabilities.

CG10

The primary duty of the Caldicott guardian in any NHS trust is:

A. To conduct workshops for patients' awareness of their rights
B. To make sure regular clinical audits are happening
C. To protect staff interests
D. To protect patient confidentiality issues
E. To provide litigation support to patients who feel unfairly treated

Part II

SBA: Answers

Antenatal Care: Answers and Explanations

15

ANC1

Answer: E

Explanation Screening for gestational diabetes using risk factors is recommended in a healthy population. At the booking appointment, the following risk factors for gestational diabetes should be determined:

- Body mass index above 30 kg/m^2
- Previous macrosomic baby weighing 4.5 kg or above
- Previous gestational diabetes
- Family history of diabetes (first-degree relative with diabetes)
- Family origin with a high prevalence of diabetes: South Asian (specifically women whose country of family origin is India, Pakistan or Bangladesh), black, Caribbean and Middle Eastern (specifically women whose country of family origin is Saudi Arabia, United Arab Emirates, Iraq, Jordan, Syria, Oman, Qatar, Kuwait, Lebanon or Egypt)

Women with any one of these risk factors should be offered testing for gestational diabetes. If she has type 2 diabetes, she will be treated as pregestational diabetes and does not need any screening for GDM.

References 1. Antenatal care NICE guideline no 62.
2. Diabetes in pregnancy NICE guideline CG63.

ANC2

Answer: C

Explanation There is no evidence that passenger air travel increases the risk of pregnancy complications such as preterm labour, rupture of membranes or abruption. The radiation dose to the fetus from flying is not significant unless frequent long-haul air travel occurs in pregnancy. Body scanners that utilise ionising radiation for security checks do not pose a risk to mother or fetus from radiation exposure. Flights of more than 4 h of duration are associated with a small increase in the relative risk of venous thrombosis, but overall the absolute risk is very small. The presence of specific risk factors for thrombosis would be expected to increase the risk, and therefore a specific risk assessment should be made for thrombosis in pregnant women who are travelling by air. Specific measures that are likely to be of benefit are graduated elastic compression stockings for women who are pregnant and flying medium- to long-haul flights lasting more than 4 h and LMWH for those with significant risk factors such as previous thrombosis or morbid obesity. Low-dose aspirin should not be used in pregnancy for thromboprophylaxis associated with air travel.

References 1. http://www.rcog.org.uk/files/rcog-corp/21.5.13SIP1AirTravel.pdf
    2. Civil Aviation Authority. Guidance for Health Professionals Information on assessing fitness to fly. http://www.caa.co.uk/default.aspx?catid=2497&pagetype=90

ANC3

Answer: B

Explanation For women who have accepted intrapartum antibiotic prophylaxis (IAP), benzylpenicillin should be administered as soon as possible after the onset of labour and given regularly until delivery. Clindamycin should be administered to those women allergic to benzylpenicillin. It is recommended that 3 g intravenous benzylpenicillin be given as soon as possible after the onset of labour and 1.5 g 4-hourly until delivery. Clindamycin 900 mg should be given intravenously 8-hourly to those allergic to benzylpenicillin.

References Green Top guideline no. 36 Early onset Group B streptococcal disease, 2012. http://www.rcog.org.uk/files/rcog-corp/GTG36_GBS.pdf

ANC4

Answer: D

Explanation Placental abruption is seen more often in gestational hypertensive disease, advanced maternal age, increasing parity, the presence of multiple gestations, polyhydramnios, chorioamnionitis, prolonged rupture of membranes, trauma and possibly thrombophilias. Potential preventable risk factors include maternal cocaine and tobacco use. Unexplained elevated maternal serum alpha-fetoprotein (MSAFP) levels in the second trimester are associated with pregnancy complications such as placental abruption.

The precise cause of abruption is unknown. Abruption arises from haemorrhage into the decidua basalis of the placenta, which results in the formation of haematoma and an increase in hydrostatic pressure leading to separation of the adjacent placenta. The resultant haematoma may be small and self-limited or may continue to dissect through the decidual layers. However, the bleeding may be in whole or in part concealed, if the haematoma does not reach the margin of the placenta and cervix for the blood loss to be revealed. Therefore the amount of revealed haemorrhage poorly reflects the degree of blood loss. The bleeding may infiltrate the myometrium resulting in the so-called Couvelaire uterus.

References Ngeh N, Bhide A. Antepartum haemorrhage. Curr Obstet Gynaecol. 2006;16:79–83.

ANC5

Answer: C

Explanation Most women in the UK will have a routine scan at 21–23 weeks (anomaly scan). The placenta will be low lying in some, necessitating a repeat scan later in pregnancy, typically at 34–36 weeks. The diagnosis of placental praevia is most commonly made on ultrasound examination. Up to 26 % of placentas are found to be low lying on ultrasound examination in the early second trimester. Several studies have demonstrated that unless the placental edge is at least reaching the internal cervical os at midpregnancy, placenta praevia at term will not be encountered. Transvaginal ultrasound is safe in the presence of placenta praevia and is more accurate than transabdominal ultrasound in locating the placental edge.

References Ngeh N, Bhide A. Antepartum haemorrhage. Curr Obstet Gynaecol. 2006;16:79–83.

ANC6

Answer: D

Explanation RCOG guidelines recommend that any women going to the operation theatre with known major placenta praevia should be attended by an experienced obstetrician and anaesthetist, with consultant presence available, especially if these women have previous uterine scars or an anterior placenta or are suspected to be associated with placenta accreta. Four units of crossmatched blood should be kept ready, even if the mother has never experienced vaginal bleeding. Delivery of women with placenta praevia should not be planned in units where blood transfusion facilities are unavailable. The choice of anaesthetic technique for caesarean sections is usually made by the anaesthetist conducting the procedure.

References RCOG Green Top guideline – Placenta Praevia, Placenta Praevia Accreta and Vasa Praevia: Diagnosis and Management (Green-Top 27).

ANC7

Answer: D

Explanation Pregnant women with complex social factors may need additional support to use antenatal care services.

  Examples of complex social factors include: substance misuse, recent arrival as a migrant, asylum seeker or refugee status, difficulty speaking or understanding English, age under 20, domestic abuse, poverty and homelessness. The NICE guideline on pregnancy and complex factors describes how access to care can be improved, how contact with antenatal carers can be maintained, the additional support and consultations that are required and the additional information that should be offered to pregnant women with complex social factors.

References NICE guideline 110, Pregnancy and complex social factors, September 2010.

ANC8

Answer: B

Explanation Diabetes when uncontrolled can cause cardiac anomalies, like transposition of great vessels, ventricular septal defect, situs inversus, single ventricle and hypoplastic left heart. A four-chamber view of the fetal heart and outflow tracts should be offered as part of routine antenatal care. Hyperglycaemia is a toxic environment for the developing embryo, and the incidence of malformation is related to glucose control. This is why optimising glycaemic control prior to pregnancy is so important, as it may be too late to reduce the teratogenic effect of hyperglycaemia by the time of the first antenatal appointment.

References 1. Lambert K, Germain S. Pre-existing type I and type II diabetes in pregnancy. Obstet Gynecol Rep Med. 20(12):353–8.
2. Nice guideline no. 63 Diabetes in pregnancy. http://www.nice.org.uk/guidance/cg63/resources/guidance-diabetes-in-pregnancy-pdf

ANC9

Answer: D

Explanation The risk of transmission of syphilis from mother to fetus is dependent on the stage of maternal infection and duration of fetal exposure. The transmission risk of early syphilis in pregnancy is up to 100 %, and 50 % of these pregnancies will result in preterm birth or perinatal death. Ten percent of infants born to women with late infection will be affected. Congenital syphilis is a multisystem infection which can result in stillbirth, neonatal death and long-term disability.

Diagnosis is by serology. Most cases of syphilis in pregnancy are detected through antenatal screening but syphilis must be considered in the differential diagnosis of women with genital ulceration in pregnancy and repeat syphilis testing should be performed. In the UK, an enzyme immunoassay, which has high sensitivity and specificity, is used for screening.

A positive enzyme immunoassay is confirmed by either a *T. pallidum* haemagglutination assay or *T. pallidum* particle agglutination assay. A non-treponemal test, either a Venereal Diseases Reference Laboratory test or reactive plasma reagin, is a quantitative assay used to monitor disease activity and treatment response.

References Allstaff S, Wilson J. The management of sexually transmitted infections in pregnancy. Obstet Gynaecol. 2012;14:25–32.

ANC10

Answer: E

Explanation Folic acid is recommended in all pregnant women to prevent neural tube defects. Folic acid at a dosage of at least 1 mg daily is recommended for women with sickle cell disease outside pregnancy in view of their haemolytic anaemia, which puts them at increased risk of folate deficiency. Folic acid 5 mg daily should be prescribed during pregnancy to reduce the risk of neural tube defect and to compensate for the increased demand for folate during pregnancy.

References Management of sickle cell disease in pregnancy. Green-Top guideline no. 61. London: RCOG Press; 2011. Available at http://www.rcog.org.uk/files/rcog-corp/GTG6111042013.pdf

ANC11

Answer: B

Explanation Neural tube defects, which are comprised of open spina bifida, anencephaly and encephalocele, complicate 1.5/1000 pregnancies in the UK. Periconceptional folic acid reduces the incidence of both occurrence and recurrence of neural tube defects. A Department of Health Expert Advisory Group has recommended that women with a history of neural tube defects should take 4 mg of folic acid preconceptionally and for the first eight weeks of pregnancy.

References Royal College of Obstetricians and Gynaecologists. Periconceptional folic acid and food fortification in the prevention of neural tube defects. Scientific impact paper no. 4. London: RCOG Press; 2003. Available at http://www.rcog.org.uk/files/rcog-corp/uploaded-files/SIP_No_4.pdf

ANC12

Answer: D

Explanation All women require follow-up imaging if the placenta covers or overlaps the cervical os at 20 weeks of gestation. Women with a previous caesarean section require a higher index of suspicion as there are two problems to exclude: placenta praevia and placenta accreta. If the placenta lies anteriorly and reaches the cervical os at 20 weeks, a follow-up scan can help identify if it is implanted into the caesarean section scar. In cases of asymptomatic women with suspected minor praevia, follow-up imaging can be left until 36 weeks of gestation. In cases with asymptomatic suspected major placenta praevia or a question of placenta accreta, imaging should be performed at around 32 weeks of gestation to clarify the diagnosis and allow planning for third-trimester management, further imaging and delivery.

References Royal College of Obstetricians and Gynaecologists. Placenta praevia, placenta praevia accreta and vasa praevia: diagnosis and management. Green-Top guideline no. 27. London: RCOG Press; 2011. Available at http://www.rcog.org.uk/files/rcog-corp/GTG27PlacentaPraeviaJanuary2011.pdf

ANC13

Answer: B

Explanation Risk factors for vasa praevia include placental anomalies such as a bilobed placenta or succenturiate lobes where the fetal vessels run through the membranes joining the separate lobes together, a history of low-lying placenta in the second trimester, multiple pregnancy and in vitro fertilisation, where the incidence of vasa praevia has been reported to be as high as one in 300. The reasons for this association are not clear, but disturbed orientation of the blastocyst at implantation, vanishing embryos and the increased frequency of placental morphological variations in in vitro fertilisation pregnancies have all been postulated.

References 1. RCOG Greentop guideline no. 27. Placenta praevia accreta and vasa praevia. https://www.rcog.org.uk/globalassets/documents/guidelines/gtg_27.pdf

2. Baulies S, et al. Prenatal ultrasound diagnosis of vasa praevia and analysis of risk factors. Prenat Diagn. 2007;27:595–9.

ANC14

Answer: A

Explanation Indomethacin had profound effects on platelet and neutrophil functioning; cerebral, renal and mesenteric haemodynamics and fetal ductus arteriosus. All these are likely to have serious effects on the fetus. It is reported to cause constriction of the ductus arteriosus, reduced urine output and frequently oligohydramnios. In the neonate born after indomethacin exposure, the reported complications include pulmonary hypertension, persistent ductus arteriosus, necrotising enterocolitis, ileal perforation and intraventricular haemorrhage.

References Tocolysis for women in preterm labour. RCOG Green Top guideline No 1B. http://www.rcog.org.uk/files/rcog-corp/GTG1b26072011.pdf

ANC15

Answer: D

Explanation Smoking remains the single largest preventable cause of fetal and infant morbidity in the UK. Potential problems during pregnancy include ectopic pregnancy, miscarriage, placental complications, premature rupture of membranes, premature birth and fetal growth restriction. Counselling sessions are effective in pregnancy and lead to a reduction in the incidence of preterm birth and low birth weight. Maternal smoking has also been associated with an overall reduced incidence of pre-eclampsia. Smoking may only be reduced in those women aged 30 years and under without pregestational hypertension. Sudden infant death syndrome describes the sudden unexplained loss of life in the first year. Data from a number of trials suggest that maternal smoking increases the risk of sudden infant death syndrome by up to fourfold compared with controls, therefore implying that many cases may be preventable. The mechanism underlying this is unclear, but some studies have suggested that exposure to a hypoxic state in the womb may diminish the normal physiological response to hypoxia in the neonate.

References Eastham R, Gosakan R. Smoking and smoking cessation in pregnancy. Obstet Gynaecol. 2010;12:103–9.

ANC16

Answer: A

Explanation Clinicians should offer a single course of antenatal corticosteroids to women between 24+0 and 34+6 weeks of gestation who are at risk of preterm birth. It is associated with a significant reduction in rates of neonatal death, RDS and intraventricular haemorrhage.

Betamethasone 12 mg given intramuscularly in two doses and dexamethasone 6 mg given intramuscularly in four doses are the steroids of choice to enhance lung maturation. A rescue course of two doses of 12 mg betamethasone or four doses of 6 mg dexamethasone should only be considered with caution in those pregnancies where the first course was given at less than 26+0 weeks of gestation and another obstetric indication arises later in pregnancy.

References Antenatal corticosteroids to reduce neonatal morbidity and mortality. RCOG Green Top guideline no. 7.

ANC17

Answer: A

Explanation External cephalic version (ECV) is the manipulation of the fetus, through the maternal abdomen, to a cephalic presentation. ECV reduces the caesarean section rate by lowering the incidence of breech presentation (RR 0.55,95 % CI 0.33–0.91, risk difference 17 %, NNT 6). Provision of an ECV service also reduces the caesarean section rates for breech presentation. This reduction is in spite of a twofold increase in intrapartum caesarean sections for successfully turned babies, when compared with babies that were not breech at term.

Women should be counselled that, with a trained operator, about 50 % of ECV attempts will be successful but this rate can be individualised for them. Results vary from 30 % up to 80 % in different series. Race, parity, uterine tone, liquor volume, engagement of the breech and whether the head is palpable and the use of tocolysis all affect the success rate.

References http://www.rcog.org.uk/files/rcog-corp/uploaded-files/GT20aExternal CephalicVersion.pdf

ANC18

Answer: B

Explanation Offer women with twin and triplet pregnancies a first-trimester ultrasound scan when crown-rump length measures from 45 mm to 84 mm (at approximately 11 to 13+6 weeks) to estimate gestational age, determine chorionicity and screen for Down syndrome (ideally, these should all be performed at the same scan).

Use the largest baby to estimate gestational age in twin and triplet pregnancies to avoid the risk of estimating it from a baby with early growth pathology.

References NICE guideline 129. Multiple pregnancy. 2011. http://www.nice.org. uk/guidance/cg129

ANC19

Answer: A

Explanation Caregivers should be aware of the higher incidence of anaemia in multiple pregnancies as compared to singleton pregnancies. Perform a full blood count at 20–24 weeks to identify women with twin and triplet pregnancies who need early supplementation with iron or folic acid, and repeat at 28 weeks as in routine antenatal care.

Booking blood test is offered to all pregnant women for screening for anaemia.

References 1. NICE guideline no 69 Multiple pregnancy, http://www.nice.org.uk/guidance/cg129

2. NICE guideline antenatal care.

ANC20

Answer: B

Explanation Inform women with uncomplicated dichorionic twin pregnancies that elective birth from 37 weeks 0 days does not appear to be associated with an increased risk of serious adverse outcomes and that continuing uncomplicated twin pregnancies beyond 38 weeks 0 days increase the risk of fetal death.

For women who decline elective birth, offer weekly appointments with the specialist obstetrician. At each appointment, offer an ultrasound scan, and perform weekly biophysical profile assessments and fortnightly fetal growth scans.

References NICE guideline no 129, Multiple pregnancy. http://www.nice.org.uk/guidance/cg129

ANC21

Answer: D

Explanation If a woman with a twin or triplet pregnancy presents after 14 weeks 0 days, determine chorionicity at the earliest opportunity by ultrasound using all of the following:

- The number of placental masses
- The lambda or T-sign
- Membrane thickness
- Discordant fetal sex

If it is not possible to determine chorionicity by ultrasound at the time of detecting the twin or triplet pregnancy, seek a second opinion from a senior ultrasonographer or offer the woman referral to a healthcare professional who is competent in determining chorionicity by ultrasound scan as soon as possible.

If it is difficult to determine chorionicity, even after referral (e.g. because the woman has booked late in pregnancy), manage the pregnancy as monochorionic until proved otherwise.

References NICE guideline no 129, Multiple pregnancy. http://www.nice.org.uk/guidance/cg129

ANC22

Answer: E

Explanation Give women with twin and triplet pregnancies the same advice about diet, lifestyle and nutritional supplements as in routine antenatal care. Be aware of the higher incidence of anaemia in women with twin and triplet pregnancies compared with women with singleton pregnancies. Perform a full blood count at 20–24 weeks to identify women with twin and triplet pregnancies who need early supplementation with iron or folic acid, and repeat at 28 weeks as in routine antenatal care.

References NICE guideline no 129 multiple pregnancy. http://www.nice.org.uk/guidance/cg129

ANC23

Answer: E

Explanation The optimal time to offer the second-trimester scan is between $18+0$ and $20+6$ weeks of gestation. If a low-lying placenta is seen on the anomaly scan, the majority of hospitals would recommend a repeat scan at 32–34 weeks of gestation. Definitive diagnosis of Down syndrome is done via amniocentesis and chromosomal analysis. Ultrasound cannot diagnose genetic conditions like inborn errors of metabolism—these will either be diagnosed by direct mutation testing or fetal metabolite analysis—both after invasive testing.

Ultrasound has low sensitivity of detection of fetal anomalies in women with high BMI due to poor tissue penetration of ultrasound waves.

Echocardiography with a four-chamber view of the heart should be done routinely in anomaly scan. Demonstration of a four-chamber view will detect 40–50 % of congenital heart disease in a low-risk population at a routine anomaly scan.

References StratOG Core training tutorial: antenatal care – ultrasound scanning of fetal anomaly.

ANC24

Answer: A

Explanation Although there is no specific risk to pregnancy associated with commercial air travel, there are conditions which may complicate the pregnancy and could lead to an increase in risk of problems. Recent haemorrhage in pregnancy (not past pregnancy haemorrhage) is a contraindication to commercial air travel.

Examples of relevant medical complications which may occur during pregnancy and which would contraindicate commercial air travel include:

- Severe anaemia with haemoglobin less than 7.5 g/dl.
- Recent haemorrhage.
- Otitis media and sinusitis.
- Serious cardiac or respiratory disease.
- Recent sickling crisis.
- Recent gastrointestinal surgery, including laparoscopic surgery, where there have been gastrointestinal procedures carried out and where suture lines on the intestine could come under stress due to the reduction in pressure and gaseous expansion.
- A fracture, where significant leg swelling can occur in flight, is particularly hazardous in the first few days of a cast being placed.

References 1. http://www.rcog.org.uk/files/rcog-corp/21.5.13SIP1AirTravel.pdf
2. Civil Aviation Authority. Guidance for health professionals information on assessing fitness to fly. http://www.caa.co.uk/default.aspx?catid=2497&pagetype=90

ANC25

Answer: D

Explanation Pregnant women should be offered screening for anaemia at booking and at 28 weeks. Women with multiple pregnancies should have an additional full blood count done at 20–24 weeks. Anaemia in pregnancy is defined as first-trimester haemoglobin (Hb) less than 110 g/l, second-/third-trimester Hb less than 105 g/l and postpartum Hb less than 100 g/l, in line with BCSH guidance.

References National Institute for Health and Clinical Excellence. Antenatal care. NICE clinical guideline 62. Manchester: NICE; 2008 RCOG Green Top guideline no. 47 Blood transfusion in obstetrics. https://www.rcog.org.uk/globalassets/documents/guidelines/gtg-47.pdf

ANC26

Answer: D

Explanation All women should be informed at the booking appointment about the importance for their own and their baby's health of maintaining adequate vitamin D stores during pregnancy and while breastfeeding. In order to achieve this, women should be advised to take a vitamin D supplement (10 µg of vitamin D per day), as found in the Healthy Start multivitamin supplement. Women who are not eligible for the Healthy Start benefit should be advised where they can buy the supplement. Particular care should be taken to enquire as to whether women at greatest risk are following advice to take this daily supplement. These include:

- Women with darker skin such as those of African, African–Caribbean or South Asian family origin
- Women who have limited exposure to sunlight, such as women who are house-bound or confined indoors for long periods or who cover their skin for cultural reasons

Vitamin D is essential for skeletal growth and bone health. Severe deficiency can result in rickets (among children) and osteomalacia (among children and adults). Dietary sources are limited. National surveys suggest that around a fifth of adults and 8–24 % of children may have low vitamin D status.

References 1. NICE guideline on Antenatal care (CG62) http://www.nice.org.uk/guidance/cg62/chapter/1-recommendations
2. NICE guideline on Vitamin D: increasing supplement use among at-risk groups (PH56) http://www.nice.org.uk/guidance/ph56

ANC27

Answer: C

Explanation Women with pre-existing medical conditions should have pre-pregnancy counselling by doctors with experience of managing their disorder in pregnancy. Women with medical disorders in pregnancy should have access to a coordinated multidisciplinary obstetric and medical clinic, thereby avoiding the need to attend multiple appointments and poor communication between senior specialists responsible for their care.

There should be adequate provision of appropriate critical care support for the management of a pregnant woman who becomes unwell. Plans should be in place for provision of critical care on delivery units or maternity care on critical care units, depending on most appropriate setting for a pregnant or postpartum woman to receive care. The deaths of all women should undergo multidisciplinary review at a local level.

References Saving lives, Improving mothers care full report 2014.

ANC28

Answer: A

Explanation Clinical care for women with twin and triplet pregnancies should be provided by a nominated multidisciplinary team consisting of a core team of named specialist obstetricians and specialist midwives and ultrasonographers, all of whom have experience and knowledge of managing twin and triplet pregnancies, and an enhanced team for referrals, which should include:

A perinatal mental health professional
A women's health physiotherapist
An infant feeding specialist
A dietician

Members of the enhanced team should have experience and knowledge relevant to twin and triplet pregnancies.

References NICE guideline no. 129, Multiple pregnancy. http://www.nice.org.uk/guidance/cg129

ANC29

Answer: B

Explanation A Cochrane systematic review in 2010 concluded that folic acid supplementation has a strong protective effect against neural tube defects (relative risk [RR] 0.28, 95 % confidence interval [CI] 0.15–0.52), supporting the current recommendation of 400 µg/day of folic acid preconceptually and for the first trimester of pregnancy. Recent meta-analyses have also reported that maternal folic acid supplementation is associated with decreased risk of other congenital anomalies, including cardiovascular defects (odds ratio [OR] 0.61, 95 % CI 0.40–0.92) and limb defects (OR 0.57, 95 % CI 0.38–0.85), and some paediatric cancers, including leukaemia, paediatric brain tumours and neuroblastomas. Although some authors have suggested a possible observed increase in twin births in women receiving periconceptional folic acid supplementation, using data from folic acid fortification studies, a large population-based study found no evidence for such an association after accounting for and confounding for in vitro fertilisation pregnancies and underreporting.

References 1. De-Regil LM, Fernandez-Gaxiola AC, Dowswell T, Pena-Rosas JP. Effects and safety of periconceptional folate supplementation for preventing birth defects. Cochrane Database Syst Rev. 2010;10:CD007950.

2. Goh YI, Bollano E, Einarson TR, Koren G. Prenatal multivitamin supplementation and rates of paediatric cancers: a meta-analysis. Clin Pharmacol Ther. 2007;81:685–91.

ANC30

Answer: E

Explanation While clinical acumen remains vitally important in suspecting and managing placenta praevia, the definitive diagnosis of most low-lying placentas is now achieved with ultrasound imaging. Clinical suspicion should, however, be raised in any woman with vaginal bleeding (classically painless bleeding or bleeding provoked by sexual intercourse) and a high presenting part or an abnormal lie, irrespective of previous imaging results.

Clinical suspicion should be raised in all women with vaginal bleeding after 20 weeks of gestation. A high presenting part, an abnormal lie and painless or provoked bleeding, irrespective of previous imaging results, are more suggestive of a low-lying placenta but may not be present, and the definitive diagnosis usually relies on ultrasound imaging.

References RCOG Greentop guideline no. 27. Placenta praevia accreta and vasa praevia. https://www.rcog.org.uk/globalassets/documents/guidelines/gtg_27.pdf

ANC31

Answer: C

Explanation Antenatal imaging techniques that can help to raise the suspicion of a morbidly adherent placenta should be considered in any situation where any part of the placenta lies under the previous caesarean section scar, *but the definitive diagnosis can be made only at surgery*. These techniques include ultrasound and magnetic resonance imaging (MRI). Antenatal sonographic imaging can be complemented by magnetic resonance imaging in equivocal cases to distinguish those women at special risk of placenta accreta.

Of those women in whom the placenta is still low at 32 weeks of gestation, the majority (73 %) will remain so at term, but 90 % of major praevias at this gestation will persist. Imaging at 32 weeks therefore seems timely in enabling a fairly definitive diagnosis to be made alongside a plan for further care, including follow-up imaging for possible accreta, counselling for delivery and planning for delivery. Women who have had a previous caesarean section who also have either placenta praevia or an anterior placenta underlying the old caesarean section scar at 32 weeks of gestation are at increased risk of placenta accreta and should be managed as if they have placenta accreta, with appropriate preparations for surgery made.

Elective delivery by caesarean section in asymptomatic women is not recommended before 38 weeks of gestation for placenta praevia or before 36–37 weeks of gestation for suspected placenta accreta.

References 1. RCOG Greentop guideline no. 27. Placenta praevia accreta and vasa praevia. https://www.rcog.org.uk/globalassets/documents/guidelines/gtg_27.pdf

2. Dashe JS, et al. Persistence of placenta previa according to gestational age at ultrasound detection. Obstet Gynecol. 2002;99:692–7.

ANC32

Answer: D

Explanation Women with no personal history or risk factors for VTE but who have a family history of an unprovoked or oestrogen-provoked VTE in a first-degree relative when aged under 50 years should be considered for thrombophilia testing. This will be more informative if the relative has a known thrombophilia.

References Reducing the risk of venous thromboembolism during pregnancy and the puerperium. Green-Top guideline no. 37a April 2015.

ANC33

Answer: B

Explanation Information about antenatal screening should be provided in a setting where discussion can take place; this may be in a group setting or on a one-to-one basis.

This guideline offers best practice advice on the care of healthy pregnant women. Women and their partners and their families should always be treated with kindness, respect and dignity. The views, beliefs and values of the woman and her partner and her family in relation to her care and that of her baby should be sought and respected at all times. Women should have the opportunity to make informed decisions about their care and treatment, in partnership with their healthcare professionals.

References Antenatal care NICE guideline no 62 (modified Dec 2014).

ANC34

Answer: C

Explanation Maternity units should adopt a process for questioning all women born in (or with recent ancestry of) those parts of the world associated with female genital mutilation. This can be based on the family origin questioning (FOQ) used for haemoglobinopathy screening.

Discussions must take into account language difficulties, psychological vulnerability and cultural differences. Healthcare workers should actively demonstrate knowledge and respect.

The consultation should include a psychological assessment, and referral to a psychologist should be discussed with the woman.

Physical examination by an obstetrician or appropriately trained midwife or nurse should be strongly recommended to identify whether antenatal surgery would be beneficial. Physical examination should also be recommended to reassess women who have had a previous defibulation, as some may have undergone a further infibulation.

A diagram or medical photography (with consent) can be used to limit repetitive examinations, to aid explanations to the woman and to communicate with a hospital or clinic that has developed expertise in the assessment and management of women with genital mutilation. A preformatted sheet, including a predrawn diagram, should be considered for the identification of the type of genital mutilation, need for antenatal defibulation and planning of intrapartum care.

Genital mutilation is not an absolute indication for caesarean birth unless the woman has such an extreme form of mutilation with anatomical distortion that makes defibulation impossible.

Decisions about delivery must take into account the psychological needs of the woman. Episiotomy should be recommended if inelastic scar tissue appears to be preventing progress, but careful placement is essential to avoid severe trauma to surrounding tissues, including bowel.

References 1. Green Top guideline no 53 FGM.
2. NICE guideline on antenatal care.

ANC35

Answer: E

Explanation Teenage pregnancy is common in the UK. Teenagers are at risk of a range of adverse pregnancy outcomes, particularly preterm birth. The reasons for this are complex and it is most likely that they reflect a combination of adverse socio-economic pressures and gynaecological and biological immaturity. While there is no evidence to date of medical interventions that can specifically improve pregnancy outcome, the obstetrician providing care for women in this age group should be aware of the potential challenges. Antenatal care should be tailored to the individual needs of this group, particularly with regard to encouraging early and regular attendance, smoking cessation programmes, counselling regarding the risk of STIs and future contraception. The high risk of adverse pregnancy outcome in the adolescent has been attributed to gynaecological immaturity and the growth and nutritional status of the mother. Gynaecological immaturity undoubtedly predisposes adolescent girls to poor pregnancy outcome in that the rates of spontaneous miscarriage and of very preterm birth (<32 weeks of gestation) are highest in girls aged 13–15 years.

References Horgan RP, Kenny LC. Management of teenage pregnancy. Obstet Gynaecol. 2007;9:153–8. doi:10.1576/toag.9.3.153.27334.

ANC36

Answer: B

Explanation Maternal anaemia and elevated haemoglobin levels are related to adverse pregnancy outcomes. Both maternal anaemia and elevated haemoglobin levels may affect the fetal supply line and cause a restricted intrauterine environment.

There is some evidence for the association between maternal iron deficiency and preterm delivery, low birth weight, possibly placental abruption and increased peripartum blood loss. Iron deficiency may contribute to maternal morbidity through effects on immune function with increased susceptibility or severity of infections, poor work capacity and performance and disturbances of postpartum cognition and emotions.

The fetus is relatively protected from the effects of iron deficiency by upregulation of placental iron transport proteins but evidence suggests that maternal iron depletion increases the risk of iron deficiency in the first 3 months of life, by a variety of mechanisms. Impaired psychomotor and/or mental development are well described in infants with iron deficiency anaemia and may also negatively contribute to infant and social emotional behaviour.

Maternal haemoglobin levels were not associated with childhood body mass index, total fat mass percentage, android/gynoid fat mass ratio, systolic blood pressure or cholesterol or insulin levels. These results do not strongly support the hypothesis that variations in maternal haemoglobin levels during pregnancy influence cardio-metabolic risk factors in childhood.

References 1. Welten M, Gaillard R, Hofman A, de Jonge LL, Jaddoe VWV. Maternal haemoglobin levels and cardio-metabolic risk factors in childhood: the generation R study. BJOG. 2015;122:805–15

2. UK guidelines on the management of iron deficiency in pregnancy British Committee for Standards in Haematology. 2011. http://www.bcshguidelines.com/documents/UK_Guidelines_iron_deficiency_in_pregnancy.pdf

3. Perez et al. Mother-infant Interactions and infant development are altered by maternal iron deficiency anemia. J Nutr. 2005;135:850–5.

ANC37

Answer: C

Explanation In this clinical situation, the most important test would be to detect fetal rhesus antigen status. If fetus is rhesus positive, it is at risk of haemolytic disease of fetus and newborn, and the pregnancy will have to be managed with active surveillance for fetal anaemia.

If the fetus is rhesus negative, the mother can be largely reassured that her isoimmunised status will not affect the fetus. Cell-free fetal DNA from maternal blood can help determine fetal rhesus status after 10 weeks of gestation.

Paternal blood group could help if it is rhesus negative but various possibilities exist if it is rhesus positive. Maternal antibody status, haemoglobin and blood group are of limited clinical value in this clinical situation.

References Non-invasive prenatal testing for chromosomal abnormality using maternal plasma DNA scientific impact paper no. 15 March 2014.

ANC38

Answer: D

Explanation A schedule of antenatal appointments should be determined by the function of the appointments. For a woman who is nulliparous with an uncomplicated pregnancy, a schedule of ten appointments should be adequate. For a woman who is parous with an uncomplicated pregnancy, a schedule of seven appointments should be adequate.

References Antenatal care NICE guideline no 62 (modified Dec 2014).

ANC39

Answer: D

Explanation There are many infectious agents but group A streptococcus is common in category 3 and 4. Category 3 = ascending genital tract infection following delivery of any type (miscarriage/abortion, termination, caesarean section, vaginal delivery). Category 4 = septic shock in a pregnant woman with intact membranes and before the onset of labour.

In category 2 (premature rupture of membranes and ascending genital tract infection), Gram-negative perineal bacilli were the most common pathogens.

References Saving lives improving mothers care report 2014.

ANC40

Answer: C

Explanation Air travel is safe during pregnancy; there is no increased risk of complication with occasional commercial air travel. There is a small increase in the absolute risk of venous thromboembolism. The key change in the environment in commercial air travel is cabin altitude.

References Scientific Impact Paper no. 1, Air Travel and Pregnancy, May 2013.

ANC41

Answer: A

Explanation Oxygen consumption is increased during pregnancy by about 20 %, and there is further increase during labour and delivery. Maternal PaO_2 increases in pregnancy to about 100–105 mm of Hg at sea level. Approximately 50 % of pregnant women experience dyspnea before 19 weeks of gestation and 76 % by 31 weeks. Reasons for experiencing the sensation during normal pregnancy may be related to the effect of progesterone on the respiratory centre, mechanical changes associated with weight gain or decreased venous return and/or the demands of the fetus. The presence of anaemia should be sought for as this is common in pregnancy. If there is no underlying disease as a cause of dyspnea, the patient can be reassured that there is no increased risk for complications during pregnancy or labour and delivery.

References Raymond P, et al. editors. De Swiet's medical disorders in pregnancy. 5th ed. Chapter 1.

ANC42

Answer: A

Explanation Blood pressure is directly proportional to systemic vascular resistance and cardiac output. Vasodilatation is perhaps the primary change in circulation in pregnancy. Before the increase in cardiac output can adequately compensate for the fall in systemic vascular resistance, blood pressure begins to decrease in early pregnancy. It continues to decrease in the second trimester of a normal pregnancy till it reaches a nadir at 22–24 weeks of gestation following that there is a steady rise till term.

Phase V (disappearance) rather than phase IV (muffling) of Korotkoff sounds should be taken as the diastolic reading. Blood pressure taken in supine position during second and third trimesters of pregnancy will be lower than that taken in sitting position due to decreased venous return to the heart.

Blood pressure usually falls immediately after delivery although it tends to rise subsequently reaching a peak in 3–6 days postpartum. Previously normotensive women may become transiently hypertensive following delivery.

References Handbook of obstetric medicine, Catherine Nelson Piercy, 5th ed. Chapter 1, p. 3.

ANC43

Answer: C

Explanation The increased cardiac output and hyperdynamic circulation of pregnancy mean that large volumes of blood can be lost rapidly, especially from the uterus, which receives 10 % of the cardiac output at term. Otherwise healthy women tolerate blood loss remarkably well and can lose up to 35 % of their circulation before becoming symptomatic. Blood loss is tolerated less well if there is a pre-existing maternal anaemia, and clotting is less efficient if there is a significant anaemia. Concealed bleeding and underestimation of loss mean that intervention is often delayed. Where signs of hypovolaemia have been subtle, hypovolaemia as the cause of maternal cardiopulmonary arrest may go unrecognised, particularly where blood loss has been concealed.

References RCOG Green Top guideline no. 56, Maternal collapse in pregnancy.

ANC44

Answer: C

Explanation The increased progesterone level in pregnancy increases the respiratory drive, leading to an increase in tidal volume and minute ventilation. Splinting of the diaphragm by the enlarged uterus reduces the functional residual capacity and also makes ventilation more difficult. These factors, along with the markedly increased oxygen consumption of the fetoplacental unit, mean that the pregnant woman becomes hypoxic much more rapidly during periods of hypoventilation. Changes in lung function, diaphragmatic splinting and increased oxygen consumption make the pregnant woman become hypoxic more readily and make ventilation more difficult.

References RCOG Green Top guideline no. 56, Maternal collapse.

ANC45

Answer: D

Explanation Carpal tunnel syndrome results from compression of the median nerve within the carpal tunnel in the hand. It is characterised by tingling, burning pain, numbness and a swelling sensation in the hand that may impair sensory and motor function of the hand.

Carpal tunnel syndrome is not an uncommon complaint among pregnant women, and estimates of incidence during pregnancy range from 21 % to 62 %. Interventions to treat carpal tunnel syndrome include wrist splints and wrist splints plus injections of corticosteroid and analgesia.

References Nice guideline antenatal care (section 7.4).

ANC46

Answer: D

Explanation Vitamin B6 is a water-soluble vitamin involved in myelin formation, synthesis of neurotransmitters and haem formation; it also decreases plasma homocysteine concentrations. Vitamin B6 levels have been found to fall in the third trimester, although it is not certain whether this represents a normal physiological response to plasma expansion or whether it is indicative of potential deficiency. There is limited evidence that vitamin B6 may reduce nausea (but not vomiting) in the first trimester and dental decay in pregnant women, but there is no convincing evidence to support routine supplementation in the UK. Similarly, there are minimal data on supplementation of the other B vitamins in pregnancy and routine supplementation is not recommended.

References Duckworth S, Mistry HD, Chappell LC. Vitamin supplementation in pregnancy. Obstet Gynaecol. 2012;14:175–8.

ANC47

Answer: A

Explanation According to health and safety executive guidelines for expectant or breastfeeding mothers about working safely with ionising radiation, many types of X-ray examinations would not pose any problem to the fetus. If you are referred for an investigation or treatment involving ionising radiation, you should inform the clinical staff that you are, or may be, pregnant so that they can advise you. It is in your own and your baby's interests that you inform your employer as soon as you know you are pregnant. Your employer needs to know if you are pregnant before they can make any changes that may be required to the protection measures. However, you are not legally required to do so and can choose to keep that information private. When you decide to inform your employer, this should be in writing. There should be no significant risk of harm to your baby from radiation at work and certainly there should never be a need to terminate a pregnancy because of radiation doses normally received at work.

Your baby will receive about 1 mSv from sources of natural radiation during pregnancy. The added exposure at work should be no more than this and in practice is likely to be considerably less. The added risk to your baby of childhood cancer from 1 mSv would, at worst, be a small percentage of that from other causes.

If you work with diagnostic X-rays, you should keep as far away as practicable from the patient and the X-ray tube while it is on, preferably behind the protective screen. If you have to be outside the protective screen during exposures, you must wear a lead apron that is comfortable to wear, fastened properly at the sides and covers your abdomen comfortably. Your employer will need to check that such protective measures do not create other risks such as back problems. Although it is not a legal requirement, it may be possible to wear an active dose monitor for additional reassurance. External radiation sources, such as X-rays, do not affect milk production or breastfeeding. You only need to consider doing anything if radioactive materials could be taken into your body or contaminate the skin, for example, by swallowing them or breathing them in.

References Health and safety executive – Working safely with ionising radiation: guidelines for expectant or breastfeeding mothers. http://www.hse.gov.uk/pubns/indg334.pdf

ANC48

Answer: C

Explanation Pregnant women should be offered an early ultrasound scan between 10 weeks 0 days and 13 weeks 6 days to determine gestational age and to detect multiple pregnancies. This will ensure consistency of gestational age assessment and reduce the incidence of induction of labour for prolonged pregnancy.

Crown-rump length measurement should be used to determine gestational age. If the crown-rump length is above 84 mm, the gestational age should be estimated using head circumference.

References Antenatal care NICE guideline 2008 (modified 2014).

ANC49

Answer: C

Explanation Giving birth in the UK is safer than ever and the risk is very small. The number of women who die during, or shortly after, pregnancy has decreased from 11 to 10 per 100,000. The latest enquiry into maternal deaths, Saving Lives, Improving Mothers' Care, reports that, in the 3 years 2009–12, 321 women died during their pregnancy or within 6 weeks of giving birth from pregnancy-related causes. This means that the chances of a woman dying in and around childbirth in the UK are smaller than ever—just 1 in every 10,000 women giving birth.

References Saving lives improving mothers care report 2014 MBRRACE-UK.

ANC50

Answer: C

Explanation Pregnant women should be offered an early ultrasound scan between 10 weeks 0 days and 13 weeks 6 days to determine gestational age and to detect multiple pregnancies. This will ensure consistency of gestational age assessment and reduce the incidence of induction of labour for prolonged pregnancy.

Crown-rump length measurement should be used to determine gestational age. If the crown-rump length is above 84 mm, the gestational age should be estimated using head circumference.

References Nice guideline of antenatal care.

ANC51

Answer: D

Explanation The UK Advisory Group on Chickenpox recommends that oral acyclovir be prescribed for pregnant women with chickenpox if they present within 24 h of the onset of the rash and if they are at more than 20 weeks of gestation.

References Green Top guideline no. 13, Chicken pox in pregnancy 2015.

ANC52

Answer: D

Explanation All women with haemoglobin level less than 105 g/L should be treated with oral iron as the first option for treatment; it is important to assess that any iron deficiency is also detected and treated with oral iron. The mean cell volume (MCV) is a good parameter to assess for iron deficiency. A haemodilution effect is common in pregnancy and assessing the MCV helps in deciding which cases need iron therapy. Haemoglobinopathies have to be ruled out prior to this. If oral iron is not tolerated or absorbed or patient compliance is in doubt, then parenteral iron is indicated.

Parenteral therapy offers a shorter duration of therapy and a quicker response than oral therapy, but it is invasive and expensive to administer. Anaemia not due to haematinic deficiency as in haemoglobinopathies and bone marrow failure should be managed by blood transfusion where appropriate in conjunction with a haematologist.

References RCOG Green Top guideline no. 47 – Blood transfusion in obstetrics.

ANC53

Answer: A

Explanation All women with APH heavier than spotting and women with ongoing bleeding should remain in hospital at least until the bleeding has stopped. At present, there is no evidence to support recommendations regarding duration of inpatient management following APH. Where the bleeding has been spotting and has settled and tests of fetal and maternal well-being are reassuring, the woman can go home.

References https://www.rcog.org.uk/globalassets/documents/guidelines/gtg63_05122011aph.pdf

ANC54

Answer: E

Explanation Ultrasound scan assessment should be undertaken as part of the preliminary investigations of a woman presenting with RFM after 28 + 0 weeks of gestation if the perception of RFM persists despite a normal CTG or if there are any additional risk factors for FGR/stillbirth.

References https://www.rcog.org.uk/globalassets/documents/guidelines/gtg_57.pdf

ANC55

Answer: A

Explanation Women who present on two or more occasions with RFM are at increased risk of a poor perinatal outcome (stillbirth, FGR or preterm birth) compared with those who attend on only one occasion (OR 1.92; 95 % CI 1.21–3.02). There are no studies to determine whether intervention (e.g. delivery or further investigation) alters perinatal morbidity or mortality in women presenting with recurrent RFM. Therefore, the decision whether or not to induce labour at term in a woman who presents recurrently with RFM when the growth, liquor volume and CTG appear normal must be made after careful consultant-led counselling of the pros and cons of induction on an individualised basis.

References https://www.rcog.org.uk/globalassets/documents/guidelines/gtg_57.pdf

ANC56

Answer: D

Explanation For any potentially sensitising event, D-negative, previously non-sensitised women should receive a minimum dose of 500 IU anti-D Ig within 72 h of the event (RCOG, 2011).

References http://onlinelibrary.wiley.com/enhanced/doi/10.1111/tme.12091/

ANC57

Answer: B

Explanation Women should be informed that expectant management is a reasonable alternative since there is a lack of direct evidence to support serial sonographic surveillance over expectant management. Furthermore, the majority of women with a history of second-trimester loss/preterm delivery will deliver after 33 weeks of gestation.

References https://www.rcog.org.uk/globalassets/documents/guidelines/gtg_60.pdf

ANC58

Answer: D

Explanation GBS bacteriuria is associated with a higher risk of chorioamnionitis and neonatal disease. It is not possible to accurately quantify these increased risks. These women should be offered IAP. Women with GBS urinary tract infection (growth of greater than 105 cfu/ml) during pregnancy should receive appropriate treatment at the time of diagnosis as well as IAP.

References https://www.rcog.org.uk/globalassets/documents/guidelines/gtg_36.pdf

ANC59

Answer: B

Explanation Poor outcome cannot currently be predicted by biochemical results and delivery decisions should not be based on results alone. No specific method of antenatal fetal monitoring for the prediction of fetal death can be recommended. Ultrasound and cardiotocography are not reliable methods for preventing fetal death in obstetric cholestasis.

References https://www.rcog.org.uk/globalassets/documents/guidelines/gtg_43.pdf

ANC60

Answer: C

Explanation Advise women with gestational diabetes to give birth no later than 40+6 weeks, and offer elective birth (by induction of labour or by caesarean section if indicated) to women who have not given birth by this time. Consider elective birth before 40+6 weeks for women with gestational diabetes if there are maternal or fetal complications.

References https://www.nice.org.uk/guidance/ng3

ANC61

Answer: E

Explanation Diagnose gestational diabetes if the woman has either a fasting plasma glucose level of 5.6 mmol/l or above or a 2-h plasma glucose level of 7.8 mmol/l or above.

References https://www.nice.org.uk/guidance/ng3

ANC62

Answer: B

Explanation Any woman with four or more current risk factors shown in Appendix I (other than previous VTE or thrombophilia) should be considered for prophylactic low-molecular-weight heparin (LMWH) throughout the antenatal period and will usually require prophylactic LMWH for 6 weeks postnatally but a postnatal risk reassessment should be made.

References https://www.rcog.org.uk/globalassets/documents/guidelines/gtg-37a. pdf

ANC63

Answer: C

Explanation Pregnant women with one *major* risk factor for SGA should be offered serial growth scans with umbilical artery Doppler from 26 weeks of gestation. Uterine artery Dopplers are offered to women with *three or more minor* risk factors and the gestation age recommended is 20–24 weeks.

Abdominal palpation has limited accuracy for the prediction of an SGA neonate and thus should not be routinely performed in this context.

Low PAPP-A levels (<0.4 MoMs) is a major risk factor for developing SGA.

Antiplatelet agents may be effective in preventing SGA in women at high risk of pre-eclampsia although the effect size is small. In women at high risk of pre-eclampsia, *antiplatelet agents should be commenced at, or before, 16 weeks* of pregnancy.

References SGA fetus – RCOG Green Top guideline no: 31. Feb 2013. Minor revisions Jan 2014. http://www.rcog.org.uk/files/rcog-corp/GTG31SGA23012013.pdf

ANC64

Answer: A

Explanation:

Major risk factors for developing SGA are maternal age >40, smoker >11 cigarettes per day, cocaine abuse, daily vigorous exercise, previous SGA baby, previous stillbirth, maternal SGA, chronic hypertension, diabetes and vascular disease, renal impairment, antiphospholipid syndrome, heavy bleeding similar to menses, echogenic bowel, pre-eclampsia, severe PIH, unexplained APH, low maternal weight and low PAPP-A levels (<0.4 MoMs).

Minor risk factors for developing SGA are maternal age more than or equal to 35 years, nulliparity, BMI less than 20, BMI 25–29.9, smoker-1–10 cigarettes per day, low pre-pregnancy fruit intake, pregnancy interval<6 months, pregnancy interval>30 months and paternal SGA.

References SGA fetus – RCOG Green Top guideline no: 31. Feb 2013. Minor revisions Jan 2014. http://www.rcog.org.uk/files/rcog-corp/GTG31SGA23012013.pdf

ANC65

Answer: C

Explanation All women should be offered a bone density scan to document pre-existing osteoporosis. Serum vitamin D concentrations should be optimised with supplements if necessary. Osteoporosis is a common finding in adults with thalassaemia. The pathology is complex but thought to be due to a variety of factors including underlying thalassaemic bone disease, chelation of calcium by chelation drugs, hypogonadism and vitamin D deficiency.

Most women with thalassaemia syndromes are vitamin D deficient and often osteoporotic as well. All women should have vitamin D levels optimised before pregnancy and thereafter maintained in the normal range.

All women should be assessed by a cardiologist with expertise in thalassaemia and/or iron overload prior to embarking on a pregnancy. An echocardiogram and an electrocardiogram (ECG) should be performed as well as T2* cardiac MRI. It is important to determine how well the cardiac status of the woman will support a pregnancy as well as the severity of any iron-related cardiomyopathy. Cardiac arrhythmias are more likely in older patients who have previously had severe myocardial iron overload and are now clear of cardiac iron.

Pancreas may be affected such that diabetes is common in women with thalassaemia. Women with established diabetes mellitus should ideally have serum fructosamine concentrations<300 nmol/l for at least 3 months prior to conception. This is equivalent to an HbA1c of 43 mmol/mol.

Thyroid function should be determined. The woman should be euthyroid pre-pregnancy. Hypothyroidism is frequently found in patients with thalassaemia.

Untreated hypothyroidism can result in maternal morbidity, as well as perinatal morbidity and mortality. Patients should be assessed for thyroid function as part of the preconceptual planning and, if known to be hypothyroid, treatment initiated to ensure that they are clinically euthyroid.

References Beta thalassemia in pregnancy – RCOG Green Top guideline no: 66. Mar 2014. http://www.rcog.org.uk/files/rcog-corp/GTG_66_Thalassaemia.pdf

Maternal Medical Disorders: Answers and Explanations

16

MMD1

MMD1 Answer: B

Explanation Clinical signs suggestive of sepsis include one or more of the following: pyrexia, hypothermia, tachycardia, tachypnoea, hypoxia, hypotension, oliguria, impaired consciousness and failure to respond to treatment. These signs, including pyrexia, may not always be present and are not necessarily related to the severity of sepsis.

References RCOG Green Top guideline No: 64a. Bacteria sepsis in pregnancy-Apr 2012. http://www.rcog.org.uk/files/rcog-corp/25.4.12GTG64a.pdf

MMD2

MMD2 Answer: C

Explanation Women who are transfused regularly or intermittently are at risk of transfusion-transmitted infections. It is therefore important to ascertain infectivity and manage the common transfusion-related viral infections appropriately.

The majority of women with thalassaemia major will have been immunised against hepatitis B, but some women with thalassaemia intermedia may not.

Hepatitis C is a common and often asymptomatic virus, so all women who are transfused require hepatitis C antibody testing. If a woman has a positive hepatitis C test, RNA titres should be determined with referral to a hepatologist.

Women who have undergone splenectomy are at risk of infection from encapsulated bacteria such as *Neisseria meningitidis*, *Streptococcus pneumoniae* and

© Springer India 2016
C. Ratha, J. Gupta, *SBAs and EMQs for MRCOG II*,
DOI 10.1007/978-81-322-2689-5_16

Haemophilus influenzae type b. UK guidance is that daily penicillin prophylaxis is given to all high-risk splenectomised patients.

Women who are allergic to penicillin should be recommended erythromycin. In addition, women should be given *Haemophilus influenzae* type b and the conjugated meningococcal C vaccine as a single dose if they have not received it as part of primary vaccination. The pneumococcal vaccine (such as Pneumovax RII, Sanofi Pasteur MSD Limited, Maidenhead, UK) should be given every 5 years.

References   Beta thalassemia in pregnancy – RCOG Green Top guideline No: 66. Mar 2014. http://www.rcog.org.uk/files/rcog-corp/GTG_66_Thalassaemia.pdf

---

MMD3

MMD3 Answer: E

Explanation   Acute fatty liver of pregnancy (AFLP) in most cases needs to be differentiated from HELLP syndrome. Both conditions are common in primiparous women. HELLP is characterised by hypertension, proteinuria and epigastric pain with or without vomiting.

Vomiting is seen more commonly in AFLP. Coagulopathy is seen more commonly in AFLP and may cause severe and life-threatening postpartum haemorrhage. The other changes that may help differentiate these two conditions are haematological—thrombocytopenia occurs in HELLP, whereas raised WBC counts are more common in AFLP. AFLP carries a high maternal and fetal mortality of between 2–18 % and 7–58 % respectively. Other complications include renal failure, pancreatitis and (transient) diabetes insipidus. There is also a risk of progression to hepatic encephalopathy and fulminant liver failure.

References   Cuckson C, Germain S. Hyperemesis, gastrointestinal and liver disorders in pregnancy. Obstet Gynaecol Reprod Med. 2013;21:3.

MMD4

MMD4 Answer: D

Explanation   Wernicke's encephalopathy is a complication of hyperemesis gravidarum which occurs due to lack of thiamine (vitamin B1). It can occur following any condition leading to imbalanced nutrition lasting for 2–3 weeks. It carries a mortality of 10–15 % and if uncorrected may lead to Korsakoff's encephalopathy where the patient develops antegrade and retrograde amnesia and confabulation. The management of hyperemesis includes thiamine replacement 50 mg po tds or

100 mg IV daily for 3 days. Another option especially in moderate to severe vomiting is to administer Pabrinex which is multivitamin intravenous supplement containing 250 mg of thiamine along with riboflavin, pyridoxine, nicotinamide and vitamin C.

References Cuckson C, Germain S. Hyperemesis, gastrointestinal and liver disorders in pregnancy. Obstet Gynaecol Reprod Med. 2013;21:3.

MMD5

MMD4 Answer: D

Explanation Obstetric cholestasis is a pregnancy-specific condition characterised by maternal pruritus and altered liver function tests. The common abnormality seen is elevated serum bile acids, but derangement in other markers of liver function such as transaminases, bilirubin and GGT (gamma-glutamyl transferase) also occurs. Other maternal symptoms include steatorrhoea, pale stools and dark urine. The risk of stillbirth is difficult to predict despite CTG monitoring and ultrasound for fetal well-being. Studies show that the risk to fetus may be related to the level of bile acids in the scrum with a 1–2 % increase in risk of death for every 1 mmol/L increase in bile acids.

References Cuckson C, Germain S. Hyperemesis, gastrointestinal and liver disorders in pregnancy. Obstet Gynaecol Reprod Med. 2013;21:3.

MMD6

MMD6 Answer: B

Explanation The FDA has established five categories to indicate the potential of a drug to cause birth defects if used during pregnancy. The categories are determined by the reliability of documentation and the risk to benefit ratio. They do not take into account any risks from pharmaceutical agents or their metabolites in breast milk. The categories are:

Category A   Adequate and well-controlled studies have failed to demonstrate a risk to the fetus in the first trimester of pregnancy (and there is no evidence of risk in later trimesters).

Category B   Animal reproduction studies have failed to demonstrate a risk to the fetus, and there are no adequate and well-controlled studies in pregnant women.

Category C Animal reproduction studies have shown an adverse effect on the fetus, and there are no adequate and well-controlled studies in humans, but potential benefits may warrant use of the drug in pregnant women despite potential risks.

Category D There is positive evidence of human fetal risk based on adverse reaction data from investigational or marketing experience or studies in humans, but potential benefits may warrant use of the drug in pregnant women despite potential risks.

Category X Studies in animals or humans have demonstrated fetal abnormalities, and/or there is positive evidence of human fetal risk based on adverse reaction data from investigational or marketing experience, and the risks involved in use of the drug in pregnant women clearly outweigh potential benefits.

Category N FDA has not classified the drug.

Cyclophosphamide is a category D drug which is fetotoxic and teratogenic and needs to be stopped 3 months prior to conception.

References McCarthy F, Germain S. Connective tissue disorders and dermatological disorders in pregnancy. 2013;23(3):71–80.

MMD7

MMD7 Answer: E

Explanation The half-life of thyroxine-binding globulin [TBG; the main binding protein for thyroxine (T4) and triiodothyronine (T3)] is prolonged by oestrogen-driven sialylation, which results in an increased circulating concentration of both TBG and of total T4 and T3. It is for this reason that these hormones are not measured in pregnancy. Instead, freeT4 and freeT3, the biologically active hormones, are measured: these are not greatly changed in normal pregnancy, although the lower limit of normal is reduced slightly in the third trimester. Normal values for thyroid-stimulating hormone (TSH) rise slightly in the third trimester, but otherwise are unchanged compared with non-pregnant ranges.

TSH and T3 do not cross the placenta. In the first trimester, T4 does cross the placenta and is believed to play a role in fetal brain development prior to the onset of fetal thyroid activity, which occurs late in the first trimester.

References Girling J, Cotzias C. Thyroid and other endocrine disorders in pregnancy. Obstet Gynaecol Reprod Med. 17(12):349–55.

MMD8

MMD8 Answer: D

Explanation Pregnancy does not affect the long-term course of hyperthyroidism. In the first trimester, there may be deterioration in control, due to reduced absorption of medication secondary to vomiting or to hCG-driven stimulation of TSH receptors. In the second and third trimesters, typically, treatment doses can be reduced as the immune effects of pregnancy result in an increase in TSH receptor inhibitory antibodies and a fall in the stimulatory ones: one third of women will be able temporarily to discontinue treatment at this time. The majority need to return to their prepregnant doses in the puerperium to prevent a disease flare. The drugs usually used propylthiouracil (PTU) and carbimazole, are safe in pregnancy and should not be stopped because of concerns about teratogenicity.

Older studies have linked carbimazole with aplasia cutis—a very rare condition resulting in deficits in the scalp and hair growth, but larger more recent studies show that either this link is spurious or at worst that the risk of the fetus developing this condition is extremely small. Both agents cross the placenta in similar amounts and, rarely, can cause fetal hypothyroidism: this risk can be minimised by ensuring that the patient takes the lowest doses of treatment to keep her clinically euthyroid and biochemically at the upper limit of the normal range. Fetal hypothyroidism rarely manifests clinically, in part because of the opposing stimulatory effect of transplacental TSH receptor antibodies.

References Girling J, Cotzias C. Thyroid and other endocrine disorders in pregnancy. Obstet Gynaecol Reprod Med. 17(12):349–55.

MMD9

MMD9 Answer: C

Explanation Presentation of hypopituitarism is with lethargy, hypothyroidism, failure to lactate, amenorrhoea and adrenocortical insufficiency. Women need hormone replacement therapy (hydrocortisone, thyroxine and oestrogen) to maintain normal metabolism and response to stress. Women will need ovulation induction to conceive in the future, and glucocorticoid and thyroxine replacement must continue throughout pregnancy, with extra hydrocortisone to cover the stress of labour or intercurrent illnesses. Mineralocorticoid replacement is often not needed as aldosterone production is not solely ACTH dependent. Untreated, those women who manage to conceive have a very poor pregnancy prognosis, with high rates of miscarriage, stillbirths and maternal death, all of which can be normalised with adequate therapy.

References Girling J, Cotzias C. Thyroid and other endocrine disorders in pregnancy. Obstet Gynaecol Reprod Med. 17(12):349–55.

MMD10

MMD10 Answer: B

Explanation Hypothyroidism is a common cause of hyperprolactinemia. The hyperprolactinemia of hypothyroidism is related to several mechanisms. In response to the hypothyroid state, a compensatory increase in the discharge of central hypothalamic thyrotropin-releasing hormone results in increased stimulation of prolactin secretion.

Furthermore, prolactin elimination from the systemic circulation is reduced, which contributes to increased prolactin concentrations. Primary hypothyroidism can be associated with diffuse pituitary enlargement, which will reverse with appropriate thyroid hormone replacement therapy

The causes of hyperprolactinemia are represented in this image

References 1. Serri O, et al. CMAJ. 2003;169:575–81.
2. Girling J, Cotzias C. Thyroid and other endocrine disorders in pregnancy. Obstet Gynaecol Reprod Med. 17(12):349–55.

MMD11

MMD11 Answer: A

Explanation Carbohydrate metabolism, especially in the third trimester, is directed towards providing the growing fetus with glucose and amino acids and liberating more free fatty acids, ketone bodies and glycerol as substrates for maternal energy. In normal pregnancy, hyperplasia of the islet cells of the pancreas results in increased levels of circulating insulin with an early increase in insulin sensitivity followed by resistance as pregnancy progresses. Thus, fasting glucose levels are 10–20 % lower due to increased glucose uptake from the maternal circulation by the growing fetus, reduced hepatic gluconeogenesis, increased peripheral glucose uptake and increased glycogenesis. Maternal insulin resistance results from placental production of diabetogenic hormones: growth hormone, placental lactogen, corticotrophin-releasing hormone and progesterone. In women with established diabetes, insulin requirements increase substantially as pregnancy progresses and until the third stage of labour when resistance falls rapidly following expulsion of the placenta.

References Chaudry R, Gilby P, Carroll PV. Pre-existing (type 1 and type 2) diabetes in pregnancy. Obstet Gynaecol Reprod Med. 17(12):339–44.

MMD12

MMD12 Answer: B

Explanation Women with diabetes should be delivered in consultant-led maternity units with access to senior medical, obstetric and neonatal staff. The progress of labour should be monitored closely as for any other high-risk woman with continuous electrical fetal monitoring and regular glycaemic checks. Good glycaemic control should be maintained during labour and delivery to reduce the risk of neonatal hypoglycaemia. The target range for blood glucose concentration during labour and delivery recommended by Diabetes UK is 4–6 mmol/L. Intravenous insulin is commenced in women taking subcutaneous insulin when labour is anticipated and NPH insulin is discontinued. Normoglycaemia can be achieved using concomitant saline; however, at the start of active labour, insulin requirements fall rapidly, and therefore glucose must be given with insulin to prevent maternal hypoglycaemia (infusion rate of around 2.55 mg dextrose/kg/min). Capillary blood glucose must be checked at least hourly and the rate of insulin-adjusted accordingly.

References Chaudry R, Gilby P, Carroll PV. Pre-existing (type 1 and type 2) diabetes in pregnancy. Obstet Gynaecol Reprod Med. 17(12):339–44.
    NICE guideline. Diabetes in pregnancy. CG 63.

MMD13

MMD13 Answer: A

Explanation Metformin is used in some cases in early pregnancy possibly due to increased use in women with polycystic ovarian syndrome. The FDA has classified the drug as a pregnancy category B medication, meaning that it does not appear to cause harm to the fetus in animal studies. No adverse outcomes have been reported in pregnancy. It may be safe and effective, but currently no oral agents are licensed for use in pregnancy. Ideally, women with Type 2 DM on oral agents should be switched to insulin prior to pregnancy so that glycaemic control is not jeopardised. The most serious potential side effect of metformin use is lactic acidosis; this complication is very rare, and the vast majority of these cases seem to be related to comorbid conditions, such as impaired liver or kidney function, rather than to the metformin itself.

References Chaudry R, Gilby P, Carroll PV. Pre-existing (type 1 and type 2) diabetes in pregnancy. Obstet Gynaecol Reprod Med. 17(12):339–44.

   NICE guideline. Diabetes in pregnancy. CG 63.

MMD14

MMD14 Answer: B

Explanation HAPO (Hyperglycaemia And Pregnancy Outcomes) study in which more than 23, 000 women had a 75 g glucose tolerance test (GTT), and in those with a fasting plasma glucose below 5.8 or a 2-h value below 11.1 mmol/L, were blinded to the clinicians and women.

   The four primary outcomes for which the study was powered included macrosomia (birth weight >90th centile for gestational age, gender, parity, ethnicity and field centre), primary caesarean delivery, clinical neonatal hypoglycaemia and hyperinsulinemia (cord serum C-peptide > 90th centile for the study group as a whole). A number of secondary outcomes were also considered. These included preterm birth; shoulder dystocia and/or birth injury; sum of skinfold thicknesses >90th centile for gestational age, gender, ethnicity, parity and field centre; percent body fat >90th centile for gestational age; admission for neonatal intensive care; hyperbilirubinemia; and pre-eclampsia. Results indicate strong, continuous associations of maternal glucose levels below those diagnostic of diabetes with increased birth weight and increased cord-blood serum C-peptide levels and the other primary outcomes. There was an association with the secondary outcomes as well but not as strong.

References Hyperglycemia and adverse pregnancy outcomes. The HAPO study cooperative research group. N Engl J Med. 2008;358:1991–2002.

MMD15

MMD15 Answer: A

Explanation One of the major determinants of the risk for development of subsequent type 2 diabetes is ethnic origin. Thus, GDM may affect as many as 15 % of south Asian women in different populations, while for Caucasian women overall risk of type 2 diabetes is lower. In addition to ethnic origin, of the many potential risk factors, maternal age and body mass index appear to be among the strongest predictors of GDM. The other risk factors include previous history of GDM, previous history of still birth/congenital abnormality or a family history of diabetes. However, even a combination of risk factors does not reliably predict the likelihood of developing GDM, missing up to 50 % of cases in population-based studies.

References Fraser R, Heller S. Gestational diabetes: aetiology and management. Obstet Gynaecol Reprod Med. 17(12):345–48.

MMD16

MMD16 Answer: B

Explanation Maternal obesity is associated with a significant risk of thromboembolism during both the antenatal and postnatal period. Case-control studies assessing the risk show a significant association between venous thromboembolism and BMI ≥30 with odds ratio of 2.7–5.

The RCOG Clinical Green Top Guideline No. 37 advises that:

- A woman with a BMI ≥30 who also has two or more additional risk factors for thromboembolism should be considered for prophylactic low molecular weight heparin (LMWH) antenatally. This should begin as early in pregnancy as practically possible.
- All women receiving LMWH antenatally should usually continue prophylactic doses of LMWH until 6 weeks postpartum, but a postnatal risk assessment should be made.
- Women with a booking BMI ≥30 requiring pharmacological thromboprophylaxis should be prescribed doses appropriate for maternal weight.

References RCOG guideline No. 37a. Reducing risk of thrombosis and embolism in pregnancy and peurperium. RCOG /CMACE joint guideline– management of women with obesity in pregnancy – March 2010.

MMD17

MMD17 Answer: B

Explanation Serum ferritin is a stable glycoprotein which accurately reflects iron stores in the absence of inflammatory change. It is the first laboratory test to become abnormal as iron stores decrease, and it is not affected by recent iron ingestion. It is generally considered the best test to assess iron deficiency in pregnancy, although it is an acute phase reactant and levels will rise when there is active infection or inflammation. During pregnancy, in women with adequate iron stores at conception, the serum ferritin concentration initially rises, followed by a progressive fall by 32 weeks to about 50 % pre-pregnancy levels. This is due to haemodilution and mobilisation of iron. The levels increase again mildly in the third trimester. Even though the ferritin level may be influenced by the plasma dilution later in pregnancy, a concentration below 15 µg/l indicates iron depletion in all stages of pregnancy. In women of reproductive age, a level <15 μg/l has shown specificity of 98 % and sensitivity of 75 % for iron deficiency, as defined by no stainable bone marrow iron.

There are a variety of levels for treatment, quoted in different studies, but in general, treatment should be considered when serum ferritin levels fall below 30 μg/l, as this indicates early iron depletion which will worsen unless treated. Van den Broek et al. found that serum ferritin is the best single indicator of storage iron provided a cut-off point of 30 μg/l is used, with sensitivity of 90 % and specificity 85 %. Concurrent measurement of the C-reactive protein (CRP) may be helpful in interpreting higher levels, where indicated. The CRP concentration seems to be independent of pregnancy and gestational age, although some studies describe a mild increase.

References 1. UK guidelines on the management of iron deficiency in pregnancy British committee for standards in haematology 2011. http://www.bcshguidelines. com/documents/UK_Guidelines_iron_deficiency_in_pregnancy.pdf

2. Van den Broek NR, Letsky EA, White SA, Shenkin A. Iron status in pregnant women: Which measurements are valid? British J Haemat. 1998;103:817–24.

MMD18

MMD18 Answer: B

Explanation The overall incidence of UTI in pregnancy is 8 %. The increased susceptibility to UTI is thought to be due to various physiological changes, which include changes in bladder volume, decreased bladder tone and ureteric dilatation, all of which lead to the development of urinary stasis. Urinary tract infection during pregnancy can cause significant potential morbidity for both mother and baby, including:

– Chorioamnionitis
– Endometritis
– Fetal growth restriction
– Stillbirth
– Preterm labour and delivery
– Increased perinatal mortality
– Mental retardation
– Developmental delay

Early recognition and treatment can reduce maternal and fetal morbidity. The risk of recurrent UTI in pregnancy is around 4–5 %. Long-term, low-dose antimicrobial cover and single-dose antimicrobial cover in intercourse-related UTI may be considered as prophylactic measures.

References Asali F, Mahfouz I, Phillips C. The management of urogynaecological problems in pregnancy and the early postpartum period. Obstet Gynaecol. 2012;14:153–8.

MMD19

MMD19 Answer: D

Explanation The rate of mother-to-child transmission (MTCT) is almost 25 % without any interventions but with uptake of interventions, especially HAART (highly active retroviral therapy), the MTCT is reduced to <1 %. For women taking HAART, a decision regarding recommended mode of delivery should be made after review of plasma viral load results at 36 weeks.

Vaginal delivery is recommended for women on HAART with an HIV viral load <50 HIV RNA copies/mL plasma. For women with a plasma VL of >50 HIV RNA copies/mL at 36 weeks, prelabour CS (PLCS) should be considered. In women in whom a vaginal delivery has been recommended and labour has commenced, obstetric management should follow the same guidelines as for the uninfected population.

References http://www.bhiva.org/documents/Guidelines/Pregnancy/2012/hiv1030_6.pd

MMD20

MMD20 Answer: C

Explanation Women considered at high risk of pre-eclampsia include those with any of the following:

- Hypertensive disease during a previous pregnancy
- Chronic kidney disease
- Autoimmune disease such as systemic lupus erythematosus or antiphospholipid syndrome
- Type 1 or type 2 diabetes
- Chronic hypertension

Risk factor	Unadjusted relative risk (95 % confidence interval):
Age>40 years, primiparae	1.68
Age>40 years, multiparae	1.96
Family history	2.90

Risk factor	Unadjusted relative risk (95 % confidence interval):
Nulliparity	2.91
Multiple pregnancy	2.93
Pre-existing diabetes	3.56
Pre-pregnancy body mass index >35	4.29
Previous pre-eclampsia	7.19
Antiphospholipid syndrome	9.72

References McCarthy FP, Kenny LC. Hypertension in pregnancy. Obstet Gynaecol Reprod Med. 22(6):141–6.

MMD21

MMD21 Answer: B

Explanation Women considered at high risk of pre-eclampsia include those with any of the following:

– Hypertensive disease during a previous pregnancy
– Chronic kidney disease
– Autoimmune disease such as systemic lupus erythematosus or antiphospholipid syndrome
– Type 1 or type 2 diabetes
– Chronic hypertension

Risk factor	Unadjusted relative risk (95 % confidence interval):
Age>40 years, primiparae	1.68
Age>40 years, multiparae	1.96
Family history	2.90
Nulliparity	2.91
Multiple pregnancy	2.93
Pre-existing diabetes	3.56
Pre-pregnancy body mass index >35	4.29
Previous pre-eclampsia	7.19
Antiphospholipid syndrome	9.72

References McCarthy FP, Kenny LC. Hypertension in pregnancy. Obstet Gynaecol Reprod Med. 22(6):141–6.

MMD22

MMD22 Answer: B

Explanation In pre-eclampsia/eclampsia, magnesium sulphate is indicated as the first-line anticonvulsant. Formal clinical review should occur every 4 h, observing for side effects (motor paralysis, absent reflexes, respiratory depression and cardiac arrhythmia).

Key points in the management of the severe pre-eclamptic patient:

- Insert an indwelling catheter and measure urine output until stable (measured four hourly).
- When present, central venous pressure (CVP) and arterial lines should be measured continuously and charted with the blood pressure.
- Neurological assessment should be performed hourly using either the AVPU or GCS scales.
- Fetal well-being should be monitored using a cardiotocography.
- Blood tests should be repeated at least every 12 h while on the magnesium sulphate protocol. In the event of complications such as haemorrhage or abnormal or deteriorating haematological and/or biochemical parameters, more frequent blood tests should be taken, e.g. every 4–8 h.
- Record blood pressure and pulse every 15 min until stable and then half hourly.
- Oxygen saturation should be measured continuously and charted with the blood pressure. If saturation falls below 95 %, then medical review is essential to rule out pulmonary oedema and other complications.
- Strict fluid balance should be recorded with detailed input and output measurements.
- Respiratory rate should be measured hourly. A reducing respiratory rate may indicate magnesium toxicity.

References McCarthy FP, Kenny LC. Hypertension in pregnancy. Obstet Gynaecol Reprod Med. 22(6): 141–6.

MMD23

MMD23 Answer: A

Explanation Women who are hypertensive and pregnant must be subdivided into those with:

A. New-onset hypertension and/or proteinuria in pregnancy
   - Gestational hypertension (without proteinuria)
   - Gestational proteinuria (without hypertension)
   - Pre-eclampsia (hypertension with proteinuria)

B. Chronic hypertension and renal disease
   – Chronic hypertension without proteinuria
   – Chronic renal disease (proteinuria with or without hypertension)
   – Chronic hypertension with superimposed pre-eclampsia (i.e. with new-onset proteinuria in pregnancy)

C. Unclassified
   – Hypertension and/or proteinuria noted when first presentation is after 20 weeks.
   – As above, when noted for the first time during pregnancy, labour or puerperium and there are insufficient background data to permit a diagnosis from category A or B above.

Chronic hypertension is defined as hypertension preceding pregnancy. Blood pressure falls in the first and second trimesters. Therefore, women with high blood pressure before the 20th week of pregnancy are assumed to have pre-existing or essential hypertension. As many women of reproductive age only present for the first time when pregnant, chronic hypertension is often revealed in the first half of pregnancy.

References McCarthy FP, Kenny LC. Hypertension in pregnancy. Obstet Gynaecol Reprod Med. 22(6):141–6.

MMD24

MMD24 Answer: A

Explanation Chicken pox, or varicella, the primary infection with varicella zoster virus (VZV; human herpesvirus 3), in pregnancy may cause maternal mortality or serious morbidity. Clinicians should be aware of the increased morbidity associated with varicella infection in adults, including pneumonia, hepatitis and encephalitis. Rarely, it may result in death.

Although varicella infection is much less common in adults than in children, it is associated with a greater morbidity, namely, pneumonia, hepatitis and encephalitis. As recently as the 1990s, chickenpox resulted in the deaths of 25 people per year in England and Wales; 80 % of these deaths occurred in adults. Between 1985 and 1999, there were nine indirect maternal deaths and one late maternal death reported in the UK from complications of maternal varicella infection, suggesting a low case fatality rate. There has been no maternal death from varicella reported in the subsequent confidential enquiries. Pneumonia may be more severe at later gestational ages due to the effects of the gravid uterus on respiratory function.

References 1.https://www.rcog.org.uk/globalassets/documents/guidelines/gtg13.pdf

2. Rawson H, et al. Deaths from chickenpox in England and Wales 1995-7: analysis of routine mortality data. BMJ. 2001;323:1091–3.

MMD25

MMD25 Answer: B

Explanation Due to increase in morbid obesity in the reproductive age, it is increasingly common to see patients who have had bariatric surgery before getting pregnant. It is advisable that pregnancy is delayed for at least 1 year following bariatric surgery. GWG should be restricted to 5–7 kg while doing GTT; we must be vigilant as dumping syndrome can be provoked. In the case series reported, there is no increased risk of preterm deliveries or congenital anomalies.

References Pregnancy outcome following bariatric surgery. TOG. 2013;15:37–43.

MMD26

MMD26 Answer: C

Explanation Asthma is a widespread condition that affects about 10 % of pregnant women. The severity of asthma during pregnancy remains unchanged, worsens or improves in equal proportions. Inhaled corticosteroids are the standard anti-inflammatory therapy for asthma. They are safe in pregnancy. Asthma does not usually affect labour or delivery with less than a fifth of women experiencing an exacerbation during labour. In the postpartum period, there is not an increased risk of asthma exacerbations, and within a few months after delivery, a woman's asthma severity typically reverts to its pre-pregnancy level.

References Goldie MH, Brightling CE. Asthma in pregnancy. Obstet Gynaecol. 2013;15:241–5.

MMD27

MMD 27 Answer: C

Explanation Offer immediate treatment with insulin, with or without metformin, as well as changes in diet and exercise, to women with gestational diabetes who have a fasting plasma glucose level of 7.0 mmol/l or above at diagnosis.

References https://www.nice.org.uk/guidance/ng3

MMD28

MMD28 Answer: B

Explanation Any woman with three current risk factors shown in Appendix I (other than previous VTE or thrombophilia) should be considered for prophylactic LMWH from 28 weeks and will usually require prophylactic LMWH for 6 weeks postnatally, but a postnatal risk reassessment should be made.

References https://www.rcog.org.uk/globalassets/documents/guidelines/gtg-37a.pdf

MMD29

MMD29 Answer: D

Explanation Consider glibenclamide for women with gestational diabetes in whom blood glucose targets are not achieved with metformin but who decline insulin therapy or who cannot tolerate metformin.

References http://onlinelibrary.wiley.com/enhanced/doi/10.1111/dme.12376/

MMD30

MMD30 Answer: B

Explanation Advise women with a fasting plasma glucose level between 6.0 and 6.9 mmol/l that they are at high risk of developing type 2 diabetes. Advise women with an HbA1c level between 39 and 47 mmol/mol (5.7 % and 6.4 %) that they are at high risk of developing type 2 diabetes.

References https://www.nice.org.uk/guidance/ng3

MMD31

MMD31 Answer: C

Explanation It is recognised that mothers with epilepsy are at higher risk of breakthrough seizures at this time (Walker, Permezel et al. 2009). Reasons for this are varied, including sleep deprivation, stress and altered treatment compliance, and it seems likely that in some women biological changes (e.g. hormonal or neurochemical factors) may also be relevant.

Women with epilepsy and their families should be specifically advised of the risks of epilepsy in the postpartum period and ways to mitigate these risks, including not sleeping or bathing alone.

References 1. Walker SP, Permezel M, Berkovic SF. The management of epilepsy in pregnancy. BJOG. 2009;116(6):758–76.
2. Saving lives improving mothers care report 2014.

MMD32

MMD32 Answer: A

Explanation Pheochromocytoma is bilateral in about 10 % cases and also familial in 10 % cases. Hypertension is seen in most cases. Other presenting features are palpitations, headache, attacks of perspiration and even arrhythmias. Patient should be first started on alpha-blockers as a single agent, and later beta-adrenergic blockers may be added. Medical management is preferred during pregnancy.

References James D, Steer PJ, Weiner CP. High risk pregnancy management options, 4th edn.

MMD33

MMD33 Answer: D

Explanation Hypertensive disorders in pregnancy, which include pre-eclampsia, gestational hypertension and chronic hypertension, complicate 2–8 % of pregnancies and confer risk to the health of mother and fetus. Pre-eclampsia is one of the three leading causes of maternal death in the UK and can result in substantial maternal morbidity, including intracranial haemorrhage, HELLP (haemolysis, elevated liver enzymes and low platelet count) syndrome and disseminated intravascular coagulation.

References Nathan HL, Duhig K, Hezelgrave NL, Chappell LC, Shennan AH. Blood pressure measurement in pregnancy. Obstet Gynaecol. 2015;17:91–8.

MMD34

MMD34 Answer: D

Explanation LMWH should be given in doses titrated against the woman's booking or early pregnancy weight. There is insufficient evidence to recommend whether the dose of LMWH should be given once daily or in two divided doses.

References https://www.rcog.org.uk/globalassets/documents/guidelines/gtg-37b. pdf

MMD35

MMD35 Answer: C

Explanation Electrocardiograms (ECGs) are classically the first-line test in making a diagnosis of AMI in any patient presenting with chest pain. The most sensitive and specific ECG marker is ST elevation, which normally appears within a few minutes of onset of symptoms. Cardiac-specific troponin I and troponin T are the biomarkers of choice for diagnosing myocardial infarction. Different hospitals will use either troponin I or troponin T, and recommended sampling times vary depending on the assay, so clinicians should check their local hospital guidelines. A negative troponin at presentation does not exclude cardiac damage as it can take 12 h for the level to peak. Troponin is never increased above the upper limit of normal in healthy pregnant women and is not affected by anaesthesia, a prolonged labour or caesarean section, and therefore is the investigation of choice. In contrast, other cardiac markers—myoglobin, creatinine kinase, creatinine kinase isoenzyme MB— can be increased significantly in labour. The troponin levels can be raised in pre-eclampsia, gestational hypertension and pulmonary embolism in the absence of significant coronary disease. It is important to note that in pre-eclampsia the troponin level is never above standard threshold set for MI.

References 1. Wuntakal R, Shetty N, Ioannou E, Sharma S, Kurian J. Myocardial infarction and pregnancy. Obstet Gynaecol. 2013;15:247–55.
2. Nelson-Piercy C. Heart disease. In: Handbook of obstetric medicine. 3rd edn. London: Informa Healthcare; 2006. p. 23–45.

MMD36

MMD36 Answer: D

Explanation Ideally the patient with prolactinoma should be thoroughly evaluated pre-pregnancy. This includes serum prolactin levels and radiology, MRI preferred. Pre-pregnancy, those with microadenoma, should be started on dopamine agonist, and macroadenoma should preferably be treated with surgery.

During pregnancy, patient should be under the care of a multidisciplinary team including obstetrician, endocrinologist and ophthalmologist.

For asymptomatic microadenoma, there is less than 5 % chance of sudden symptomatic enlargement. Medication can be safely stopped for these patients. They should be educated for self-referral in case of any warning signs like headache or visual disturbance. If any symptoms suggestive of enlargement are seen, it warrants urgent MRI. Headache is caused due to pressure over the dura and visual disturbance due to compression of optic nerve both as a consequence of tumour enlargement.

For asymptomatic macroadenomas, risk of symptomatic exacerbation is 30–35 %. Regarding continuation of medical treatment with bromocriptine, the decision must be individualised. These patients must be evaluated every 3 months with visual testing. Those with symptomatic macroadenoma should be evaluated monthly. Cabergoline is used in refractory cases.

Bromocriptine/cabergoline has not been found to be teratogenic; however, long-term use of both has been associated with a small increased risk of mother developing heart valve fibrosis. Echocardiogram should be considered in women who have significant murmur.

References James D, Steer PJ, Weiner CP. High risk pregnancy management options, 4th edn.

MMD37

MMD37 Answer: C

Explanation Acute hepatitis C is a rare event in pregnancy. The most common scenario is chronic hepatitis C virus (HCV) infection in pregnancy.

Observations regarding serum HCV-RNA concentration have been variable. In some women, HCV-RNA levels rise towards the end of pregnancy. In general, pregnancy does not have a negative effect on HCV infection. Conversely, chronic hepatitis does not appear to have an adverse effect on the course of pregnancy or the birth weight of the newborn infant. The role of spontaneous abortion is approximately the same as in the general population. The overall rate of mother-to-child transmission for HCV is 3–5 % if the mother is known to be anti-HCV positive. Co-infection with human immunodeficiency virus (HIV) increases the rate of mother-to-child transmission up to 19.4 %. Numerous risk factors for vertical transmission have been studied. In general, high viral load defined as at least 2.5×106 viral RNA copies/mL, HIV co-infection and invasive procedures are the most important factors.

(Please note: HCV is a RNA virus, not DNA.)

Both interferon and ribavirin are contraindicated during pregnancy. Viral clearance prior to pregnancy increases the likelihood that a woman remains non-viremic in pregnancy with a consequent reduced risk of vertical transmission.

References Floreani A. Hepatitis C and pregnancy. World J Gastroenterol. 2013 Oct 28;19(40):6714–20. doi:10.3748/wjg.v19.i40.6714.

MMD38

MMD38 Answer: C

Explanation In pregnancy, there is a progressive rise in D-dimer levels with advancing gestation and levels become 'abnormal' at term and in the postnatal period in most healthy pregnant women. D-dimer levels are increased further in multiple pregnancies, following caesarean section and in major postpartum haemorrhage and if there is concomitant pre-eclampsia. Thus, a 'positive' D-dimer test in pregnancy is not necessarily consistent with VTE. The role of D-dimer testing in the investigation of acute VTE in pregnancy remains controversial.

References https://www.rcog.org.uk/globalassets/documents/guidelines/gtg-37b.pdf

MMD39

MMD39 Answer: C

Explanation Pregnant women with an uncertain or no previous history of chickenpox, or who come from tropical or subtropical countries, who have been exposed to infection, should have a blood test to determine VZV immunity or non-immunity. If the pregnant woman is not immune to VZV and she has had a significant exposure, she should be offered VZIG as soon as possible. VZIG is effective when given up to 10 days after contact (in the case of continuous exposures, this is defined as 10 days from the appearance of the rash in the index case).

References https://www.rcog.org.uk/globalassets/documents/guidelines/gtg13.pdf

MMD40

MMD40 Answer: C

Explanation The postmortem process in maternal sepsis: Thorough examination and histological sampling of all organs (including bone marrow) is important. If the placenta is available, that must be examined also. Information on the status of the fetus may be informative. Blood cultures as soon as possible after death; these must be taken from the heart or neck veins, *not from below the umbilicus*, and before the body is opened; if this is not possible, a clean sample of spleen parenchyma may be cultured.

References Saving lives and improving mother's care report 2014.

MMD41

MMD41 Answer: C

Explanation Pituitary insufficiency is usually seen in cases of autoimmune lymphocytic infiltration, pituitary apoplexy (Sheehan's syndrome), tumour and surgery. Massive postpartum haemorrhage leading to hypo-perfusion of hyper plastic pituitary and ischemic necrosis is the pathology behind Sheehan's syndrome. There is no correlation though between the amount of PPH (blood lost) and the occurrence of Sheehan's syndrome.

It may present in postpartum period with failure to lactate, but in many cases, it has insidious course over months to years. There is an average delay of 7 years from the onset to diagnosis. Late-onset disease may present with loss of pubic hair, oligo-/amenorrhoea, senile vaginal atrophy, hypothyroidism, etc. These women are usually infertile but may conceive spontaneously.

During pregnancy, these patients require supplementation of thyroxine 100–200 micrograms/day and steroids, prednisolone 5 mg in the morning and 2.5 mg in the evening. Mineralocorticoid replacement is usually not required. Postpartum dosages need to be readjusted.

References James D, Steer PJ, Weiner CP. High risk pregnancy management options, 4th edn.

MMD42

MMD42 Answer: C

Explanation Severe nausea and vomiting occurs in up to 30 % of pregnant women, and it can cause significant morbidity. There are over 25 000 admissions per year for hyperemesis gravidarum in England. Safe, effective treatments for severe nausea and vomiting of pregnancy are available. Early treatment is important to prevent the development of hyperemesis gravidarum. Treatment algorithms have been developed in other countries. Severe nausea and vomiting of pregnancy often occurs after midday, so the term 'morning sickness' is inappropriate.

Although nausea and vomiting of pregnancy (NVP) is now rarely life threatening, it can have a profound effect on the quality of women's lives. Severe NVP can cause feelings of depression, difficulties between partners, less effective parenting and concern for the health of the unborn child. Some women have such severe NVP that they are less likely to have another child, or they consider terminating subsequent pregnancies. In some women, the condition is so intolerable that they actually elect to have a termination of the current pregnancy.

References Gadsby R, Barnie-Adshead T. Severe nausea and vomiting of pregnancy: should it be treated with appropriate pharmacotherapy? Obstet Gynaecol. 2011;13:107–11.

MMD43

MMD43 Answer: A

Explanation If female patients become unexpectedly pregnant during anti-HBV therapy, treatment indications should be re-evaluated. The same treatment indications apply to women who are first diagnosed to have CHB during pregnancy. Patients with advanced fibrosis or cirrhosis should definitely continue to be treated, but the treating agent should be reconsidered.

(PEG-)IFN must be stopped, and the patients should continue on a NA, while FDA category C NAs, particularly adefovir and entecavir, should be changed to a FDA category B NA. Among FDA category B NAs, tenofovir is preferred because of its high potency, high genetic barrier and available safety data in pregnancy.

The prevention of HBV perinatal transmission, which is considered to occur mainly at delivery, is traditionally based on the combination of passive and active immunisation with hepatitis B immunoglobulin (HBIg) and HBV vaccination. Such a strategy, however, may not be effective in a proportion of newborns from highly viremic (serum HBV DNA >106–7 IU/ml), mostly HBeAg-positive, mothers, who carry a >10 % risk of vertical HBV transmission despite HBIg and vaccination. Mothers with these high concentrations of HBV DNA should be informed that utilising a NA to reduce their viral loads could add to the effectiveness of HBIg and vaccination. Lamivudine and recently telbivudine therapy during the last trimester of pregnancy in pregnant HBsAg-positive women with high levels of viremia have been shown to be safe and to reduce the risk of intrauterine and perinatal transmission of HBV if given in addition to passive and active vaccination by HBIg and HBV vaccination. Thus, telbivudine, lamivudine or tenofovir (as a potent FDA category B agent) may be used for the prevention of perinatal and intrauterine HBV transmission in the last trimester of pregnancy in HBsAg-positive women with high levels of viremia (serum HBV DNA >106–7 IU/ml). No controlled clinical trial of tenofovir to prevent perinatal transmission has been conducted. If NA therapy is given only for the prevention of perinatal transmission, it may be discontinued within the first 3 months after delivery.

References EASL clinical practice guidelines: Management of chronic hepatitis B virus infection.

(EASL = European Association for the Study of the Liver) http://www.easl.eu/medias/cpg/issue8/Report.pdf.

MMD44

MMD44 Answer D

Explanation In cases of primary pituitary disease (Cushings disease) with adrenal hyperplasia, there is increase in androgen production from adrenals which inhibit pituitary gonadotrophin leading to amenorrhoea and infertility. In adrenal adenomas, there is overproduction of cortisol only, and these are less likely to impair fertility. Therefore, primary adrenal disease, i.e. adrenal adenomas, is more commonly encountered during pregnancy. Clinically, many clinical features of Cushing's syndrome mimic signs and symptoms of normal pregnancy like weakness, weight gain, oedema, striae, hypertension and impaired GTT. The distinguishing features of Cushing's syndrome would be early-onset hypertension, easy bruising and features of proximal myopathy.

Preferred screening test in a suspected case is 24 h urine free cortisol measurement. Serum cortisol levels are raised. Pregnancy-specific range for plasma and urine cortisol should be used. Further diagnostic tests which may be useful include ACTH levels, high-dose dexamethasone suppression test, USG and MRI of adrenals and MRI of pituitary.

References James D, Steer PJ, Weiner CP. High risk pregnancy management options, 4th edn.

MMD45

MMD45 Answer: E

Explanation Tell women who had pre-eclampsia that their risk of developing:

- Gestational hypertension in a future pregnancy ranges from about 1 in 8 (13 %) pregnancies to about 1 in 2 (53 %) pregnancies.
- Pre-eclampsia in a future pregnancy is up to about 1 in 6 (16 %) pregnancies.
- Pre-eclampsia in a future pregnancy is about 1 in 4 (25 %) pregnancies if their pre-eclampsia was complicated by severe pre-eclampsia, HELLP syndrome or eclampsia and led to birth before 34 weeks and about 1 in 2 (55 %) pregnancies if it led to birth before 28 weeks.

References http://www.nice.org.uk/guidance/cg107/chapter/1-guidance

MMD46

MMD46 Answer: B

Explanation If maternal infection occurs in the last 4 weeks of a woman's pregnancy, there is a significant risk of varicella infection of the newborn. A planned delivery should normally be avoided for at least 7 days after the onset of the maternal rash to allow for the passive transfer of antibodies from mother to child, provided that continuing the pregnancy does not pose any additional risks to the mother or baby.

References https://www.rcog.org.uk/globalassets/documents/guidelines/gtg13.pdf

MMD47

MMD47 Answer: C

Explanation The condition is cystic fibrosis.

- The women are amenorrhoeic if the BMI is low, but once the menstruation starts, they are usually fertile.
- FEV1 >50 % or even >70 % is an essential prerequisite for safely embarking on pregnancy.
- Prematurity is seen in 25 % of pregnancies.
- 14–20 % of women with cystic fibrosis develop either gestational diabetes or have pre-existing diabetes.
- As a background risk, if the partner does not carry the mutation, then the risk of having affected child is 1:250

References Goddard J, Bourke SJ. Cystic fibrosis and pregnancy. Obstet Gynaecol. 2009;11:19–24.

MMD48

MMD48 Answer: E

Explanation Healthcare practitioners must ensure that LFTs return to normal, pruritus resolves, all investigations carried out during the pregnancy have been reviewed and the mother has fully understood the implications of obstetric cholestasis. The latter will include reassurance about the lack of long-term sequelae for mother and baby and discussion of the high recurrence rate (45–90 %), contraceptive choices (usually avoiding estrogen containing methods) and the increased incidence of obstetric cholestasis in family members.

References https://www.rcog.org.uk/globalassets/documents/guidelines/gtg_43. pdf

MMD49

MMD49 Answer: D

Explanation Prior to pregnancy, up-to-date checks should be made of the woman's serology for hepatitis B and C, HIV and rubella, and relevant measures taken, accordingly. She should be up-to-date with pneumococcal and hepatitis B immunisations.

Assessments should be made of cardiac function (with electrocardiography and echocardiography), retinal screening (for sickling infarctions) and renal function (with blood pressure and urine protein checks). There may be general health issues which need to be addressed before pregnancy for the individual woman, such as advising smoking cessation.

She also needs to be made aware of what the arrangements will be for her pregnancy care, so that she is prepared for these practicalities.

References Eissa AA, Tuck SM. Sickle cell disease and β-thalassaemia major in pregnancy. Obstet Gynaecol. 2013;15:71–8.

MMD50

MMD50 Answer: C

Explanations

A   Haemoglobinopathies are one of the most common inherited disorders. More than 70 000 babies are born with thalassaemia worldwide each year, and there are 100 million individuals who are asymptomatic thalassaemia carriers.

B   The basic defect in the thalassaemia syndromes is reduced globin chain synthesis with the resultant red cells having inadequate haemoglobin content.

C   Thalassaemia major (homozygous β-thalassaemia) results from the inheritance of a defective β-globin gene from each parent. This results in a severe transfusion-dependent anaemia and not iron deficiency anaemia.

D   The heterozygous state, β-thalassaemia trait (thalassaemia minor) causes mild to moderate microcytic anaemia with no significant detrimental effect on overall health.

E   Thalassaemia intermedia is defined as a group of patients with β-thalassaemia whose disease severity varies. At the severe end of the clinical spectrum of thalassaemia intermedia, patients are usually diagnosed between the ages of 2 and 6 years, and, although they survive without regular blood transfusions, growth and development are impaired. At the other end of the spectrum, there are patients who are completely asymptomatic until adulthood, when they present with mild anaemia and splenomegaly often found by chance during haematological examinations or family studies

References Beta thalassemia in pregnancy – RCOG Green Top guideline No: 66. Mar 2014. http://www.rcog.org.uk/files/rcog-corp/GTG_66_Thalassaemia.pdf

MMD51

MMD51 Answer: C

Explanation LMWH should be given in doses titrated against the woman's booking or early pregnancy weight. There is insufficient evidence to recommend whether the dose of LMWH should be given once daily or in two divided doses.

References https://www.rcog.org.uk/globalassets/documents/guidelines/gtg-37b.pdf

MMD52

MMD52 Answer: D

Explanation

Table 2. Adjustments in the infusion rate of unfractionated heparin according to the APTT

APTT ratio	Dose change (units/kg/hour)	Additional action	Next APTT (hour)
< 1.2	+ 4	Re-bolus 80 units/kg	6
1.2–1.5	+ 2	Re-bolus 40 units/kg	6
1.5–2.5	no change		24
2.5–3.0	– 2		6
> 3.0	– 3	Stop infusion 1 hour	6

References https://www.rcog.org.uk/globalassets/documents/guidelines/gtg-37b.pdf

MMD53

MMD53 Answer: A

Explanation

Table 2 Management of pregnancy with pre-eclampsia

Degree of hypertension	Mild hypertension (140/90 to 149/99 mmHg)	Moderate hypertension (150/100 to 159/109 mmHg)	Severe hypertension (160/110 mmHg or higher)
Admit to hospital	Yes	Yes	Yes
Treat	No	With oral labetalol[†] as first-line treatment to keep: • diastolic blood pressure between 80–100 mmHg • systolic blood pressure less than 150 mmHg	With oral labetalol[†] as first-line treatment to keep: • diastolic blood pressure between 80–100 mmHg • systolic blood pressure less than 150 mmHg

References http://www.nice.org.uk/guidance/cg107/chapter/1-guidance

---

MMD54

MMD54 Answer: E

Explanation The benefits of UFH are that it has a shorter half-life than LMWH and there is more complete reversal of its activity by protamine sulphate. The required interval between UFH and regional analgesia or anaesthesia is less (4 h) than with LMWH (12 h), and there is less concern regarding neuraxial haematomas with UFH. Any exposure to UFH is associated with an increased risk of heparin-induced thrombocytopenia (HIT). If UFH is used after caesarean section (or other surgery), the platelet count should be monitored every 2–3 days from days 4–14 or until heparin is stopped.

References RCOG GTG 37a reducing the risk of venous thromboembolism during pregnancy and the puerperium April 2015. https://www.rcog.org.uk/globalassets/documents/guidelines/gtg-37a.pdf

MMD55

MMD55 Answer: B

Explanation   The UK incidence of antenatal PE calculated in the UKOSS study is 1.3 per 10 000 maternities. The relative risk of VTE in pregnancy is increased four- to sixfold, and this is increased further postpartum; the absolute risk is low with an overall incidence of VTE in pregnancy and the puerperium of 1–2 per 1000. Many fatal antenatal VTE events occur in the first trimester, and therefore prophylaxis for women with previous VTE should begin early in pregnancy. The risk for VTE increases with gestational age, reaching a maximum just after delivery

References   RCOG GTG 37a.

MMD56

MMD56 Answer: B

Explanations

A   The cornerstones of modern treatment in β-thalassaemia are blood transfusion and iron chelation therapy.

B   Patients with severe forms of β-thalassaemia intermedia and those patients with thalassaemia major who had poor access to blood were previously offered sple- nectomy to help reduce transfusion requirements. *Splenectomy is no longer the mainstay of treatment* for these conditions, but a considerable number of both thalassaemia major and intermedia patients have undergone splenectomy.

C   The anterior pituitary is very sensitive to iron overload, and evidence of dys- function is common. Puberty is often delayed and incomplete, resulting in low bone mass.

D   Cardiac failure is the primary cause of death in over 50 % of cases. Improved transfusion techniques and effective chelation protocols have improved the quality of life and survival of individuals with thalassaemia.

E   The mortality from cardiac iron overload has reduced significantly since the development of magnetic resonance imaging (MRI) methods for monitoring cardiac (cardiac T2*) and hepatic iron overload (liver T2*) and FerriScanR liver iron assessment (FerriScanR, Resonance Health, Australia). These meth- ods are now available in most large centres looking after patients with haemoglobinopathies.

References   Beta thalassemia in pregnancy – RCOG Green Top guideline No: 66. Mar 2014. http://www.rcog.org.uk/files/rcog-corp/GTG_66_Thalassaemia.pdf

Fetal Medicine: Answers and Explanations

17

FM1

FM1 Answer: C

Explanation It is estimated that around 5 % of the pregnant population (approximately 30 000 women per annum in the UK) are offered a choice of invasive prenatal diagnostic tests (most commonly amniocentesis or chorionic villus sampling). The type of diagnostic test available and offered is likely to vary depending upon the timing of any initial screening test that is performed.

References Green Top guideline no 8, June 2010, Amniocentesis and CVS http://www.rcog.org.uk/files/rcog-corp/GT8Amniocentesis0111.pdf

FM2

FM2 Answer: E

Explanation Amniocentesis in the third trimester is carried out for a number of indications, most commonly, for late karyotyping and detection of suspected fetal infection in prelabour preterm rupture of the membranes (PPROM). Serious complications are rare.

Women should be informed that third-trimester amniocentesis does not appear to be associated with a significant risk of emergency delivery [C].

Women should be informed that, compared with mid-trimester procedures, complications including multiple attempts and bloodstained fluid are more common in third-trimester procedures [C].

© Springer India 2016
C. Ratha, J. Gupta, *SBAs and EMQs for MRCOG II*,
DOI 10.1007/978-81-322-2689-5_17

There is a suggestion that culture failure rates may be higher following third-trimester amniocentesis with a rate of 9.7 % reported in the series of O'Donoghue et al.

References 1. Green Top guideline no 8, June 2010, Amniocentesis and CVS http://www.rcog.org.uk/files/rcog-corp/GT8Amniocentesis0111.pdf
2. O'Donoghue K, et al. Amniocentesis in the third trimester of pregnancy. Prenat Diagn. 2007;11:1000–4.

FM3

FM3 Answer: D

Explanation Decontamination of ultrasound probes between patients is variable, and there are practical difficulties in balancing the need for cleaning with prevention of degradation of the probe. Severe sepsis, including maternal death, has been reported following invasive prenatal procedures.

The level of risk cannot be quantified as case report literature does not provide denominator information, but the risk of severe sepsis is likely to be less than 1/1000 procedures. Infection can be caused by inadvertent puncture of the bowel, skin contaminants or organisms present on the ultrasound probe or gel.

Maternal RhD status should be available or obtained in every case. Prophylaxis with anti-D immunoglobulin must be offered following each procedure in line with national recommendations. Ultrasound gel may contain organisms, and many departments have mechanisms to minimise the risks including the use of sterile ultrasound gel when performing invasive procedures.

In case of maternal HIV infection, the risk of transmission should be discussed and consideration given to starting antiretroviral therapy to reduce the viral load prior to the procedure. Review viral load and treatment regimens prior to invasive prenatal testing in women with HIV and consider delaying the procedure until there is no detectable viral load if the woman is already on treatment.

Consider antiretroviral therapy prior to prenatal invasive procedures in women not yet on treatment for HIV.

References 1. Green Top guideline no 8, June 2010, Amniocentesis and CVS http://www.rcog.org.uk/files/rcog-corp/GT8Amniocentesis0111.pdf
2. Backhouse S. Establishing a protocol for the cleaning and sterilisation/disinfection of ultrasound transducers. Br Med Ultrasound Soc Bull. 2003;11:37–9.

FM4

FM4 Answer: A

Explanation Ultrasound diagnosis of chorionicity was based on demonstration of the 'lambda' or 'twin peak' sign (dichorionic) or 'T-sign' (monochorionic) at the membrane–placenta interface.

When the gender of the twins is dicscordant—it indicates they are dizygotic (arising from different zygotes) and hence dichorionic (two placentae)

Two separate placental masses are obviously 'dichorionic'. The option 'bicornuate uterus' is a simple distractor.

References Green-Top guideline No. 51, December 2008, Management of monochorionic twin pregnancy http://www.rcog.org.uk/files/rcog-corp/uploadedfiles/T51ManagementMonochorionicTwinPregnancy2008a.pdf

FM5

FM5 Answer: B

Explanation Chorionicity in multifetal pregnancy is established by assessment of placental signs like the 'twin peak' sign (lambda sign) indicating dichorionicity and 'T-sign' indicating monochorionicity. Chorionicity is better assessed by ultrasound before 14 weeks than after 14 weeks. The optimal time for chorionicity determination is 11–14 weeks as very early in pregnancy, while for 5–6 weeks, the placental masses are not well developed.

References Green-Top guideline No. 51, December 2008, Management of monochorionic twin pregnancy http://www.rcog.org.uk/files/rcog-corp/uploadedfiles/T51ManagementMonochorionicTwinPregnancy2008a.pdf

FM6

FM6 Answer: C

Explanation Twin to twin transfusion is a complication of monochorionic pregnancies. The diagnosis of TTTS is based on ultrasound criteria: the presence of a single placental mass, concordant gender, oligohydramnios with maximum vertical pocket [MVP] less than 2 cm in one sac and polyhydramnios in other sac (MVP $\geq$ 8 cm) (some would say $\geq$ 8 cm at $\leq$ 20 weeks and $\geq$ 10 cm over 20 weeks) 12, discordant bladder appearances, severe TTTS, haemodynamic and cardiac compromise, severe TTTS.

The option B—discordant gender—represents dichorionicity and hence is not a criteria to diagnose TTTS.

References Green-Top guideline No. 51, December 2008, Management of monochorionic twin pregnancy http://www.rcog.org.uk/files/rcog-corp/uploadedfiles/T51ManagementMonochorionicTwinPregnancy2008a.pdf

FM7

FM7 Answer: C

Explanation TTTS complicates 10–15 % of MC pregnancies; the placentas are more likely to have unidirectional artery–vein anastomoses and less likely to have bidirectional artery–artery anastomoses.

TTTS is unique to monochorionic placentae.

Do not monitor for feto-fetal transfusion syndrome in the first trimester. Start diagnostic monitoring with ultrasound for feto-fetal transfusion syndrome (including to identify membrane folding) from 16 weeks. Repeat monitoring fortnightly until 24 weeks.

Ultrasound examinations between 16 and 24 weeks focus primarily on detection of TTTS. After 24 weeks, when first presentation of TTTS is uncommon, the main purpose is to detect fetal growth restriction, which may be concordant or discordant.

Severe twin–twin transfusion syndrome presenting before 26 weeks of gestation should be treated by laser ablation rather than by amnioreduction or septostomy (grade A recommendation)

References 1. NICE clinical guidelines 129, multiple pregnancy: The management of twin and triplet pregnancies in the antenatal period issued: September 2011 guidance.nice.org.uk/cg129 http://www.nice.org.uk/nicemedia/live/13571/56422/56422.pdf

2. Green-Top guideline No. 51, December 2008, Management of monochorionic twin pregnancy http://www.rcog.org.uk/files/rcog-corp/uploadedfiles/T51ManagementMonochorionicTwinPregnancy2008a.pdf

FM8

FM8 Answer: C

Explanantion With regard to noninvasive prenatal testing for fetal aneuploidies, published data indicate extremely good results for trisomy 21 and trisomy 18 prediction when sequencing is successful. For trisomy 21 and 18, the detection rates in large series using different technologies have reported (after successful sequencing) sensitivity and specificity close to 100 %. However, there are few possible sources of error in this technology, and these include:

(a) Early gestational age (not late GA)—The amount of cffDNA in maternal blood increases with gestational age, and if the samples are taken too early in pregnancy, false-negative results become more likely.
(b) Maternal obesity (not low BMI)—Increased maternal weight is associated with lower fetal DNA percentage. The reason is unclear, but could be high adipose cell turnover increasing maternal plasma DNA or increasing blood volume and so a dilutional effect.
(c) Multiple pregnancies—When twins are dichorionic, and so may be discordant, maternal plasma DNA testing would, in theory, not be as straightforward.
(d) Placental mosaicism—There is good evidence that the source of the cffDNA is the placenta. It is known from chorionic villus sampling (CVS) that abnormal cell lines can be present in the placenta that are not present in the fetus (in approximately 1 % of CVS samples), a phenomenon often called 'confined placental mosaicism'. The most likely explanation for the so-called 'false' (discordant) positives is confined placental mosaicism: i.e. NIPT is detecting mosaic abnormal colonies of cells in the placenta.
(e) Maternal conditions—Maternal chromosomal abnormalities, including mosaicism or malignant disease, could be very rare causes of discordant results.

Maternal heart disease and placenta previa are simple distractors.

References http://www.rcog.org.uk/files/rcog-corp/SIP_15_04032014.pdf

---

FM9

FM9 Answer: A

Explanation Multifetal pregnancy is a condition with two or more foetuses in the uterus. The three important features of multifetal pregnancy are 'zygosity', 'chorionicity' and amnionicity. Each zygote can form its own placenta (chorion) and sac (amnion).

However, if a zygote divides with 1–3 days of fetulisation, it can form two separate placenta and two separate sacs—dichorionic diamniotic. Some other possibilities are as follows:

– Monochorionic diamniotic—Single placenta, two sacs (cleavage day 4–8)
– Monochorionic monoamniotic—Single placenta, one sac (cleavage day 8–13)
– Dichorionic monoamniotic—Two placentas but only one sac (physiologically not possible!!)

– Dichorionic triamniotic—Two placentas, three sacs. This can happen if there are triplets with a monochorionic pair
– Dichorionic quadriamniotic—two placentas, four sacs, quadruplets with two MCDA pairs

As a general rule, the number of sacs should be equal to or more than the number of placentae; hence, combinations like dichorionic, monoamniotic are not physiologically possible.

Suggested Reading Dewhurst's textbook of obstetrics and gynaecology, 7th edn, edited by Keith Edmonds, Chapter on Multiple pregnancy (p. 166–76)

FM10

FM10 Answer: B

Explanation A medical pedigree is a graphic presentation of a family's health history and genetic relationships.
Example of a pedigree drawing.
Each family member is represented by a square (male) or a circle (female). Individuals with unspecified gender are represented by 'diamonds'. They are connected to each other by lines (relationship lines). Vertical lines connect generations. Horizontal lines are 'mating lines' and consanguineous mating is represented by two horizontal lines. Usually 3 generations are depicted in a standard pedigree, and this helps in establishing the pattern of inheritance and assists in identifying persons at risk of an inherited disorder.

References Benett et al. Standardized human pedigree nomenclature: Update and assessment of the recommendations of the national society of genetic counselors. J Genet Counsel. 2008;17:424–33.
Link to article: http://geneticcounselingtoolkit.com/cases/pedigree

FM11

FM11 Answer: C

Explanation Change in AC or EFW may improve the prediction of wasting at birth (neonatal morphometric indicators) and adverse perinatal outcome suggestive of FGR.
When using two measurements of AC or EFW to estimate growth velocity, they should be at least 3 weeks apart to minimise false-positive rates for diagnosing

FGR. More frequent measurements of fetal size may be appropriate where birth weight prediction is relevant outside of the context of diagnosing SGA/FGR.

References SGA fetus – RCOG Green Top guideline No. 31. Feb 2013. Minor revisions Jan 2014 http://www.rcog.org.uk/files/rcog-corp/GTG31SGA23012013.pdf

FM12

FM12 Answer: A

Explanation Achondroplasia has an autosomal-dominant (AD) mode of inheritance, while others have an autosomal recessive (AR) mode of inheritance. Hence, the recurrence risk for achondroplasia is 50 %, while for the conditions inherited in AR manner, it is 25 %.

Autosomal recessive inheritance

Suggested Reading Davidson's principles and practice of medicine, 22nd edn. Chapter 3: Molecular and genetic factors in disease.

FM13

FM13 Answer: A

Explanation Monochorionicity confers major increases in perinatal morbidity and mortality when compared to dichorionic gestations. Chorionicity may be accurately determined by ultrasound between 10 and 14 weeks gestation. A number of methods are widely used, including the presence of the lambda or 'twin peak sign' for dichorionicity and the 'T-sign' for monochorionicity. In addition, the thickness of the intertwin membrane may be determined—a membrane thickness of less than 2 mm is suggestive of monochorionicity. Other indicators in the second trimester may be the presence of two separate placental masses or discordant fetal sex. If it is difficult to determine chorionicity, even after senior referral, the pregnancy should be managed as monochorionic until proven otherwise.

References Bonney E, Rathod M, Cohen K, Ferriman E. Twin pregnancy. Obstet Gynaecol Reprod Med. 2013;23:6.

FM14

FM14 Answer: C

Explanation Congenital adrenal hyperplasia (CAH) is a spectrum of autosomal recessive conditions in which there is a mutation in the coding of one of the many enzymes responsible for cortisol synthesis from cholesterol in the adrenal gland, resulting in defective enzyme production. About 1 in 60 of the Northern Europe population is a carrier of CAH. All affected families—either homozygous mothers planning a pregnancy or families with a child previously affected—should be offered genetic counselling. The family with a previously affected child has a 1 in 4 chance of having a subsequently affected offspring and a 1 in 8 chance that the child will be a virilised female.

References Girling J, Cotzias C. Thyroid and other endocrine disorders in pregnancy. Obstet Gynaecol Reprod Med. 17(12):349–55.

FM15

FM15 Answer: C

Explanation Dexamethasone readily crosses the placenta. It should be started prior to 7 weeks gestation (when the external genitalia begin to differentiate) to suppress fetal ACTH excretion and androgen overproduction. This dexamethasone regimen, 1–1.5 mg daily, reduces the need for corrective surgery for virilisation but is not always successful. Early fetal sexing by identification of cell-free DNA in maternal blood identifies a male fetus and means that dexamethasone can be stopped appropriately early. Alternatively a CVS at 11 weeks can be used to determine whether the female fetus is affected or not and therefore helps to time the cessation of dexamethasone therapy.

References Girling J, Cotzias C. Thyroid and other endocrine disorders in pregnancy. Obstet Gynaecol Reprod Med. 17(12):349–55.

FM16

FM16 Answer: E

Explanation The commonest enzyme deficiency is 21-hydroxylase (responsible for about 90 % of CAH), and therefore 17-hydroxy progesterone is not converted into 11-deoxycortisol. Failure to produce cortisol causes increased ACTH secretion, and overstimulation and hyperplasia of the adrenals, which in turn overproduce steroid precursors that are shunted along the androgen pathway.

Classic CAH occurs in about 1 in 15 000 births and produces either:

- A simple virilising condition with normal aldosterone production in 25 % of cases (thought to be when enzymes with 1–2 % of normal activity are produced)
- A severe salt-wasting condition when aldosterone is also not produced (enzyme activity is totally ablated by the genetic mutation)

There is also a milder, nonclassic or late-onset CAH which produces signs of androgen excess later in life (associated with 20–60 % normal enzyme activity).

References Girling J, Cotzias C. Thyroid and other endocrine disorders in pregnancy. Obstet Gynaecol Reprod Med. 17(12):349–55.

FM17

FM17 Answer: E

Explanation Chromosomal abnormalities are thought to account for two thirds of sporadic first trimester miscarriages. These defects may be structural, such as Robertsonian translocations, or be caused by single gene abnormalities. In couples with recurrent miscarriage 4 % are found to have abnormal karyotypes. In couples with low maternal age, multiple miscarriages and a family history of recurrent miscarriage, the presence of carrier status for a structural chromosomal abnormality should be suspected. Increasing pregnancy losses caused by fetal aneuploidy are seen with advancing maternal age, where the rate of karyotypic abnormality is 52 % in women under 35 years, rising to 82 % in women older than 35 years.

References Morley L, Shillito J, Tang T. Preventing recurrent miscarriage of unknown aetiology. Obstet Gynaecol. 2013;15:99–105.

FM18

FM18 Answer: B

Explanation The recommended strategy for Down syndrome screening at 12 weeks gestation is the combined test (maternal serum and nuchal translucency scan). Key requisites for the combined test are crown-rump length to estimate fetal gestational age, measurement of the nuchal translucency space at the back of the fetal neck and maternal blood to measure the serum markers of pregnancy-associated plasma protein A (PAPP-A) and human chorionic gonadotrophin hormone (hCG). The quadruple test (maternal serum) is recommended for those presenting later from 14 weeks+2 days to 20 weeks+0 days. Chorionic villus sampling (CVS) or amniocentesis under direct ultrasound guidance is recommended for a 'higher-risk' result (greater than 1 in 150 at term).

References NHS Fetal Anomaly Screening Programme. Screening for Down's syndrome: UK NSC Policy recommendations. 2011–2014 Model of Best Practice. Exeter, NHS evidence: 2011. Available at: file:///C:/Users/User/Downloads/Model-of-Best-Practice-Web-v5-FASP75.pdf

FM19

FM19 Answer: C

Explanation Because the fetal blood volume is around 80–100 ml/kg, the loss of relatively small amounts of blood can have major implications for the fetus; thus, rapid delivery and aggressive resuscitation including the use of blood transfusion if required are essential.

References 1. RCOG GreenTop guideline No. 27. Placenta praevia accreta and vasa praevia https://www.rcog.org.uk/globalassets/documents/guidelines/gtg_27.pdf
  2. Oyelese Y, et al. Vasa previa: The impact of prenatal diagnosis on outcomes. Obstet Gynecol. 2004;103:937–42.

FM20

FM20 Answer: D

Explanation Maternal syphilis is a well-established cause of fetal congenital defects, and treatment of syphilis helps prevent the teratogenicity. The other pathogens do not fulfil the criteria.

References Fetal infections, high risk pregnancy.

FM21

FM21 Answer: B

Explanation As maternal cardiac defects are known to be associated with maternal diabetes, a normal anomaly scan and fetal echocardiography at 20 weeks will help reassure the mother regarding fetal anatomy.

References Diabetes and pregnancy, NICE guideline 2015.

FM22

FM22 Answer: B

Explanation Severe twin–twin transfusion syndrome presenting before 26 weeks of gestation should be treated by laser ablation rather than by amnioreduction or septostomy. Anastomoses may be missed at laser ablation, and TTTS can recur later in up to 14 % of pregnancies treated by laser ablation. Septostomy is the deliberate creation of a hole in the dividing septum with the intention of improving amniotic fluid volume in the donor sac. There seems to be no significant difference in outcome between amnioreduction and septostomy. Some women request termination of pregnancy when severe TTTS is diagnosed, and this should be discussed as an option. Another option is to offer selective termination of pregnancy using bipolar diathermy of one of the umbilical cords, with inevitable sacrifice of that baby. This may be appropriate if there is severe hydrops fetalis in the recipient or evidence of cerebral damage in either twin.

References Green Top guideline No. 51. Management of monochorionic twin pregnancy.

FM23

FM23 Answer: C

Explanation There are several broad causes for stillbirth. Fetal causes include chromosomal problems and fetal structural abnormalities. Maternal associations include obesity, smoking and diseases of the endocrine, renal cardiac and haematological systems. Infection accounts for some fetal losses. Morphological placental complications account for 12 % of stillbirths. These involve marginal insertions (present in 5–7 % of pregnancies), and velamentous insertions parvovirus causes a mild disease in children but is an important cause of stillbirth through development of severe anaemia and hydrops, as well as through direct viral attack of the fetal myocardium.

References   Vais A, Kean L. Stillbirth – is it a preventable public health problem in the twenty-first century? Obstet Gynaecol Reprod Med. 22:5 130–5.

FM24

FM24 Answer: D

Explanation   SGA birth is defined as an estimated fetal weight (EFW) or abdominal circumference (AC) less than the 10th centile and severe SGA as an EFW or AC less than the third centile. Fetal growth restriction (FGR) is not synonymous with SGA. Some, but not all, growth-restricted fetuses/infants are SGA, while 50–70 % of SGA fetuses are constitutionally small, with fetal growth appropriate for maternal size and ethnicity. The likelihood of FGR is higher in severe SGA infants.

Growth restriction implies a pathological restriction of the genetic growth potential. As a result, growth restricted fetuses may manifest evidence of fetal compromise (abnormal Doppler studies, reduced liquor volume).

References   The Investigation and Management of the Small–for–Gestational–Age Fetus. RCOG Green Top guideline No. 31.

FM25

FM 25 Answer: C

Explanation   There is evidence that antenatal corticosteroids are effective not only in reducing respiratory distress syndrome (RDS) but also in reducing other complications of prematurity such as intraventricular haemorrhage (IVH). Clinicians should offer a single course of antenatal corticosteroids to women between 24+0 and 34+6 weeks of gestation who are at risk of preterm birth. It is associated with a significant reduction in rates of neonatal death, RDS and intraventricular haemorrhage. Betamethasone 12 mg given intramuscularly in two doses or dexamethasone 6 mg given intramuscularly in four doses are the steroids of choice to enhance lung maturation

References   Antenatal corticosteroids to reduce neonatal morbidity and mortality. RCOG Green Top guideline No. 7.

FM26

FM26 Answer: B

Explanation At least seven case reports of adverse pregnancy outcome associated with a daily intake of vitamin A of 25,000 IU or more have been published. Almost all of the FDA cases are brief, retrospective reports of malformed infants or fetuses exposed to supplements of 25,000 IU/day or more of vitamin A during pregnancy. Some of these infants have malformations similar to those found among isotretinoin-exposed infants; the malformations of the others were quite different.

The malformations mainly involved craniofacial structures.

References http://teratology.org/pubs/vitamina.htm

FM27

FM 27 Answer: C

Explanation Monozygotic twins result from the splitting of a single zygote. The earliest separation occurs at the two-cell stage, in which two separate placentas and amniotic cavities result (dichorionic diamniotic). In the majority of monozygotic twins, separation takes place at the early blastocyst stage when the resulting two embryos have a common placenta and two amniotic cavities (monochorionic diamniotic). Uncommonly, embryonic splitting occurs late at the stage of bilaminar germ disc and results in monoamniotic twins with a single placenta and a common amniotic cavity.

Rarely, incomplete splitting of the embryo from later zygotic division results in conjoined twinning.

References Green Top guideline No. 51. Management of monochorionic twin pregnancy.

FM28

FM28 Answer: A

Explanation Human parvovirus B19 has a predilection for rapidly dividing cells, mainly the erythroid cell precursors, thereby interrupting red cell production. Approximately 60 % of adults have serological evidence of prior infection, and the presence of human parvovirus IgG appears to confer lasting immunity. The primary infection rate in pregnant women, as measured by the frequency of seroconversion, is about 1.1 % per year. Transplacental transmission occurs in 15 % of cases before 15 weeks of gestation and 25 % between 15 and 20 weeks: this rises to 70 % towards term.

References 1. To M, Kidd M, Maxwell D. Prenatal diagnosis and management of fetal infections. Obstet Gynaecol, 2009;11:108–16. doi:10.1576/ toag.11.2.108.27484.

    2. Ismail KM, Kilby MD. Human parvovirus B19 infection and pregnancy. Obstet Gynaecol. 2003;5:4–9. doi:10.1576/toag.5.1.4.

FM29

FM29 Answer: A

Explanation Congenital CMV infection is one of the most common congenital infections, with a reported incidence of 0.5–2 %. The primary parvovirus infection rate in pregnant women, as measured by the frequency of seroconversion, is about 1.1 % per year. In the UK, 90 % of women of childbearing age are susceptible to toxoplasma infection, and the incidence of maternal infection is approximately 2 per 1000 pregnancies. Infection in pregnancy is rare, but the proportion of women of childbearing age thought to be susceptible to the rubella virus is in the region of 1–2 %. Varicella zoster virus is endemic in the UK, and >90 % of the antenatal population are seropositive for varicella zoster virus IgG. For this reason, primary infection is uncommon in pregnancy and is estimated to occur in 3 per 1000 pregnancies.

References To M, Kidd M, Maxwell D. Prenatal diagnosis and management of fetal infections. Obstet Gynaecol. 2009;11:108–16. doi:10.1576/ toag.11.2.108.27484.

FM30

FM30 Answer: C

Explanation Women should be informed that the additional risk of miscarriage following amniocentesis is around 1 %.

References https://www.rcog.org.uk/globalassets/documents/guidelines/gt8am- niocentesis0111.pdf

FM31

FM31 Answer: D

Explanation An anti-D level of > 4 iu/ml but < 15 iu/ml correlates with a moderate risk of HDFN, and an anti-D level of > 15 iu/ml can cause severe HDFN. Referral for a fetal medicine opinion should therefore be made once anti-D levels are > 4 iu/ml.

References https://www.rcog.org.uk/globalassets/documents/guidelines/rbc_gtg65.pdf

FM32

FM 32 Answer: D

Explanation Vertical transmission in Rubella infection occurs during maternal viraemia; the risk of fetal infection is 90 % before 12 weeks of gestation, about 55 % at 12–16 weeks, and it declines to 45 % after 16 weeks. The risk of congenital defects in infected fetuses is 90 % before 12 weeks, 20 % between 12 and 16 weeks and, thereafter, deafness is a risk up until 20 weeks. Reinfection can occur and is more likely after prolonged or intense exposure and with vaccine-induced, rather than natural, immunity. It is usually subclinical, however, and the risk to the fetus is thought to be <5 %.

FM33

FM33 Answer: C

Explanation Conjoined twins are very rare, occurring in around one in 90 000–100 000 pregnancies worldwide. The underlying pathogenic mechanism remains uncertain, with theories including incomplete separation of the developing embryo, development of codominant axes and embryonic fusion.

Most cases are now prenatally diagnosed and delivered by elective caesarean section, but vaginal deliveries of conjoined twins are reported. Risk of dystocia and uterine rupture has been reported in association with prenatally undiagnosed cases.

References Green Top guideline No. 51 Management of monochorionic twins.

FM34

FM34 Answer: D

Explanations

A. Antenatal CTG has been compared with no intervention in a Cochrane systematic review of RCTs. There was no clear evidence that antenatal CTG improved perinatal mortality.
B. Amniotic fluid volume is usually estimated by the single deepest vertical pocket (SDVP) or amniotic fluid index (AFI) methods; although both correlate poorly with actual amniotic fluid volume. However, compared to a SDVP < 2 cm, when an AFI ≤ 5 cm was used, more cases of oligohydramnios were diagnosed and more women had induction of labour without an improvement in perinatal outcome.
C. The biophysical profile (BPP) includes four acute fetal variables (breathing movement, gross body movement, tone and CTG, and amniotic fluid volume each assigned a score of 2 (if normal) or 0 (if abnormal). Reducing BPP score is associated with lower antepartum umbilical venous pH and increasing perinatal mortality. The BPP is time consuming and the incidence of an equivocal result (6/10) is high (15–20 %) in severely SGA foetuses, although this rate can be reduced if cCTG is used instead of conventional CTG.
D. In the preterm SGA fetus, middle cerebral artery (MCA) Doppler has limited accuracy to predict acidaemia and adverse outcome and should not be used to time delivery. *It is reasonable to use MCA Doppler to time delivery in **the term SGA fetus** with normal umbilical artery Doppler.*
E. The ductus venosus (DV) Doppler flow velocity pattern reflects atrial pressure–volume changes during the cardiac cycle. As FGR worsens, velocity reduces in the DV a wave owing to increased afterload and preload, as well as increased end-diastolic pressure, resulting from the direct effects of hypoxia/acidaemia and increased adrenergic drive.

References SGA fetus – RCOG Green Top guideline No. 31. Feb 2013. Minor revisions Jan 2014. http://www.rcog.org.uk/files/rcog-corp/GTG31SGA23012013.pdf

FM35

FM35 Answer: C

Explanation Meckel–Gruber syndrome is associated with the classical combination of occipital encephalocele, polydactyly and bilateral polycystic kidneys. Arnold–Chiari malformation affects the posterior fossa of the fetal brain, Beckwith–Wiedemann syndrome has macrosomia with anterior wall hernias. Noonan syndrome has cardiac defects and unusual facial facies. Seckel syndrome is microcephalic primordial dwarfism.

References Twinnings Text book of fetal anomalies.

FM36

FM36 Answer: C

Explanation
The quintero classification system stage classification

I. There is a discrepancy in amniotic fluid volume with oligohydramnios of a maximum vertical pocket (MVP)$\leq$2 cm in one sac and polyhydramnios in other sac (MVP$\geq$8 cm). The bladder of the donor twin is visible and Doppler studies are normal.
II. The bladder of the donor twin is not visible (during length of examination, usually around 1 h), but Doppler studies are not critically abnormal.
III. Doppler studies are critically abnormal in either twin and are characterised as abnormal or reversed end-diastolic velocities in the umbilical artery, reverse flow in the Ductus venosus or pulsatile umbilical venous flow.
IV. Ascites, pericardial or pleural effusion, scalp oedema or overt hydrops present.
V. One or both babies are dead.

References GTG MC twins.

FM37

FM37 Answer: D

Explanation Hydrops fetalis is accumulation of fluid in two or more fetal compartments, and this can be diagnosed with certainty on antenatal ultrasound. Down syndrome and Edward syndrome are chromosomal abnormalities and require fetal karyotyping for definite diagnosis. The other two options are metabolic, genetic disorders which can be diagnosed by molecular analysis of DNA.

References Fetology.

FM38

FM38 Answer: E

Explanation   Stillbirth is common, with 1 in 200 babies born dead. This compares with one sudden infant death per 10 000 live births. There were 4037 stillbirths in the UK and crown dependencies in 2007, at a rate of 5.2 per 1000 total births. The overall adjusted stillbirth rate was 3.9 per 1000.

Rates ranged from 3.1 in Northern Ireland to 4.6 in Scotland. Scotland had a significantly higher stillbirth rate than the other nations. Overall, over one third of stillbirths are small-for-gestational age fetuses with half classified as being unexplained. The stillbirth rate has remained generally constant since 2000. It has been speculated that rising obesity rates and average maternal age might be behind the lack of improvement; a systematic review identified these as the more prevalent risk factors for stillbirth.

Auscultation and cardiotocography should not be used to investigate suspected IUFD. Real-time ultrasonography is essential for the accurate diagnosis of IUFD. Ideally, real-time ultrasonography should be available at all times. A second opinion should be obtained whenever practically possible.

References   Green Top guideline No. 55 Late IUFD.

FM39

FM39 Answer: D

Explanation   VZV DNA can be detected in amniotic fluid by PCR. The presence of VZV DNA has a high sensitivity but a low specificity for the development of FVS. Given that amniocentesis has a strong negative predictive value but a poor positive predictive value in detecting fetal damage that cannot be detected by non-invasive methods, women who develop varicella infection during pregnancy should be counselled about the risks versus benefits of amniocentesis to detect varicella DNA by polymerase chain reaction (PCR). Amniocentesis should not be performed before the skin lesions have completely healed.

References   Green Top guideline, Chickenpox in pregnancy.

FM40

FM40 Answer: D

Explanation TTTS complicates 10–15 % of MC pregnancies; the placentas are more likely to have unidirectional artery–vein anastomoses and less likely to have bidirectional artery–artery anastomoses in MCDA pregnancies than MCMA pregnancies, possibly reflecting that there are more protective artery–artery anastomoses in the latter. Rarely (in approximately 5 % of cases), the transfusion may reverse during pregnancy, with the donor fetus demonstrating features of a recipient fetus and vice versa. Anastomoses may be missed at laser ablation, and TTTS can recur later in up to 14 % of pregnancies treated by laser.

References Ref: GTG 51 December 2008.

FM41

Explanations

A. In the preterm SGA fetus with umbilical artery AREDV detected prior to 32 weeks of gestation, delivery is recommended when DV Doppler becomes abnormal or UV pulsations appear, provided the fetus is considered viable and after completion of steroids.
B. When umbilical artery Doppler flow indices are normal, it is reasonable to repeat surveillance every 14 days. Therefore, there is no indication for immediate LSCS.
C. Static growth for 3 weeks is an indication to deliver.
D. Umbilical Dopplers are normal; there is no indication for 'immediate LSCS'.
E. Umbilical Dopplers are normal; there is no indication for 'immediate LSCS' (*flowchart in Appendix III of the SGA GTG*).

Even when venous Doppler is normal, delivery is recommended by 32 weeks of gestation and should be considered between 30 and 32 weeks of gestation.

If MCA Doppler is abnormal, delivery should be recommended no later than 37 weeks of gestation.

In the SGA fetus detected after 32 weeks of gestation with an abnormal umbilical artery Doppler, delivery no later than 37 weeks of gestation is recommended.

In the SGA fetus detected after 32 weeks of gestation with normal umbilical artery Doppler, a senior obstetrician should be involved in determining the timing and mode of birth of these pregnancies.

References SGA fetus – RCOG Green Top guideline No. 31. Feb 2013. Minor revisions Jan 2014. http://www.rcog.org.uk/files/rcog-corp/GTG31SGA23012013.pdf

FM42

FM42 Answer: A

Explanation There is little consensus on the appropriate timing of induction of labour, and decisions have to be based on the specific needs of each pregnancy. Each case should be examined individually, and maternal discomfort and requests, parity and suitability for induction, and presence or absence of pregnancy complications should all be taken into account.

Local legal and ethical practice need also to be given due consideration. Early induction of labour where the fetus has a lethal anomaly is not an option in the UK; it may in some jurisdictions be considered termination of pregnancy and not be legally possible. If early induction is planned, then the woman should be fully aware of the potential for failure, which may necessitate repeat attempts at induction at a later date or even caesarean section. Consideration also needs to be given to the location of labour. Ideally women should be given the opportunity to labour in private, in a single room. A senior midwife who has had experience in dealing with pregnancies complicated by lethal fetal anomaly should be present. This helps to reduce both parental and staff stress and anxiety at this crucial time.

All usual forms of analgesia should be available—entonox, pethidine, diamorphine, epidural analgesia. Also if polyhydramnios has been an issue or maternal pre-eclampsia is present, it may be necessary to site an intravenous cannula, check haematology and biochemistry indices and have blood crossmatched, in anticipation of the increased risk of postpartum haemorrhage.

Flexibility when seeing these families for antenatal care is hugely important. Some women will request to be seen outside of the usual antenatal clinic times, when there are fewer pregnant women in the clinical areas, and this request should be accommodated wherever possible. Women will often need to be seen for more frequent visits than the usual antenatal care schedule. This is both for ongoing reassurance that the fetus is alive, and for early diagnosis of any developing pregnancy complications.

References McNamara K, O'Donoghue K, O'Connell O, Greene RA. Antenatal and intrapartum care of pregnancy complicated by lethal fetal anomaly. Obstet Gynaecol. 2013;15:189–94.

FM43

FM43 Answer: C

Explanation Do not use abdominal palpation or symphysis-fundal height measurements to predict intrauterine growth restriction in twin or triplet pregnancies. Estimate fetal weight discordance using two or more biometric parameters at each ultrasound scan from 20 weeks. Aim to undertake scans at intervals of less than 28 days. Consider a 25 % or greater difference in size between twins or triplets as a clinically important indicator of intrauterine growth restriction and offer referral to a tertiary level fetal medicine centre. Do not use umbilical artery Doppler ultrasound to monitor for intrauterine growth restriction or birthweight differences in twin or triplet pregnancies.

References NICE guideline No. 69 multiple pregnancy.

FM44

FM44 Answer: A

Explanation Selective feticide by intracardiac injection of potassium chloride is not an option in MC pregnancies because of the presence of anastomoses. A series of 80 MC pregnancies (twin and triplet) with severe discordant abnormalities, twin reversed arterial perfusion (TRAP) sequence or severe TTTS, underwent cord coagulation by bipolar diathermy or intrafetal laser ablation.

References Green Top guideline No. 51, Management of monochorionic twins.

FM45

FM45 Answer: D

Explanation Duodenal atresia is a condition in which the first part of the small bowel (the duodenum) has not developed properly. It is not open and cannot allow the passage of stomach contents. The cause of duodenal atresia is unknown, but it is thought to result from problems during an embryo's development in which the duodenum does not normally change from a solid to a tubelike structure. Duodenal atresia is seen in more than 1 in 10,000 live births. Approximately 20–30 % of infants with duodenal atresia have Down syndrome. Duodenal atresia is often associated with other birth defects. The double bubble sign is seen in infants and represents dilatation of the proximal duodenum and stomach. It is seen in both radiographs and ultrasound and can be identified antenatally.

References Jeffrey T. The double bubble sign. Radiology 220, No. 2 (2001): 463–4. doi:VL – 220.

FM46

FM46 Answer: B

Explanation Women should be advised that the risk of spontaneous miscarriage does not appear to be increased if chickenpox occurs in the first trimester. If the pregnant woman develops varicella or shows serological conversion in the first 28 weeks of pregnancy, she has a small risk of FVS and she should be informed of the implications. FVS is characterised by one or more of the following: skin scarring in a dermatomal distribution, eye defects (microphthalmia, chorioretinitis or cataracts), hypoplasia of the limbs and neurological abnormalities (microcephaly, cortical atrophy, mental retardation or dysfunction of bowel and bladder sphincters). It does not occur at the time of initial fetal infection but results from a subsequent herpes zoster reactivation in utero and only occurs in a minority of infected fetuses. FVS has been reported to complicate maternal chickenpox occurring as early as 3 weeks and as late as 28 weeks of gestation. The risk appears to be lower in the first trimester (0.55 %).

The negative predictive value of the combination of amniotic fluid PCR testing and ultrasound is good, but the positive predictive value is poor.

References Green Top guideline, Chicken pox in pregnancy 2015.

FM47

FM47 Answer: B

Explanation The MCA Doppler is currently the main tool for surveillance for fetal anaemia in cases of red cell alloimmunisation disease. The MCA has revolutionised the management of fetal anaemia and is as good if not better than the Delta OD 450 from amniotic fluid, which was once the traditional method of surveillance. The MCA PSV can predict the existence of moderate-to-severe fetal anaemia with a sensitivity of 100 % and a false-positive rate of 12 %. An MCA PSV greater than 1.5 MoM may prompt the optimum time to perform cordocentesis and intrauterine transfusion.

Maternal uterine artery Dopplers are predictive of pre-eclampsia. Amniotic fluid is obtained through an invasive method (amniocentesis).

References 1. Mone F, McAuliffe FM, Ong S. The clinical application of Doppler ultrasound in obstetrics. Obstet Gynaecol 2015;17:13–9.

2. Mari G, Deter RL, Carpenter RL, Rahman F, Zimmerman R, Moise KJ. Noninvasive diagnosis by Doppler ultrasonography of fetal anaemia due to maternal red-cell alloimunization. Collaborative Group for Doppler Assessment for the Blood Velocity in Anemic Fetuses. New Engl J Med 2000;343:9–14.

FM48

FM48 Answer: E

Explanation

Booking assessment
(first trimester)

Minor risk factors

Maternal age ≥35 years
IVF singleton pregnancy
Nulliparity
BMI <20
BMI 25–34.9
Smoker 1–10 cigarettes per day
Low fruit intake pre–pregnancy
Previous pre–eclampsia
Pregnancy interval <6 months
Pregnancy interval ≥60 months

Major risk factors

Maternal age >40 years
Smoker ≥11 cigarettes per day
Paternal SGA
Cocaine
Daily vigorous exercise
Previous SGA baby
Previous stillbirth
Maternal SGA
Chronic hypertension
Diabetes with vascular disease
Renal impairment
Antiphospholipid syndrome
Heavy bleeding similar to menses
PAPP–A <0.4 MoM

References   https://www.rcog.org.uk/globalassets/documents/guidelines/gtg_31.
pdf

FM49

FM49 Answer: A

Explanation   In a high-risk population, the use of umbilical artery Doppler has
been shown to reduce perinatal morbidity and mortality. Umbilical artery Doppler
should be the primary surveillance tool in the SGA fetus. When umbilical artery
Doppler flow indices are normal, it is reasonable to repeat surveillance every 14
days.

References   https://www.rcog.org.uk/globalassets/documents/guidelines/gtg_31.
pdf

FM50

FM50 Answer: D

Explanation   An anti-c level of > 7.5 iu/ml but < 20 iu/ml correlates with a moderate risk of HDFN, whereas an anti-c level of > 20 iu/ml correlates with a high risk of
HDFN. Referral for a fetal medicine opinion should therefore be made once anti-c
levels are > 7.5 iu/ml.

References   https://www.rcog.org.uk/globalassets/documents/guidelines/rbc_
gtg65.pdf

Labour and Delivery: Answers and Explanations

18

LD1

LD1 Answer: C

Explanation Shoulder dystocia should be managed systemically and the manoeuvres should be attempted in order as per the algorithm suggested by the RCOG.

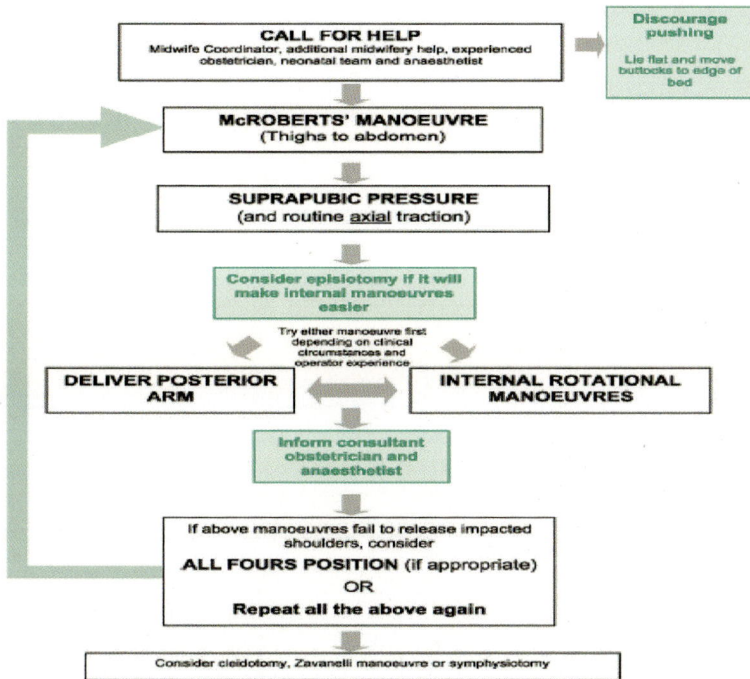

References Green Top guideline no 42, March 2012, Shoulder dystocia. http://www.rcog.org.uk/files/rcog-corp/GTG42_25112013.pdf

LD2

LD2 Answer: B

Explanation Shoulder dystocia is difficult to predict or prevent. Conventional risk factors predicted only 16 % of shoulder dystocia that resulted in infant morbidity.

PPROM is not a known risk factor for shoulder dystocia.

Previous shoulder dystocia cases can be offered either vaginal delivery or elective LSCS based on discussions with the woman although it is known that women with previous shoulder dystocia have a higher risk of the same in future pregnancies. There is no requirement to recommend elective caesarean birth routinely, but factors such as the severity of any previous neonatal or maternal injury, predicted fetal size and maternal choice should all be considered and discussed with the woman and her family when making plans for the next delivery.

There is no recommendation for elective LSCS in nondiabetic women with suspected macrosomia to prevent shoulder dystocia or morbidity thereof. Infants of diabetic mothers have a two- to fourfold increased risk of shoulder dystocia compared with infants of the same birth weight born to nondiabetic mothers. Elective caesarean section should be considered to reduce the potential morbidity for pregnancies complicated by pre-existing or gestational diabetes, regardless of treatment, with estimated fetal weight of greater than 4.5 kg.

Having two previous caesarean births is not known to be a risk factor for shoulder dystocia and neither is it an absolute indication for elective caesarean section.

References Green Top guideline No. 42, March 2012, Shoulder dystocia. http://www.rcog.org.uk/files/rcog-corp/GTG42_25112013.pdf

LD3

LD3 Answer: C

Explanation Offer women with uncomplicated monochorionic twin pregnancies elective birth from 36 weeks 0 days, after a course of antenatal corticosteroids has been offered. Offer women with uncomplicated triplet pregnancies elective birth from 35 weeks 0 days, after a course of antenatal corticosteroids has been offered.

Offer women with uncomplicated dichorionic twin pregnancies elective birth from 37 weeks 0 days. It is appropriate to aim for vaginal birth of monochorionic twins unless there are accepted, specific clinical indications for caesarean section, such as twin one lying breech or previous caesarean section.

Most monochorionic, monoamniotic twins have cord entanglement and are best delivered at 32 weeks, by caesarean section, after corticosteroids.

References 1. NICE clinical guideline 129, Multiple pregnancy: the management of twin and triplet pregnancies in the antenatal period issued: September 2011 guidance. nice.org.uk/cg129. http://www.nice.org.uk/nicemedia/live/13571/56422/56422.pdf
2. Green-Top guideline no. 51, December 2008, Management of monochorionic twin pregnancy. http://www.rcog.org.uk/files/rcog-corp/uploadedfiles/T51ManagementMonochorionicTwinPregnancy2008a.pdf

LD4

LD4 Answer: A

Explanation Conventional risk factors predicted only 16 % of shoulder dystocia that resulted in infant morbidity:

- Either caesarean section or vaginal delivery can be appropriate after a previous shoulder dystocia. The decision should be made jointly by the woman and her carers.
- While managing shoulder dystocia, fundal pressure should not be used. McRoberts' manoeuvre is a simple, rapid and effective intervention and should be performed first. Suprapubic pressure should be used to improve the effectiveness of the McRoberts' manoeuvre.
- There is a relationship between fetal size and shoulder dystocia, but it is not a good predictor partly because fetal size is difficult to determine accurately and also because the large majority of infants with a birth weight of ≥4500 g do not develop shoulder dystocia. Equally important, 48 % of births complicated by shoulder dystocia occur with infants who weigh less than 4000 g.
- Induction of labour does not prevent shoulder dystocia in nondiabetic women with a suspected macrosomic fetus.

References Shoulder dystocia – RCOG Green Top guideline No. 42. Mar 2012. http://www.rcog.org.uk/files/rcog-corp/GTG42_25112013.pdf

LD5

LD5 Answer: C

Explanation Evidence reports mediolateral episiotomy (favoured in UK and European practice) to have a significantly lower risk of sphincter injury compared with a midline episiotomy (favoured in the USA) at 2 versus 12 %. Published evidence on the role of episiotomy is contradictory. Traditional teaching is that episiotomy protects the perineum from uncontrolled trauma during delivery.

Although several authors have demonstrated a protective effect against sphincter injury with mediolateral episiotomy, others have reported the converse. The differences between medical and midwifery staff in conducting a mediolateral episiotomy have been studied, with doctors performing episiotomies that are longer and at a wider angle compared with midwives. An important learning point is that current evidence is unable to support the routine use of episiotomy to prevent anal sphincter injury. The type of episiotomy is important.

References Fowler G. Risk factors & management of obstetric anal sphincter injury. Obstet Gynaecol Reprod Med. 2013;23(5): 131–6.

LD6

LD6 Answer: B

Explanation There should be a clear local protocol for massive obstetric haemorrhage. Massive blood loss is defined as a loss of one blood volume in 24 h or loss of 50 % of blood volume within three hours. Another definition is blood loss at a rate of 150 ml/min. Normal blood volume in the adult is defined as 7 % of ideal body weight. Major haemorrhage should involve a consultant obstetrician, anaesthetist and haematologist and the blood bank with training drills and regular practice. Women should have group and save or crossmatch sample taken according to local protocol, if a major haemorrhage is anticipated as in placenta previa/accreta.

References RCOG Green Top guideline No. 47 – Blood transfusion in obstetrics.

LD7

LD7 Answer: A

Explanation An abnormal cardiotocograph is the most consistent finding in uterine rupture and is present is 55–87 % of these events. Hence, continuous electronic fetal monitoring is generally used in women during planned VBAC. Other signs of uterine rupture include cessation of previously efficient uterine activity, maternal hypotension or shock and loss of station of the presenting part. None of these are pathognomic but the presence of any of the above should raise the concern of the possibility of this event. Early diagnosis of scar rupture followed by expeditious laparotomy and resuscitation is essential to reduce associated morbidity in mother and infant.

References RCOG Green Top guideline No 45. Birth after previous caesarean birth.

LD8

LD8 Answer: D

Explanation A number of factors are associated with successful VBAC. Previous vaginal birth, particularly previous VBAC, is the single best predictor for successful VBAC. Risk factors for unsuccessful VBAC are induced labour, no previous vaginal birth, body mass index greater than 30 and previous section for dystocia. Other factors associated with a decreased likelihood of successful VBAC are VBAC at or after 41 weeks, birth weight greater than 4000 g, previous preterm caesarean birth, less than 2 years from previous caesarean birth, advanced maternal age, non-white ethnicity, short stature and a male infant. Counselling a woman should include appropriate risk assessment and counselling to ensure safe delivery and successful outcome.

References RCOG Green Top guideline No. 45. Birth after previous caesarean birth.

LD9

LD9 Answer: D

Explanation Delay in the first stage is suspected if the cervix is dilated <2 cm in 4 h. If delay in the established first stage of labour is suspected, amniotomy should be considered for all women with intact membranes, after explanation of the procedure and advice that it will shorten her labour by about an hour and may increase the strength and pain of her contractions.

Whether or not a woman has agreed to an amniotomy, advise all women with suspected delay in the established first stage of labour to have a vaginal examination 2 h later, and diagnose delay if progress is less than 1 cm.

References https://www.nice.org.uk/guidance/cg190/chapter/1-Recommendations

LD10

LD10 Answer: E

Explanation Planned VBAC carries a risk of uterine rupture of 22–74/10,000. There is virtually no risk of uterine rupture in women undergoing ERCS. Uterine rupture in an unscarred uterus is extremely rare at 0.5–2.0/10,000 deliveries; this risk is mainly confined to multiparous women in labour. If women with a previous scar undergo induced and/or augmented labours, this risk increases by two- to three-fold. There is also a 1.5-fold increased risk of caesarean section in induced and/or augmented labours compared with spontaneous labours. There is higher risk of uterine rupture with induction of labour with prostaglandins.

References Birth after previous Caesarean birth. RCOG Green Top guideline No. 45

LD11

LD11 Answer: B

Explanation NICE guidelines recommend delivery at 37–38 weeks for dichorionic twins and 36–37 weeks for monochorionic diamniotic twins, but marked variability in policy exists in practice. There is growing evidence that perinatal mortality rates increase after 38 weeks even in uncomplicated twin pregnancies. Additionally, intervention at 37 weeks does not appear to be associated with a significant difference in mode of delivery or maternal complications when compared to expectant management.

Regarding preterm birth, evidence suggests that progesterone supplementation does not prevent early preterm labour in twin pregnancies and the use of untargeted single or multiple courses of corticosteroids is not recommended. The Twin Birth Study suggests that there is no advantage to a policy of planned caesarean section for twins with respect to both maternal and neonatal morbidity. Current practice supports the policy of planned vaginal birth in uncomplicated pregnancies with a cephalic first twin, unless the mother prefers caesarean delivery.

References Bonney E, Rathod M, Cohen K, Ferriman E. Twin pregnancy. Obstet Gynaecol Reprod Med. 23(6):165–70.

LD12

LD12 Answer: A

Explanation Steps in active management of the third stage of labour:

- Oxytocin is given within 1 min of birth of the baby (oxytocin 10 units im).
- Deliver the placenta by controlled cord traction:
- When the uterus becomes rounded or the cord lengthens, a gentle pull is applied downwards on the cord to deliver the placenta. Countertraction is applied to the uterus with the other hand. This prevents uterine inversion. After the placenta is delivered, it is examined to ensure it is completely expelled.
- The fundus of the uterus is massaged through the woman's abdomen until the uterus is contracted. This is repeated every 15 min for the first 2 h.

References http://www.who.int/maternal_child_adolescent/documents/postpartum/en/

LD13

LD13 Answer: C

Explanation The 1996 guidelines from AAP and ACOG for HIE indicate that all of the following must be present for the designation of perinatal asphyxia severe enough to result in acute neurological injury:

- Profound metabolic or mixed academia (pH<7) in an umbilical artery blood sample
- Persistence of an APGAR score of 0–3 for longer than 5 min
- Neonatal neurologic sequelae (e.g. seizures, coma, hypotonia)
- Multiple organ involvement (e.g. kidneys, lungs, liver, heart, intestines)

References [Guideline] Committee on fetus and newborn, American Academy of Pediatrics and Committee on obstetric practice, American College of Obstetrics and Gynecology. Use and abuse of the APGAR score. Pediatrics. 1996;98:141–2.

LD14

LD14 Answer: E

Explanation When negotiating the birth canal, the fetus undergoes a series of manoeuvres. As the fetus descends through the different planes of the pelvis, it needs to move into the position of best fit.

Engagement

The pelvis is widest in the transverse diameter at the pelvic inlet. The fetal head will therefore usually engage in the OT (occipito-transverse) position. The head is engaged when the widest part (the biparietal diameter) has passed the pelvic brim (2/5 palpable per abdomen).

Descent and Flexion

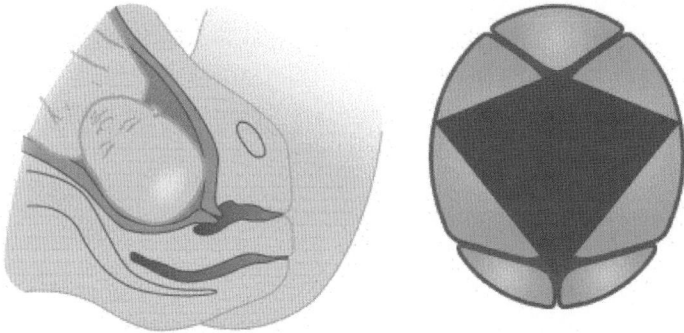

As labour progresses, the fetal head is forced downwards on to the cervix, and this flexes the head so that the vertex is leading.

Internal Rotation

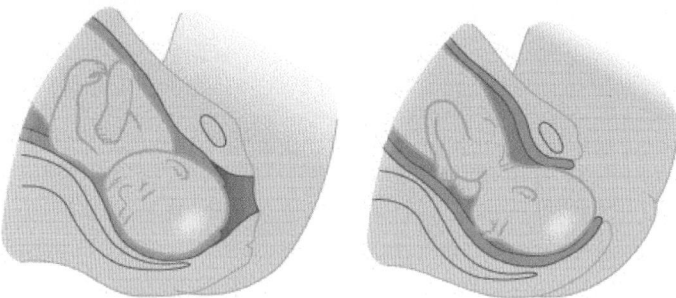

The fetus continues to descend and, on reaching the levator ani muscles, it rotates, usually to the OA (occipito-anterior) position.

Further Descent and Crowning

The occiput comes to lie below the symphysis pubis. The head continues to descend and distend the perineum. The head crowns when the widest part of the head is through the pelvic outlet. The head distends the vulva and doesn't move backwards when the mother stops pushing.

Extension

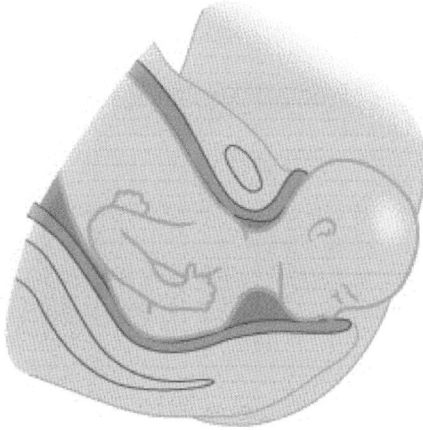

As the head delivers, it extends upwards around the pubic bone (following the curve of the pelvis).

Restitution (External Rotation)

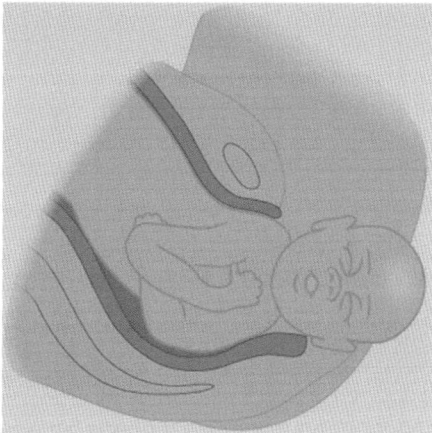

After the head has delivered, it rotates to come in line with the fetal shoulders—restitution.

Delivery

Gentle downward traction is applied to the fetal head to aid delivery of the anterior shoulder (under the symphysis pubis). Following the delivery of the anterior shoulder, the posterior shoulder can be delivered with upward traction.

References http://www.rcog.org.uk/stratog/page/mechanism-labour

LD15

LD15 Answer: A

Explanation Pregnancy itself affects the immune system, and conditions such as anaemia, impaired glucose tolerance or diabetes mellitus reduce resistance to infection. Obesity, an increasing problem in the developed world, is a risk factor for sepsis, as is multiparity. Antibiotic prophylaxis plays an important role in preventing surgical-site infection. Therapy should be directed towards likely offending organisms endogenous in the lower genital tract including: *Escherichia coli*, other Gram-negative rods, *Streptococcus* species, *Staphylococcus aureus*, coagulase-negative staphylococci, *Enterococcus faecalis*, *Gardnerella vaginalis* and anaerobes including *Bacteroides* species and *Peptostreptococcus* species. To optimise intraoperative tissue concentration, prophylactic antibiotics should be given at the time of induction. Repeated doses confer no further benefit and increase the risk of adverse effects and antibiotic resistance. The antibiotic of choice should be well tolerated and safe to use and will be determined by local microbial population and their known sensitivities.

References Glackin K, Harper M. Postpartum pyrexia. Obstet Gynaecol Reprod Med. 22(11):327–31.

LD16

LD16 Answer: D

Explanation Safe operative vaginal delivery requires a careful assessment of the clinical situation, clear communication with the mother and healthcare personnel and expertise in the chosen procedure. Since this primigravida had been actively pushing for 2 h (without an epidural), it will be acceptable to resort to instrumental delivery.

The definition of inadequate progress is: for nulliparous women, lack of continuing progress for 3 h (total of active and passive second-stage labour) with regional anaesthesia or 2 h without regional anaesthesia, while for multiparous women, lack of continuing progress for 2 h (total of active and passive second-stage labour) with regional anaesthesia or 1 h without regional anaesthesia.

References Operative vaginal delivery. RCOG Green Top guideline No. 26.

LD17

LD17 Answer: D

Explanation Safe operative vaginal delivery requires a careful assessment of the clinical situation, clear communication with the mother and healthcare personnel and expertise in the chosen procedure. Even though this primigravida had been actively pushing for 1 h (without an epidural), it will be acceptable to expedite delivery as the CTG shows complicated fetal tachycardia. Since the vaginal examination findings fulfil the criteria for an instrumental delivery, it would be reasonable to do so.

Full abdominal and vaginal examination findings that are prerequisite for safe vaginal delivery: the head is ≤1/5th palpable per abdomen and vertex presentation.

Cervix is fully dilated and the membranes ruptured.

Exact position of the head can be determined so proper placement of the instrument can be achieved.

Assessment of caput and moulding.

Pelvis is deemed adequate. Irreducible moulding may indicate cephalo-pelvic disproportion.

References Operative vaginal delivery. RCOG Green Top guideline No. 26.

LD18

LD18 Answer: B

Explanation Spinal cord injury during pregnancy has a higher risk to both the mother and fetus. Maternal resuscitation and preventing supine hypotension in the mother are paramount. Once stabilised, women are cared for as inpatients, usually for several months.

Thromboprophylaxis is strongly recommended, as the risk of a thrombotic event is greatest in the first 3 months of injury. In labour, regional anaesthesia is offered. If general anaesthesia is required, rocuronium would be the muscle relaxant of choice. Suxamethonium is the usual muscle relaxant, for mandatory rapid sequence induction in pregnancy of more than 16 weeks. However, in lesions between 3 days and 9 months post-injury, suxamethonium is not used because of the risk of hyperkalaemia leading to cardiac arrest and death.

Breastfeeding is normal in women with SCI. In women with complete SCI above T4, the initiation of breastfeeding is delayed and requires additional stimulation such as visual stimulation or oxytocin nasal spray.

References Dawood R, Altanis E, Ribes-Pastor P, Ashworth F. Pregnancy and spinal cord injury. Obstet Gynaecol. 2014;16:99–107.

LD19

LD19 Answer: B

Explanation At 38 weeks of antenatal visit, all women should be offered information about the risks associated with pregnancies that last longer than 42 weeks and their options. The information should cover:

- Membrane sweeping:
  - That membrane sweeping makes spontaneous labour more likely and so reduces the need for formal induction of labour to prevent prolonged pregnancy
  - What a membrane sweep is
  - That discomfort and vaginal bleeding are possible from the procedure
- Induction of labour between 41 + 0 and 42 + 0 weeks
- Expectant management

Women should be informed that most women will go into labour spontaneously by 42 weeks. Women with uncomplicated pregnancies should be given every opportunity to go into spontaneous labour. Women with uncomplicated pregnancies should usually be offered induction of labour between 41 + 0 and 42 + 0 weeks to avoid the risks of prolonged pregnancy. The exact timing should take into account the woman's preferences and local circumstances.

If induction fails, the subsequent management options include:

- A further attempt to induce labour (the timing should depend on the clinical situation and the woman's wishes)
- Caesarean section (refer to 'Caesarean Section')

References NICE guideline No. 70, Induction of labour.

LD20

LD20 Answer: C

Explanation Induction of labour is not generally recommended if a woman's baby is in the breech presentation. If external cephalic version is unsuccessful, declined or contraindicated and the woman chooses not to have an elective caesarean section, induction of labour should be offered, if delivery is indicated, after discussing the associated risks with the woman.

In PPROM, delivery should be considered at 34 weeks of gestation. Where expectant management is considered beyond this gestation, women should be informed of the increased risk of chorioamnionitis and the decreased risk of respiratory problems in the neonate. If a woman has preterm prelabour rupture of membranes after 34 weeks, the maternity team should discuss the following factors with her before a decision is made about whether to induce labour, using vaginal PGE2:

- Risks to the woman (e.g. sepsis, possible need for caesarean section)
- Risks to the baby (e.g. sepsis, problems relating to preterm birth)
- Local availability of neonatal intensive care facilities

If there is severe fetal growth restriction with confirmed fetal compromise, induction of labour is not recommended.

Induction of labour should not routinely be offered on maternal request alone. However, under exceptional circumstances (e.g. if the woman's partner is soon to be posted abroad with the armed forces), induction may be considered at or after 40 weeks.

References NICE guideline No. 70, Induction of labour.

LD21

LD21 Answer: B

Explanation Antenatal steroids are associated with a significant reduction in rates of neonatal death, RDS and intraventricular haemorrhage and are safe for the mother.

References Antenatal corticosteroids GTG7.

LD22

LD22 Answer: B

Explanation Women with recurrent genital herpes should be informed that the risk of neonatal herpes is low, even if lesions are present at the time of delivery (0–3 % for vaginal delivery).

References https://www.rcog.org.uk/globalassets/documents/guidelines/management-genitalherpes. pdf

LD23

LD23 Answer: B

Explanation Explain to both multiparous and nulliparous women that they may choose any birth setting (home, free-standing midwifery unit, alongside midwifery unit or obstetric unit), and support them in their choice of setting wherever they choose to give birth:

Advise low-risk multiparous women that planning to give birth at home or in a midwifery-led unit (free standing or alongside) is particularly suitable for them because the rate of interventions is lower and the outcome for the baby is no different compared with an obstetric unit.

Advise low-risk nulliparous women that planning to give birth in a midwifery-led unit (free standing or alongside) is particularly suitable for them because the rate of interventions is lower and the outcome for the baby is no different compared with an obstetric unit. Explain that if they plan birth at home, there is a small increase in the risk of an adverse outcome for the baby.

Do not perform cardiotocography on admission for low-risk women in suspected or established labour in any birth setting as part of the initial assessment.

In the third stage of labour, do not clamp the cord earlier than 1 min from the birth of the baby unless there is concern about the integrity of the cord or the baby has a heartbeat below 60 beats/min that is not getting faster.

Clamp the cord before 5 min in order to perform controlled cord traction as part of active management. If the woman requests that the cord is clamped and cut later than 5 min, support her in her choice.

References NICE guideline No. 190, Intrapartum care: care of healthy women and their babies during childbirth.

LD24

LD 24: A

Explanation Women considering their options for birth after a single previous caesarean should be informed that, overall, the chances of successful planned VBAC
are 72–76 %. A number of factors are associated with successful VBAC. Previous
vaginal birth, particularly previous VBAC, is the single best predictor for successful
VBAC and is associated with an approximately 87–90 % planned VBAC success
rate.

References GTG VBAC.

LD25

LD25 Answer: A

Explanation An abnormal cardiotocograph (CTG) is the most consistent finding
in uterine rupture and is present in 55–87 % of these events.

References https://www.rcog.org.uk/globalassets/documents/guidelines/
gtg4511022011.pdf

LD26

LD26 Answer: E

Explanation In women with PPROM between 24 and 34 weeks of gestation and
without evidence of infection or preterm labour, delayed removal of the cerclage for
48 h can be considered, as it may result in sufficient latency that a course of prophylactic steroids for fetal lung maturation is completed and/or in utero transfer
arranged. Delayed suture removal until labour ensues or delivery is indicated is
associated with an increased risk of maternal/fetal sepsis and is not recommended.

References https://www.rcog.org.uk/globalassets/documents/guidelines/gtg_60.pdf

LD27

LD27 Answer: D

Explanation Women presenting in established preterm labour with intact membranes with no other risk factors for GBS should not routinely be offered IAP unless they are known to be colonised with GBS. IAP should be offered to women who are pyrexial in labour (>38 °C).

Women who are pyrexial in labour should be offered broad-spectrum antibiotics including an antibiotic for prevention of neonatal EOGBS disease.

The evidence for IAP for women with term prelabour rupture of membranes is unclear, and NICE recommends that it is not given, unless there are other risk factors.

Antibiotic prophylaxis for GBS is unnecessary for women with preterm rupture of membranes. IAP should be offered to women with a previous baby with neonatal GBS disease.

References RCOG Green Top guideline No. 36. The prevention of early-onset neonatal Group B Streptococcal disease. 2012.

LD28

LD 28 Answer: B

Explanation If delay in the established first stage is suspected, take the following into account:

- Parity
- Cervical dilatation and rate of change
- Uterine contractions
- Station and position of presenting part
- The woman's emotional state
- Referral to the appropriate healthcare professional
  Offer the woman support, hydration and appropriate and effective pain relief.

References NICE guideline No. 190. Intrapartum care: care of healthy women and their babies during childbirth.

LD29

LD29 Answer: C

Explanation Antenatal steroids are associated with a significant reduction in rates of neonatal death, RDS and intraventricular haemorrhage and are safe for the mother. Antenatal corticosteroids have no known benefits for the mother.

References RCOG Green Top guideline No. 7. 2010.

LD30

LD30 Answer: C

Explanation Prelabour rupture of membranes at term is defined as rupture of the membranes prior to the onset of labour in women at or over 37 weeks of gestation with an overall incidence of 8–10 % of all pregnancies. Infection of the lower genital tract and/or amniotic cavity is one of the most important aetiologies of prelabour rupture of membranes at term. Women with prelabour rupture of membranes at term (at or over 37 weeks) should be offered a choice of induction of labour with vaginal PGE2 or expectant management.

Induction of labour is appropriate approximately 24 h after prelabour rupture of the membranes at term. Vaginal PGE2 is less invasive than oxytocin, which requires intravenous access and continuous EFM, thus reducing women's mobility during induction. On balance, the GDG reached a consensus that a vaginal PGE2 regimen is the preferred method of induction of labour for women with prelabour rupture of membranes at term.

References NICE guideline No. 70, Induction of labour.

LD31

LD31 Answer: B

Explanation Offer women with uncomplicated triplet pregnancies elective birth from 35 weeks 0 days, after a course of antenatal corticosteroids has been offered. Inform women with triplet pregnancies that about 75 % of triplet pregnancies result in spontaneous birth before 35 weeks 0 days. Inform women with twin and triplet pregnancies that spontaneous preterm birth and elective preterm birth are associated with an increased risk of admission to a special care baby unit.

References NICE guideline No. 69, Multiple pregnancy.

LD32

LD32 Answer: C

Explanation PPROM complicates only 2 % of pregnancies but is associated with 40 % of preterm deliveries and can result in significant neonatal morbidity and mortality. The diagnosis of spontaneous rupture of the membranes is best achieved by maternal history followed by a sterile speculum examination. The diagnosis is made by a history suggestive of spontaneous rupture of membranes followed by a sterile speculum examination demonstrating pooling of fluid in the posterior vaginal fornix; a Nitrazine test is not necessary. Digital vaginal examination is best avoided unless there is a strong suspicion that the woman may be in labour. This is because microorganisms may be transported from the vagina into the cervix leading to intrauterine infection, prostaglandin release and preterm labour.

Delivery should be considered at 34 weeks of gestation. Where expectant management is considered beyond this gestation, women should be informed of the increased risk of chorioamnionitis and the decreased risk of respiratory problems in the neonate.

References Green Top guideline No. 44. Preterm prelabour rupture of membranes.

LD33

LD33 Answer: E

Explanation Misoprostol should only be offered as a method of induction of labour to women who have intrauterine fetal death or in the context of a clinical trial.

Misoprostol is currently unlicensed for use in pregnancy in the UK. Oral and vaginal misoprostol is used in women with an undefined, variable and unfavourable cervix:

- Misoprostol is not licensed for induction of labour in the UK.
- If misoprostol is given orally, the dose should not exceed 50 micrograms.
- Higher doses are associated with higher rates of uterine hyperstimulation.
- Misoprostol 25 microgram vaginal tablet is not superior to vaginal PGE2 for induction of labour.
- When the cervix is unfavourable, doses above 25 micrograms are associated with higher rates of successful induction of labour but at the expense of higher rates of uterine hyperstimulation.

For vaginal misoprostol (favourable cervix), there were insufficient data comparing this route with other regimens to reach a conclusion.

For buccal/sublingual misoprostol (both unfavourable and favourable cervix), there were insufficient data comparing this route with other regimens to reach a conclusion.

References NICE guideline (CG70). Induction of labour.

LD34

LD34 Answer: A

Explanation Obstetric anal sphincter injury encompasses both third- and fourth-degree perineal tears. The overall risk of obstetric anal sphincter injury is 1 % of all vaginal deliveries. With increased awareness and training, there appears to be an increase in detection of anal sphincter injury.

Obstetricians who are appropriately trained are more likely to provide a consistent, high standard of anal sphincter repair and contribute to reducing the extent of morbidity and litigation associated with anal sphincter injury.

References Green Top guideline third and fourth degree perineal tears.

LD35

LD34 Answer: D

Explanation In women with amniotic fluid embolism, perimortem caesarean section should be carried out within five minutes or as soon as possible after cardiac arrest and is carried out for the benefit of the woman; there is no need to confirm fetal viability, since to do so wastes valuable time.

Pregnant women become hypoxic more quickly than non-pregnant women and irreversible brain damage can ensue after 4–6 min. Delivery of the fetus and placenta facilitates resuscitation; the procedure is performed primarily in the interests of maternal, not fetal, survival (Royal College of Obstetricians and Gynaecologists 2011c).

The basic principles are:

- Take the decision to perform a caesarean section if there is no cardiac output after 4 min of collapse.
- When resuscitation is ongoing, the uterus should be emptied even if there has been delay.
- Aim to deliver the fetus and placenta within 1 min.
- Do it on the spot—do not move to theatre.

- No anaesthetic is necessary.
- A scalpel is the only essential equipment (A pre-mounted scalpel blade and two cord clamps should be kept available on the resuscitation trolley to ensure that there are no delays if perimortem caesarean section is necessary.).
- Use the incision that will give most rapid access (A midline abdominal incision and a classical uterine incision will give the most rapid access, but a transverse approach can be used if the operator is more comfortable with that incision.).
- If resuscitation is successful following delivery, the uterus and abdomen can be closed in the usual manner and the woman transferred to a more appropriate environment.

References Saving lives improving mothers care report 2014.

LD36

LD36 Answer: D

Explanation Clinicians should offer IAP to women with GBS bacteriuria identified during the current pregnancy. GBS bacteriuria is associated with a higher risk of chorioamnionitis and neonatal disease. It is not possible to accurately quantify these increased risks. These women should be offered IAP. Women with GBS urinary tract infection (growth of greater than 105 cfu/ml) during pregnancy should receive appropriate treatment at the time of diagnosis as well as IAP.

References https://www.rcog.org.uk/globalassets/documents/guidelines/gtg36_gbs.pdf

LD37

LD37 Answer: B

Explanation Recent evidence suggests that women with suspected accreta demonstrated significantly reduced short-term morbidity (intensive care unit admission, massive blood transfusion, coagulopathy, urological injury, re-laparotomy) if the placenta was left in place and hysterectomy performed electively compared with attempting to remove the placenta first (36 % compared with 67 %, P=0.038). If the placenta is retained in situ, the woman should be warned of the risks of bleeding and infection postoperatively, and prophylactic antibiotics may be helpful in the immediate post-partum period to reduce this risk. Neither methotrexate nor arterial embolisation reduces these risks and neither is recommended routinely.

References https://www.rcog.org.uk/globalassets/documents/guidelines/gtg_27.pdf

LD38

LD38 Answer: B

Explanation Clinicians should be aware, however, that risk factors do not allow the accurate prediction of OASIS.

The following risk factors have been identified:

Asian ethnicity (OR 2.27, 95 % CI 2.14–2.41)
Nulliparity (relative risk [RR] 6.97, 95 % CI 5.40–8.99)
Birth weight greater than 4 kg (OR 2.27, 95 % CI 2.18–2.36) and shoulder dystocia
    (OR 1.90, 95 % CI 1.72–2.08)
Occipito-posterior position (RR 2.44, 95 % CI 2.07–2.89), duration of second stage
    between 2 and 3 h (RR 1.47, 95 % CI 1.20–1.79), duration of second stage
    between 3 and 4 h (RR 1.79, 95 % CI 1.43–2.22) and duration of second stage
    more than 4 h (RR 2.02, 95 % CI 1.62–2.51)
Ventouse delivery without episiotomy (OR 1.89, 95 % CI 1.74–2.05)
Ventouse delivery with episiotomy (OR 0.57, 95 % CI 0.51–0.63)
Forceps delivery without episiotomy (OR 6.53, 95 % CI 5.57–7.64)
Forceps delivery with episiotomy (OR 1.34, 95 % CI 1.21–1.49).

References https://www.rcog.org.uk/globalassets/documents/guidelines/gtg-29.pdf

LD39

LD 39 Answer: B

Explanation The android type of pelvis favours oblique occipito-posterior position as there is a narrow forepelvis and a roomy hind pelvis which accommodates the occiput. Anthropoid pelvis favours direct occipito-posterior position, whereas platypelloid pelvis favours transverse position of the occiput.

References Arulkumaran et al. Essentials of obstetrics, 2004. 38, p. 307

LD40

LD40 Answer: A

Explanation IAP should be offered to women with a previous baby with neonatal GBS disease. Subsequent infants born to these women are likely to be at increased risk of GBS disease, although this has not been accurately quantified. The probable increase in risk may be attributable to persistence of low levels of maternal anti-GBS antibodies. Vaginal or rectal swabs are not helpful, as IAP would be recommended even if these swabs were negative for GBS.

References https://www.rcog.org.uk/globalassets/documents/guidelines/gtg_36.pdf

LD41

LD 41 Answer: D

Explanation As per NICE

Advise women presenting with prelabour rupture of the membranes at term that:

- 60 % of women with prelabour rupture of the membranes will go into labour within 24 h
- Induction of labour is appropriate approximately 24 h after rupture of the membranes

References https://www.nice.org.uk/guidance/cg190/chapter/1-Recommendations

LD42

LD42 Answer: C

Explanation Recommended methods of induction of labour: membrane sweeping and vaginal PGE2
The following should not be used for induction of labour:

- Oral PGE2
- Intravenous PGE2
- Extra-amniotic PGE2
- Intracervical PGE2
- Intravenous oxytocin alone
- Hyaluronidase
- Corticosteroids
- Oestrogen
- Vaginal nitric oxide donors

Non-pharmacological methods
Healthcare professionals should inform women that the available evidence does not support the following methods for induction of labour:

- Herbal supplements
- Acupuncture
- Homeopathy
- Castor oil
- Hot baths
- Enemas
- Sexual intercourse

Surgical methods

Amniotomy, alone or with oxytocin, should not be used as a primary method of induction of labour unless there are specific clinical reasons for not using vaginal PGE2, in particular the risk of uterine hyperstimulation.

Mechanical methods

Mechanical procedures (balloon catheters and laminaria tents) should not be used routinely for induction of labour.

References NICE guideline (CG70) Induction of labour.

LD43

LD43 Answer: C

Explanation The incidence of breech presentation decreases from about 20 % at 28 weeks of gestation to 3–4 % at term, as most babies turn spontaneously to the cephalic presentation. This appears to be an active process whereby a normally formed and active baby adopts the position of 'best fit' in a normal intrauterine space.

References www.rcog.org.uk/globalassets/documents/guidelin es/gtg-no-20b-breech-presentation.pdf

LD44

LD44 Answer: D

Explanation Antenatal treatment with benzylpenicillin is not recommended. Antenatal prophylaxis with oral benzylpenicillin for vaginal/rectal colonisation does not reduce the likelihood of GBS colonisation at the time of delivery and so is not indicated in this situation. IAP (intrapartum antibiotic prophylaxis) should be offered to GBS-colonised women.

References https://www.rcog.org.uk/globalassets/documents/guidelines/gtg36_gbs.pdf

LD45

LD45 Answer: D

Explanation   Where episiotomy is indicated, the mediolateral technique is recommended, with careful attention to ensure that the angle is 60° away from the midline when the perineum is distended.

References   https://www.rcog.org.uk/globalassets/documents/guidelines/gtg-29.pdf

LD46

LD46 Answer: C

Explanation   Advise women presenting with prelabour rupture of the membranes at term that:

- The risk of serious neonatal infection is 1 %, rather than 0.5 % for women with intact membranes
- Induction of labour is appropriate approximately 24 h after rupture of the membranes

References   https://www.nice.org.uk/guidance/cg190/chapter/1-Recommendations

LD47

LD47 Answer: A

Explanation   As per NICE guidelines

References   https://www.nice.org.uk/guidance/cg190/chapter/1-Recommendations

LD48

LD48 Answer: C

Explanation   Caesarean section should be recommended to all women presenting with primary-episode genital herpes lesions at the time of delivery or within 6 weeks of the expected date of delivery, in order to reduce exposure of the fetus to HSV, which may be present in maternal genital secretions. There is some evidence to suggest that the benefit of caesarean section reduces if the membranes have been ruptured for greater than 4 h. However, there may be some benefit in performing a caesarean section even after this time interval. Where primary-episode genital herpes lesions are present at the time of delivery and the baby is delivered vaginally, the risk of neonatal herpes is estimated to be 41 %.

References https://www.rcog.org.uk/globalassets/documents/guidelines/management-genitalherpes.pdf

LD49

LD49 Answer: D

Explanation Antenatal corticosteroids are most effective in reducing RDS in pregnancies that deliver 24 h after and up to 7 days after administration of the second dose of antenatal corticosteroids.

Antenatal corticosteroid use reduces neonatal death within the first 24 h and therefore should still be given even if delivery is expected within this time.

References RCOG Green Top guideline No. 7. 2010.

LD50

LD 50 Answer: A

Explanation In cases of high fetal head, the operator should consider why the fetal head is high. Attempts should be made to keep the lie longitudinal and the assistant should apply fundal pressure.

Forceps may be required to achieve delivery. Routine use of forceps at caesarean section should be avoided. Again, breech extraction should be considered as a method of achieving delivery.

References Strat OG labour and delivery. https://stratog.rcog.org.uk/tutorial/caesarean-section---teaching-resource/delivery---model-answer-7434

Postpartum Issues: Answers and Explanations

19

PP1

PP1 Answer: E

Explanation Mastitis can occur as a result of milk stasis from engorgement or blocked milk duct or as a consequence of unresolved nipple trauma. Inflammation is typically localised, confined to one lobe, often the upper outer quadrant of the breast. The inflammatory response can lead to localised redness and tenderness, extreme malaise, flu-like symptoms and muscular aching. Local treatment with hot and cold compresses and gentle hand expression can alleviate symptoms, and analgesics and antipyretics are helpful. Women should be advised to not restrict feeding, as good breast drainage will usually alleviate the problem. Antibiotic therapy is rarely necessary, as most cases are non-infective, benign and self-limiting. Infective mastitis should be diagnosed by microbiological techniques to ensure correct treatment. In all cases mothers should be managed symptomatically. Where antibiotic therapy is indicated, prolonged treatment (10–14 days) may be necessary to avoid recurrence.

References Fraser DM, Cullen L. Postnatal management and breastfeeding. Curr Obstet Gynaecol. 2006;16:65–71.

PP2

PP2 Answer: C

Explanation Stress incontinence is the most common urinary problem to occur after childbirth, and studies have demonstrated that the problem can persist for months or even years. Incidence does not appear to be associated with mode of

© Springer India 2016
C. Ratha, J. Gupta, *SBAs and EMQs for MRCOG II*,
DOI 10.1007/978-81-322-2689-5_19

delivery. However, it can affect the physical, psychological and social well-being, and women therefore should be asked about this postnatally. Training in the use of pelvic floor exercises appears to be effective in reducing stress incontinence, and referral to a physiotherapist is recommended.

Detrusor instability is the second most common cause of urinary incontinence in postpartum women. This can be a problem for postnatal mothers, although studies suggest it is more problematic during pregnancy.

The incidence of urinary tract infection after childbirth is around 2–4 %. Risk factors include previous history, caesarean section, instrumental birth, bladder catheterisation and epidural analgesia. A good aseptic technique will reduce the risks. Management consists of appropriate antibiotic therapy and analgesia.

Vesicovaginal fistula is rare in the developed world but should be suspected in women who complain of continuous leakage of urine, particularly if they give a history of traumatic childbirth.

References Fraser DM, Cullen L. Postnatal management and breastfeeding. Curr Obstet Gynaecol. 2006;16:65–71.

PP3

PP3 Answer: D

Explanation The symptoms and signs of VTE include leg pain and swelling (usually unilateral), lower abdominal pain, low-grade pyrexia, dyspnoea, chest pain, haemoptysis and collapse. It is up to ten times more common in pregnant women than in nonpregnant women of the same age and can occur at any stage of pregnancy, but the puerperium is the time of highest risk. When suspected, objective testing should be performed expeditiously and treatment with low-molecular-weight heparin (LMWH) started until the diagnosis is excluded by objective testing, unless treatment is strongly contraindicated. Where there is clinical suspicion of acute PTE, a chest X-ray should be performed. Compression duplex Doppler should be performed where this is normal. If both tests are negative with persistent clinical suspicion of acute PTE, a ventilation–perfusion (V/Q) lung scan or a computed tomography pulmonary angiogram (CTPA) should be performed.

References RCOG Green-Top guideline No. 37b. The acute management of thrombosis and embolism during pregnancy and the puerperium.

PP4

PP4 Answer: E

Explanation Early diagnosis of a uterine scar rupture followed by expeditious laparotomy and resuscitation is essential to reduce associated morbidity and mortality in the mother and infant. There is no single pathognomonic clinical feature that is indicative of uterine rupture, but the presence of any of the following peripartum should raise the concern of the possibility of this event:

- Abnormal CTG
- Severe abdominal pain, especially if persisting between contractions
- Chest pain or shoulder tip pain and sudden onset of shortness of breath
- Acute-onset scar tenderness
- Abnormal vaginal bleeding or haematuria
- Cessation of previously efficient uterine activity
- Maternal tachycardia, hypotension or shock
- Loss of station of the presenting part

The diagnosis is ultimately confirmed at emergency caesarean section or postpartum laparotomy.

References RCOG Green-Top guideline No. 45 – Birth after previous Caesarean birth.

PP5

PP5 Answer: C

Explanation The Royal College of Obstetricians and Gynaecologists (RCOG) guidelines on PPH refer to a blood loss of more than 1000 ml as PPH. This is further subclassified into 'moderate PPH' (1000–2000 ml) and 'severe PPH' (>2000 ml). Loss of >2 L of blood and/or the presence of haemodynamic instability would necessitate a blood transfusion to replace volume and oxygen carrying capacity. In addition, to compensate for the 'washout phenomenon', blood products (clotting factors, fibrinogen and platelets) should be administered. The management of PPH identifies four components, all of which must be undertaken simultaneously.

These are effective communication, resuscitation, monitoring and investigation as well as arresting of bleeding. In addition to these, prompt diagnosis of the aetiology, a 'multidisciplinary' approach, appropriate post-PPH care in ITU or HDU setting and communication with relatives and debriefing of patient form the cornerstones of good clinical care to optimise outcome.

References Moore J, Chandraharan E. Management of massive postpartum haemorrhage and coagulopathy. Obstet Gynaecol Rep Med. 20(6):174–80.

PP6

PP6 Answer: C

Explanation After delivery, the placental bed, caesarean section and episiotomy wounds and cervical and vaginal lacerations are all susceptible to bacterial infection. Prolonged rupture of membranes, prolonged labour, operative vaginal delivery, caesarean section, pre-existing vaginal infection or history of group B streptococcal (GBS) infection, postpartum haemorrhage, wound haematoma, retained pieces of placenta, membranes or intrauterine clot and retained swabs all increase the risk of postpartum infection. The condition presents with lower abdominal pain, fever and offensive vaginal discharge or secondary postpartum haemorrhage. Management consists of broad-spectrum antibiotics with coverage for anaerobic organisms as well.

References Glackin K, Harper M. Postpartum pyrexia. Obstet Gynaecol Rep Med. 22(11):327–31.

PP7

PP7 Answer: C

Explanation A depressive disorder is the single most common psychiatric disorder and affects one in five women over the course of a lifetime and one in ten women during pregnancy. It is just as common in pregnancy as it is postnatal. It is characterised by a depressed mood, decreased lack of interest or enjoyment in things and loss of energy and tiredness. In pregnancy, these last symptoms are less helpful for diagnosis, and NICE promotes the use of the 'Whooley' questions to screen for depression at booking and subsequent antenatal contacts.

References Kent A. Psychiatric disorders in pregnancy. Obstet Gynaecol Rep Med. 21(11):317–22.

PP8

PP8 Answer: D

Explanation If secondary postpartum haemorrhage is significant enough to result in admission into the hospital, treatment falls into two broad categories—drug treatment or surgery or both. The rationale appears to be that the uterus failed to contract adequately to prevent bleeding from the placental site, the underlying cause of this being retained products or intrauterine infection or both. However, the underlying cause is often not known. Drug therapy consists of antibiotics, syntocinon or both; hormonal preparations may be used to regulate cycles. Surgical management may involve evacuation of retained products of conception, repair of cervical tear or uterine rupture, treatment of molar pregnancy or, rarely, hysterectomy.

References Alexander J, Thomas PW, Sanghera J. Treatments for secondary post partum haemorrhage. Cochrane database of systematic reviews 2002. Issue 1. Art no: CD002867.

PP9

PP9 Answer: C

Explanation Mature breast milk contains 3–5 % fat, 0.8–0.9 % protein and 6.9–7.2 % carbohydrate with energy content of 65–75 kCal/100 ml. Protein content is markedly higher and carbohydrate content lower in colostrum than in mature milk. Fat content does not vary consistently during lactation.

References Jenness R. The composition of human milk. Semin Perinatol. 1979;3(3):225–39. Subject: Postpartum problems.

PP10

PP10 Answer: D

Explanation Caloric needs vary depending on age, just as nutrient needs. Healthy full-term neonates require, on average, 120 Kcal/day to meet energy needs and sustain growth. On a per kilogram basis, requirement reduces with age. Once growth has ceased, caloric requirements are impacted by age, activity and other health factors but can be approximated at 1500 Kcal/m^2/day.

References http://www.nichd.nih.gov/health/topics/breastfeeding/conditioninfo/pages/dga.aspx

PP11

PP11 Answer: A

Explanation Anaemia in pregnancy is defined as first trimester haemoglobin (Hb) less than 110 g/l, second/third trimester Hb less than 105 g/l and postpartum Hb less than 100 g/l, in line with the British Committee for Standards in Haematology (BCSH) guidance.

References Green-Top guideline No. 47. Blood transfusion in obstetrics. https://www.rcog.org.uk/globalassets/documents/guidelines/gtg-47.pdf

PP12

PP12 Answer: C

Explanation The most likely diagnosis is a degree of altered perineal/vaginal architecture as a result of childbirth trauma. Her psychological or psychosexual history may be relevant. Management depends on the findings during genital examination. The use of lubricants is likely to be of benefit in this woman's case as she is breastfeeding. If there is no localised tenderness, the vagina may be atrophic and local oestrogen application can be tried empirically. Localised scar tenderness can be treated by application of lidocaine ointment approximately 30 min prior to intercourse . Vaginal dilators may be used with lidocaine ointment if there is some degree of stenosis; if this fails, injection of a steroid, such as depot medrone, can be injected into the scar, and if necessary this can be repeated after 3 months. Surgical refashioning of the perineum is rarely indicated.

References Strat OG perineal and vaginal surgery. https://stratog.rcog.org.uk/tutorial/perineal-and-vaginal-surgery---teachingresource/model-answer-7180

PP13

PP13 Answer: D

Explanation Antepartum haemorrhage (APH) is defined as bleeding from or into the genital tract, occurring from 24+0 weeks of pregnancy and prior to the birth of the baby. The most important causes of APH are placenta praevia and placental abruption, although these are not the most common. APH complicates 3–5 % of pregnancies and is a leading cause of perinatal and maternal mortality worldwide. A number of clinical and epidemiological studies have identified predisposing risk factors for placental abruption. The most predictive is abruption in a previous pregnancy. A large observational study from Norway reported a 4.4 % incidence of recurrent abruption (adjusted OR 7.8, 95% CI 6.5–9.2). Abruption recurs in 19–25 % of women who have had two previous pregnancies complicated by abruption.

References RCOG Green-Top guideline No 63. Antepartum hemorrhage. 2011.

PP14

PP14 Answer: C

Explanation

Table 3. Tasks to be performed within the first 6 hours of the identification of severe sepsis; modified from the Surviving Sepsis Campaign Resuscitation Bundles[?]

Obtain blood cultures prior to antibiotic administration

Administer broad-spectrum antibiotic within 1 hour of recognition of severe sepsis

Measure serum lactate

In the event of hypotension and/or a serum lactate greater than 4 mmol/l:
  Deliver an initial minimum 20 ml/kg of crystalloid or an equivalent
  Apply vasopressors for hypotension not responding to initial fluid resuscitation to maintain mean arterial pressure above 65 mmHg

In the event of persistent hypotension despite fluid resuscitation (septic shock) and/or serum lactate greater than 4 mmol/l:
  Achieve a central venous pressure of ≥ 8 mmHg
  Achieve a central venous oxygen saturation ≥ 70% or mixed venous oxygen saturation ≥ 65%

References https://www.rcog.org.uk/globalassets/documents/guidelines/gtg_64b.pdf

PP15

PP15 Answer: D

Explanation For women who were diagnosed with gestational diabetes and whose blood glucose levels returned to normal after the birth:

- Offer lifestyle advice (including weight control, diet and exercise).
- Offer a fasting plasma glucose test 6–13 weeks after the birth to exclude diabetes (for practical reasons this might take place at the 6-week postnatal check).
  Do not routinely offer a 75 g 2-h OGTT.

References https://www.nice.org.uk/guidance/ng3

PP16

PP16 Answer: B

Explanation Labetelol cannot be used as she is asthmatic. In women who still need antihypertensive treatment in the postnatal period, avoid diuretic treatment for hypertension if the woman is breastfeeding or expressing milk.

Tell women who still need antihypertensive treatment in the postnatal period that the following antihypertensive drugs have no known adverse effects on babies receiving breast milk:

- labetalol
- Nifedipine
- Enalapril
- Captopril
- Atenolol
- Metoprolol

Tell women who still need antihypertensive treatment in the postnatal period that there is insufficient evidence on the safety in babies receiving breast milk of the following antihypertensive drugs:

- ARBs (angiotensin receptor blockers)
- Amlodipine
- ACE inhibitors other than enalapril and captopril.

References http://www.nice.org.uk/guidance/cg107/chapter/1-Guidance

---

PP17

PP17 Answer: D

Explanation Serum lactate should be measured within 6 h of the suspicion of severe sepsis to guide management. Serum lactate ≥4 mmol/l is indicative of tissue hypoperfusion.

References https://www.rcog.org.uk/globalassets/documents/guidelines/gtg_64b.pdf

PP18

PP18Answer: E

Explanation Administration of intravenous broad-spectrum antibiotics within 1 h of suspicion of severe sepsis, with or without septic shock, is recommended as part of the surviving sepsis resuscitation care bundle. If genital tract sepsis is suspected, prompt early treatment with a combination of high-dose broad-spectrum intravenous antibiotics may be life-saving. A combination of either piperacillin/tazobactam or a carbapenem plus clindamycin provides one of the broadest ranges of treatment for severe sepsis.

References https://www.rcog.org.uk/globalassets/documents/guidelines/gtg_64b.pdf

PP19

PP19 Answer: C

Explanation Following birth of a D-positive infant, at least 500 iu anti-D, i.m., must be administered to the woman if the FMH is ≤4 mL. Additional dose of anti-D immunoglobulin is necessary for larger FMH, and the dose to be administered by intramuscular route should be calculated as 125 i.u for each additional mL of FMH. In cases of very large FMH, i.e. in excess of 80 mLs, intravenous anti-D should be considered.

References http://www.bcshguidelines.com/documents/Anti-D_bcsh_07062006.pdf

PP20

PP20 Answer: A

Explanation Cabergoline is a dopamine agonist which decreases prolactin in circulation. Cabergoline is used to treat hyperprolactinemia which can cause symptoms such as infertility, sexual problems and bone loss in women who are not breastfeeding. Use of this drug in breastfeeding women would cause failure of lactation and is hence contraindicated. This has been shown to be more effective than bromocriptine in lowering prolactin levels, with substantially fewer adverse effects and higher patient compliance when used in hyperprolactinaemia.

References Hamoda H, Khalaf Y, Carroll P. Hyperprolactinaemia and female reproductive function: what does the evidence say? Obstet Gynaecol. 2012;14:81–6.

PP21

PP21 Answer: D

Explanation Therapeutic anticoagulant therapy should be continued for the duration of the pregnancy and for at least 6 weeks postnatally and until at least 3 months of treatment has been given in total. Before discontinuing treatment the continuing risk of thrombosis should be assessed. Women should be offered a choice of LMWH or oral anticoagulant for postnatal therapy after discussion about the need for regular blood tests for monitoring of warfarin, particularly during the first 10 days of treatment.

Postpartum warfarin should be avoided until at least the fifth day and for longer in women at increased risk of postpartum haemorrhage. Women should be advised that neither heparin (unfractionated or LMWH) nor warfarin is contraindicated in breastfeeding

References https://www.rcog.org.uk/globalassets/documents/guidelines/gtg-37b.pdf

PP22

PP22 Answer: E

Explanation The major pathogens causing sepsis in the puerperium are GAS, also known as *Streptococcus pyogenes*, *Escherichia coli*, *Staphylococcus aureus*, *Streptococcus pneumonia*, methicillin-resistant *S. aureus* (MRSA), *Clostridium septicum* and *Morganella morganii*.

References https://www.rcog.org.uk/globalassets/documents/guidelines/gtg_64b.pdf

PP23

PP23 Answer: D

Explanation Women should be advised that 60–80 % of women are asymptomatic 12 months following delivery and EAS repair.

References https://www.rcog.org.uk/globalassets/documents/guidelines/gtg-29. pdf

Early Pregnancy Care: Answers and Explanations

20

EP1

EP1 Answer: D

Explanation The incidence of clinically recognised miscarriage remains around 10–20 %, though post-implantation and biochemical pregnancy loss rates appear to be in the order of 30 %. The majority of miscarriages occur early, before 12 weeks of pregnancy. Second trimester pregnancy loss contributes to less than 4 % of pregnancy losses, and less than 5 % of miscarriages occur after identification of fetal heart activity. In the UK, miscarriage is defined as the loss of an intrauterine pregnancy before 24 completed weeks of gestation.

References 1. Saraswat L, Ashok PW, Mathur M. Medical management of miscarriage. Obstet Gynaecol. 2014;16:79–85.

2. Alberman E. Spontaneous abortions: epidemiology. In: Stabile I, Grudzinskas JG, Chard T, editors. Spontaneous abortion: diagnosis and treatment. London: Springer; 1992. p. 9–20.

EP2

EP2 Answer: A

Explanation Bleeding in early pregnancy is the most common reason for women to present to the gynaecology emergency department, and miscarriage alone accounts for 50,000 of inpatient admissions to hospitals in the UK annually

© Springer India 2016
C. Ratha, J. Gupta, *SBAs and EMQs for MRCOG II*,
DOI 10.1007/978-81-322-2689-5_20

References 1. Saraswat L, Ashok PW, Mathur M. Medical management of miscarriage. Obstet Gynaecol. 2014;16:79–85.

2. Bradley E, Hamilton-Fairley D. Managing miscarriage in early pregnancy assessment units. Hosp Med. 1998;59:451–6.

EP3

EP3 Answer: B

Explanation Routes of misoprostol administration include oral, vaginal, sublingual, buccal or rectal. This medication is not administered in injectable form. There are many studies comparing the pharmacokinetics of misoprostol in various modes of administration.

Vaginal misoprostol is associated with slower absorption, lower peak plasma levels and slower clearance, similar to an extended-release preparation.

The rectal route of administration shows a similar pattern to vaginal administration but has a lower AUC, including a significantly lower maximum peak concentration. The sublingual route of administration has an AUC similar to that of vaginal administration but more rapid absorption (higher T_{max}) and higher peak levels (C_{max}) than either vaginal or oral administration.

The buccal route is another mode of administration—the drug is placed between the teeth and the cheek and absorbed through the buccal mucosa. The absorption rate (T_{max}) after the buccal administration is the same as after vaginal administration, but the serum drug levels attained are much lower with the AUC being half that of the vaginal route.

References 1. Khan RU, El-Refaey H, Sharma S, Sooranna D, Stafford M. Oral, rectal, and vaginal pharmacokinetics of misoprostol. Obstet Gynecol. 2004;103:866–70.

2. Danielsson KG, Marions L, Rodriguez A, Spur BW, Wong PY, Bygdeman M. Comparison between oral and vaginal administration of misoprostol on uterine contractility. Obstet Gynecol. 1999;93:275–80.

EP4

EP4 Answer: A

Explanation Diagnosis of miscarriage using just one ultrasound scan cannot be guaranteed to be 100 % accurate and there is a small chance that the diagnosis may be incorrect, particularly at very early gestational ages.

According to the NICE guideline, if the crown-rump length is 7.0 mm or more with a transvaginal ultrasound scan and there is no visible heartbeat, seek a second opinion on the viability of the pregnancy and/or perform a second scan a minimum of 7 days after the first before making a diagnosis.

If the mean gestational sac diameter is less than 25.0 mm with a transvaginal ultrasound scan and there is no visible fetal pole, perform a second scan a minimum of 7 days after the first before making a diagnosis. Further scans may be needed before a diagnosis can be made.

References https://www.nice.org.uk/guidance/CG154/chapter/ 1-Recommendations#symptoms-and-signs-of-ectopic-pregnancy-and-initial- assessment-2

EP5

EP5 Answer: C

Explanation It is defined as bleeding without passage of tissue but with an open cervix. The patient may be managed by expectant, medical or surgical management. Surgical evacuation remains the treatment of choice if bleeding is excessive, vital signs are unstable or infected tissue is present in the uterine cavity (in which case surgery must be done under antibiotic cover). Fewer than 10 % of women who miscarry fall into these categories. Expectant management can be continued as long as the woman is willing and provided there are no signs of infection. For medical management, a variety of equally effective prostaglandin regimens have been described, including Gemeprost 0.5–1 mg, vaginal misoprostol and oral misoprostol. However, vaginal misoprostol is as effective as oral misoprostol, with a significant reduction in the incidence of diarrhoea. Success rates varied from 61 to 95 %, mild to moderate bleeding lasted 4–6 days, side effects were tolerable in 96 %, and satisfaction rates were 95 %.   *miso = 95%*

References Sagili H, Divers M. Modern management of miscarriage. Obstet Gynaecol. 2007;9:102–8.

EP6

EP6 Answer: B

Explanation The NICE guideline recommends offering systemic methotrexate as a first-line treatment to women who are able to return for follow-up and who have all of the following:

- No significant pain
- An unruptured ectopic pregnancy with an adnexal mass smaller than 35 mm with no visible heartbeat

– A serum hCG level less than 1500 IU/l
– No intrauterine pregnancy (as confirmed on an ultrasound scan)

References http://www.nice.org.uk/guidance/CG154/chapter/
1-Recommendations#management-of-ectopic-pregnancy

EP7

EP7 Answer: E

Explanation The serial measurement of serum hCG is particularly useful in the diagnosis of asymptomatic ectopic pregnancy (grade B recommendation) and pregnancy of unknown location. The use of a 'discriminatory zone' for serum hCG above which an intrauterine pregnancy should be expected to be seen is recommended and employed by most units. An ectopic pregnancy will usually be visualised on transvaginal ultrasound when the hCG level is above 1500 iu/L but often occurs in association with lower levels, particularly those that plateau. The absence of an intrauterine gestation sac and an hCG titre of between 1000 and 1500 iu/L has been shown to be highly predictive of ectopic pregnancy (sensitivity 0–95 %, specificity 95 %). When repeated 48 h later, the expected rise in values is >63 %, and then the possibility of a developing intrauterine pregnancy is higher (although an ectopic pregnancy cannot be excluded). For a woman with a decrease in serum hCG concentration greater than 50 % after 48 h, the pregnancy is unlikely to continue but that cannot be confirmed. A repeat pregnancy test needs to be done after 2 weeks to confirm negative.

References 1. Raine-Fenning N, Hopkisson J. Management of ectopic pregnancy: a clinical approach. Obstet Gynecol Rep Med. 19(1):19–24.
2. http://www.nice.org.uk/guidance/CG154/chapter/
1-Recommendations#management-of-ectopic-pregnancy

EP8

EP8 Answer: C

Explanation The above scenario relates to a stable patient, with a single TV scan which shows a CRL of less than 7 mm, which means the absence of a fetal heart does not indicate miscarriage. She requires a rescan in 7–10 days to confirm either miscarriage or viability. It is not appropriate to label this as a miscarriage and manage it, neither is it appropriate to scan again after only 2 days as the interval is too short.

References http://www.nice.org.uk/guidance/CG154/chapter/1-Recommendations

EP9

EP9 Answer: E

Explanation Be aware that atypical presentation for ectopic pregnancy is common. Be aware that ectopic pregnancy can present with a variety of symptoms. Even if a symptom is less common, it may still be significant. Symptoms of ectopic pregnancy include:

1. Common symptoms: abdominal or pelvic pain, amenorrhoea or missed period and vaginal bleeding with or without clots
2. Other reported symptoms: breast tenderness, gastrointestinal symptoms, dizziness, fainting or syncope, shoulder tip pain, urinary symptoms, passage of tissue, rectal pressure or pain on defecation

References http://www.nice.org.uk/guidance/CG154/chapter/1-Recommendations

EP10

EP10 Answer: D

Explanation The ultrasound diagnosis of a partial molar pregnancy is more complex; the finding of multiple soft markers, including both cystic spaces in the placenta and a ratio of transverse to anteroposterior dimension of the gestation sac of greater than 1.5, is required for the reliable diagnosis of a partial molar pregnancy.

References RCOG Green-Top guideline No. 38. Gestational trophoblastic disease. https://www.rcog.org.uk/en/guidelines-research-services/guidelines/gtg38/

EP11

EP11 Answer: B

Explanation If the crown-rump length is 7.0 mm or more with a transvaginal ultrasound scan and there is no visible heartbeat, seek a second opinion on the viability of the pregnancy and/or perform a second scan a minimum of 7 days after the first before making a diagnosis.

References https://www.nice.org.uk/guidance/cg154/chapter/1-Recommendations#diagnosis-of-viable-intrauterine-pregnancy-and-of-ectopic-pregnancy

EP12

EP12 Answer: B

Explanation Do not offer mifepristone as a treatment for missed or incomplete miscarriage. For women with a missed miscarriage, use a single dose of 800 µg of misoprostol. Offer all women receiving medical management of miscarriage pain relief and anti-emetics as needed.

References https://www.nice.org.uk/guidance/cg154/chapter/1-Recommendations#diagnosis-of-viable-intrauterine-pregnancy-and-of-ectopic-pregnancy

EP13

EP13 Answer: B

Explanation If the mean gestational sac diameter is 25.0 mm or more using a transvaginal ultrasound scan and there is no visible fetal pole:

- Seek a second opinion on the viability of the pregnancy.
- Perform a second scan a minimum of 7 days after the first before making a diagnosis.

References https://www.nice.org.uk/guidance/cg154/chapter/1-Recommendations#diagnosis-of-viable-intrauterine-pregnancy-and-of-ectopic-pregnancy

EP14

EP14 Answer: C

Expanation In pregnancies <12 weeks' gestation, anti-D Ig prophylaxis is only indicated following ectopic pregnancy, molar pregnancy, therapeutic termination of pregnancy and, in cases of uterine bleeding where this is repeated, heavy or associated with abdominal pain. The minimum dose should be 250 IU. A test for fetomaternal haemorrhage (FMH) is not required. Following potentially sensitising events, anti-D Ig should be administered as soon as possible and always within 72 h of the event. If, exceptionally, this deadline has not been met, some protection may be offered if anti-D Ig is given up to 10 days after the sensitising event.

References BCSH guideline for the use of anti-D immunoglobulin for the prevention of haemolytic disease of the fetus and newborn. http://onlinelibrary.wiley.com/enhanced/doi/10.1111/tme.12091/

EP15

EP15 Answer: C

Explanation Excessive vaginal bleeding can be associated with molar pregnancy. There is theoretical concern over the routine use of potent oxytocic agents because of the potential to embolise and disseminate trophoblastic tissue through the venous system. To control life-threatening bleeding, oxytocic infusions may be used.

References RCOG Green-Top guideline No. 38. Gestational trophoblastic disease. https://www.rcog.org.uk/en/guidelines-research-services/guidelines/gtg38/

EP16

EP16 Answer: B

Explanation hCG or serum progesterone should be not be used alone or as an adjunct to determine the location of pregnancy, as it is important to also evaluate presenting clinical signs and symptoms. Mifepristone should not be used in the cases of missed abortion or incomplete abortion. Post salpingotomy, one in five patients may need further treatment in the form of methotrexate or salpingectomy.

References NICE clinical guideline 154. Ectopic pregnancy and miscarriage. 2012. http://www.nice.org.uk/guidance/CG154/chapter/1-Recommendations

EP17

EP17 Answer: E

Explanation The revised criteria for medical management of ectopic pregnancy according to the NICE guidelines:

- Sac size <35 mm
- No cardiac activity
- hCG <1500 IU/ml

- No pain
- No intrauterine pregnancy

References NICE clinical guideline 154. Ectopic pregnancy and miscarriage. 2012. http://www.nice.org.uk/guidance/CG154/chapter/1-Recommendations

EP18

EP18 Answer: D

Explanation GTD (hydatidiform mole, invasive mole, choriocarcinoma, placental-site trophoblastic tumour) is a rare event in the UK, with a calculated incidence of 1/714 live births. There is evidence of ethnic variation in the incidence of GTD in the UK, with women from Asia having a higher incidence compared with non-Asian women (1/387 versus 1/752 live births). However, these figures may under-represent the true incidence of the disease because of problems with reporting, particularly in regard to partial moles. GTN may develop after a molar pregnancy, a non-molar pregnancy or a live birth. The incidence after a live birth is estimated at 1/50,000. Because of the rarity of the problem, an average consultant obstetrician and gynaecologist may deal with only one new case of molar pregnancy every second year.

References 1. RCOG Green-Top guideline No. 38. Gestational trophoblastic disease. https://www.rcog.org.uk/en/guidelines-research-services/guidelines/gtg38/

2. Tham BWL, et al. Gestational trophoblastic disease in the Asian population of Northern England and North Wales. BJOG. 2003;110:555–9.

EP19

EP19 Answer: A

Explanation Gestational trophoblastic disease (GTD) forms a group of disorders spanning the conditions of complete and partial molar pregnancies through to the malignant conditions of invasive mole, choriocarcinoma and the very rare placental-site trophoblastic tumour (PSTT). There are reports of neoplastic transformation of atypical placental-site nodules to placental-site trophoblastic tumour.

If there is any evidence of persistence of GTD, most commonly defined as a persistent elevation of beta human chorionic gonadotrophin (βhCG), the condition is referred to as gestational trophoblastic neoplasia (GTN).

Molar pregnancies can be subdivided into complete (CM) and partial moles (PM) based on genetic and histopathological features. Complete moles are diploid and androgenic in origin, with no evidence of fetal tissue.

Chorioangioma is a vascular malformation in the placenta unrelated to GTD

References RCOG Green-Top guideline No. 38. Gestational trophoblastic disease. https://www.rcog.org.uk/en/guidelines-research-services/guidelines/gtg38/

EP20

EP20 Answer: E

Explanation Complete moles usually (75–80 %) arise as a consequence of duplication of a single sperm following fertilisation of an 'empty' ovum. Some complete moles (20–25 %) can arise after dispermic fertilisation of an 'empty' ovum. Partial moles are usually (90 %) triploid in origin, with two sets of paternal haploid genes and one set of maternal haploid genes. Partial moles occur, in almost all cases, following dispermic fertilisation of an ovum. Ten percent of partial moles represent tetraploid or mosaic conceptions. In a partial mole, there is usually evidence of a fetus or fetal red blood cells.

References RCOG Green-Top guideline No. 38. Gestational trophoblastic disease. https://www.rcog.org.uk/en/guidelines-research-services/guidelines/gtg38/

Gynaecological Problems: Answers and Explanations

21

GYN1

GYN1 Answer: E

Explanation Compounds with both agonist and antagonist properties on the progesterone receptor (PR) and fewer antiglucocorticoid properties are classified as selective progesterone receptor modulators (SPRMs). SPRMs have been shown to have an antagonistic effect on endometrial and breast tissue PRs without influencing the effect of oestrogen on endometrial and breast tissue. Mifepristone and ulipristal acetate are the only SPRMs currently licensed for use in the UK; however, other SPRMs have been or are currently being developed and undergoing trial. Raloxifene and ormeloxifene are SERMs (selective oestrogen receptor modulators). Misoprostol and dinoprostone are prostaglandins.

References Murdoch M, Roberts M. Selective progesterone receptor modulators and their use within gynaecology. Obstet Gynaecol. 2014;16:46–50.

GYN2

GYN2 Answer: C

Explanation Uterine fibroids (leiomyomas or myomas) are benign tumours of smooth muscle cells and fibrous tissue that develop within the wall of the uterus. They are the most common tumours of the female genital tract present in 20–40 % of women in the reproductive age group. Treatment is often only required if the woman is symptomatic and is dependent on symptoms. If the woman has heavy menstrual bleeding, the National Institute for Health and Care Excellence (NICE) recommends consideration of pharmaceutical treatment when fibroids are less than 3 cm in diameter and causing no distortion of the uterine cavity

References National Institute for Health and Care Excellence. Heavy menstrual bleeding. (CG44) London: National Institute for Health and Care Excellence; 2007.

GYN3

GYN3 Answer: D

Explanation Chronic pelvic pain (CPP) is a common condition in women of reproductive age. Current data from the USA and UK suggest that it occurs in 14–24 % of women aged between 18 and 50 years. It is a common condition at the population level. Further work has indicated that rates of consultation for CPP in general practice are similar to those for asthma and migraine. The USA and UK population-based studies, together with data from UK hospital settings, demonstrate a substantial impact of CPP on health-related quality of life. The differences in estimated prevalence may be due to the design and type of study performed, for example, the use of different definitions of the condition.

References Cheong Y, Stones RW. Management of chronic pelvic pain: evidence from randomised controlled trials. Obstet Gynaecol. 2006;8:32–8.

GYN4

GYN4 Answer: D

Explanation Typical laparoscopic findings in women investigated for CPP are, in increasing order of frequency, adhesions (24 %), endometriosis (33 %) and 'no pathology' (35 %). Patterns of symptoms and received diagnosis in the population-based studies cited above suggest a broad pattern of pathophysiology, with urinary (31 %) and gastrointestinal (37 %) problems being more common than specifically gynaecological (20 %) problems.

References Cheong Y, Stones RW. Management of chronic pelvic pain: evidence from randomised controlled trials. Obstet Gynaecol. 2006;8:32–8.

GYN5

GYN5 Answer: A

Explanation Incidentally detected ovarian pathology at the time of caesarean section is rare. However, when detected, it is necessary to differentiate benign from malignant. Ultrasound is the commonly used tool, and complex, septate mass with mural nodules and papillary projections is highly suggestive of malignancy. Unilocular thin-walled anechoic cysts, measuring <5 cm in diameter, have a 90–100 % chance of regression. If suspected to be benign, a policy of 'wait and watch' can be adopted keeping in mind the complications that may occur. And these include cyst rupture, cyst haemorrhage, torsion (up to 5 %), obstructed labour and fetal malpresentation.

References Spencer CP, Robarts PJ. Management of adnexal masses in pregnancy. Obstet Gynaecol. 2006;8:14–9.

GYN6

GYN6 Answer: D

Explanation The indications for surgery will depend on the degree of suspicion of malignancy in the mass or the development of cyst complications. If there is doubt regarding the diagnosis, MRI can prove useful as a tool to help distinguish dermoids and endometriomas from malignant neoplasms. If elective surgery is embarked upon, this should be done after 14 weeks' gestation to minimise the risk of fetal loss due to miscarriage, although this risk is very small. This recommendation is based on the principle that the developing pregnancy is dependent on the corpus luteum during the first trimester and much less so after 12 weeks. The standard approach is to perform the surgery via a laparotomy, but laparoscopic surgery has been used, although it is skill dependent and more time-consuming than open surgery.

References Spencer CP, Robarts PJ. Management of adnexal masses in pregnancy. Obstet Gynaecol. 2006;8:14–9.

GYN7

GYN 7 Answer: C

Explanation Simple cysts smaller than 5 cm regress in 90–100 % of cases and can be safely observed. These cysts do not need further evaluation, and rescanning is only required if there is a clinical indication, such as pelvic pain. Adnexal masses that undergo torsion are usually dermoids or cystadenomas. If this complication occurs, it does so during the first trimester or in the immediate puerperium (up to 14 days after delivery). Ovarian dermoids that measure less than 6 cm are unlikely to grow significantly in pregnancy and can be managed conservatively as the risk of complications, such as torsion, is thought to be low. The woman should be rescanned in the postnatal period to determine further management of any ovarian dermoid that has not resolved spontaneously.

Persistent, simple, unilocular cysts without any solid elements that are larger than 10 cm can be aspirated either transvaginally or abdominally under ultrasound guidance using a fine needle (greater than 20 gauge). This procedure is only indicated if the cyst is causing pain or thought to be increasing the risks of fetal malpresentation or obstructed labour due to its location in the pelvis. Although not commonly employed, this technique seems to be a reasonable alternative to surgery in suitable women. The woman should be subsequently rescanned to determine whether cyst recurrence has taken place, and the risk of this is thought to be 33–50 %, and the mother should therefore be counselled that further aspirations can be required during the rest of the pregnancy.

References Spencer CP, Robarts PJ. Management of adnexal masses in pregnancy. Obstet Gynaecol. 2006;8:14–9.

GYN8

GYN 8 Answer: B

Explanation Nipple discharge is a common presentation to a breast clinic. In one study over 32 years, 4.8 % of women presented with nipple discharge, although only 2.6 % occurred spontaneously. Controversy surrounds the management of such patients including their initial investigations through to the requirement and type of surgery. The surgical options for the treatment of nipple discharge are either single or multiple duct excision. It is recommended that major duct excision in women over 45 years is a safe, effective procedure with good cosmesis when performed well and provision of maximal histological information. However, several studies advocate microdochectomy as the treatment of choice with minimal morbidity and few missed cases of malignancy and may be performed under local anaesthetic. Studies demonstrate that 3.8 % of patients may have associated malignancy.

References Burton S, Li W-Y, Himpson R, Sulieman S, Ball A. Microdochectomy in women aged over 50 years. Ann R Coll Surg Engl. 2003; 85:47–50

GYN9

GYN9 Answer: A

Explanation Women presenting with PCOS (particularly if they are obese, have a strong family history of type 2 diabetes or are over the age of 40 years) are at increased risk of type 2 diabetes and should be offered a glucose tolerance test. Oligo- or amenorrhoea in women with PCOS may predispose to endometrial hyperplasia and later carcinoma. It is good practice to recommend treatment with progestogens for at least 12 days to induce a withdrawal bleed at least every 3–4 months. 60–85 % of patients will ovulate on clomiphene citrate.

References Royal College of Obstetricians and Gynaecologists. Long term consequences of polycystic ovary syndrome. Green-Top guideline No. 33. London: RCOG Press. 2007. Available at http://www.rcog.org.uk/files/rcog-corp/uploaded-files/GT33_LongTermPCOS.pdf

SOGC Clinical Practice Guideline. Ovulation induction in polycystic ovary syndrome. 2010. Available at http://sogc.org/wp-content/uploads/2013/01/gui242CPG1005E_000.pdf

GYN10

GYN10 Answer: A

Explanation Pregnancy outcomes in patients post-UAE include increased preterm delivery rate up to 20 % and caesarean section rates up to 80 %. Only about 1/3 of the patients deliver vaginally. In addition there are increased chances of malpresentations and postpartum haemorrhage. There is significantly higher miscarriage rate following UAE for fibroids than for women with untreated fibroids, thought to be due to relative endometrial ischaemia and distortion of uterine cavity.

References Pregnancy outcomes after uterine artery embolisation for fibroids. TOG. 2009;11:265–70.

GYN11

GYN11 Answer: C

Explanation While the diagnosis of molar pregnancy is rare, there are two groups of women who have significantly elevated risks of developing a molar pregnancy. At the extremes of the reproductive age, girls under the age of 15 years have a risk approximately 20 times higher than women aged 20–40, while women aged over 45 have a several hundredfold higher risk than those aged 20–40. The increased risk for these groups is mainly for complete molar pregnancy, with the incidence of partial molar pregnancy changing less across the age groups.

The second group of women with an increased risk of molar pregnancy are those who have had a molar pregnancy previously. In this group, the risk appears to be approximately 1 in 55 for those with one previous molar pregnancy and 1 in 10 for those with two.

In the first few months of pregnancy, molar pregnancy is associated with a higher incidence of vaginal bleeding or discharge, abdominal pain and morning sickness. However, as these symptoms are relatively nonspecific, they rarely lead to the diagnosis being made prior to the routine first ultrasound scan.

In complete molar pregnancy, the ultrasound characteristically shows an absent gestational sac and a complex echogenic intrauterine mass with cystic spaces. In contrast, the ultrasound of a partial molar pregnancy may resemble a normal conception with an embryo visible. As the diagnosis of a partial molar pregnancy is frequently difficult to make on the initial ultrasound, a significant proportion of these women present later with early pregnancy loss, with the diagnosis achieved histologically.

References   Savage P. Molar pregnancy. Obstet Gynaecol. 2008;10:3–8.

GYN12

GYN12 Answer: E

Explanation It is recommended that ovarian cysts in postmenopausal women should be assessed using CA125 and transvaginal greyscale sonography. There is no routine role yet for Doppler, MRI, CT or PET. Serum CA125 is well established, being raised in over 80 % of ovarian cancer cases, and, if a cut-off of 30 u/ml is used, the test has a sensitivity of 81 % and specificity of 75 %. Ultrasound is also well established, achieving a sensitivity of 89 % and specificity of 73 % when using a morphology index. Ovarian cysts should normally be assessed using transvaginal ultrasound, as this appears to provide more detail and hence offers greater sensitivity than the transabdominal method. Larger cysts may also need to be assessed transabdominally.

References   https://www.rcog.org.uk/globalassets/documents/guidelines/gtg34ovariancysts.pdf

GYN13

GYN13 Answer: C

Explanation One generally accepted definition of an ovarian cyst – 'it is a fluid-containing structure more than 30 mm in diameter'. Women with simple cystic structures less than 50 mm generally do not require follow-up as these cysts are very likely to be physiological and almost always resolve within three menstrual cycles. The Society of Radiologists in Ultrasound published a consensus statement concluding that asymptomatic simple cysts 30–50 mm in diameter do not require follow-up, cysts 50–70 mm require follow-up and cysts more than 70 mm in diameter should be considered for either further imaging (MRI) or surgical intervention due to difficulties in examining the entire cyst adequately at time of ultrasound. A recent Cochrane review of the effects of the oral contraceptive pill in the treatment of functional ovarian cysts concluded that there was no earlier resolution in the treatment group compared to the control group.

References https://www.rcog.org.uk/globalassets/documents/guidelines/gtg_62.pdf

GYN14

GYN14 Answer: E

Explanation Oligo- or amenorrhoea in women with PCOS may predispose to endometrial hyperplasia and later carcinoma. It is good practice to recommend treatment with gestagens to induce a withdrawal bleed at least every 3–4 months. Transvaginal ultrasound should be considered in the absence of withdrawal bleeds or abnormal uterine bleeding. In PCOS, an endometrial thickness of less than 7 mm is unlikely to be hyperplasia. A thickened endometrium or an endometrial polyp should prompt consideration of endometrial biopsy and/or hysteroscopy. There does not appear to be an association with breast or ovarian cancer and no additional surveillance is required.

References https://www.rcog.org.uk/globalassets/documents/guidelines/gtg_33.pdf

GYN15

GYN15 Answer: C

Explanation *Actinomyces*-like organisms (ALOs) require no specific intervention in the vast majority of patients and are usually seen in patients using an intrauterine contraceptive device (including the Mirena IUS). If the patient complains of specific symptoms, the device may need to be removed, after first ensuring that the patient has not had sexual intercourse in the preceding five days. These symptoms include:

- Pelvic pain
- Deep dyspareunia
- Intermenstrual bleeding (after six months of a device being in situ)
- Vaginal discharge, dysuria or significant pelvic tenderness.

If the device is removed because the woman has any of the above symptoms:

- The device should be sent for culture and alternative contraception advised.
- A course of antibiotics (such as amoxicillin 250 mg three times daily for two weeks or erythromycin 500 mg three times daily for two weeks in penicillin-sensitive patients) should be given and a gynaecological opinion arranged to ensure that the symptoms or signs have resolved.

References http://www.cancerscreening.nhs.uk/cervical/publications/nhscsp20.pdf

GYN16

GYN16 Answer: C

Explanation Endometrial polyps are rare among women under the age of 20 years. The incidence rises steadily with increasing age, peaks in the fifth decade of life and gradually declines after the menopause. With the increased use of pelvic ultrasonography as a basic investigation for gynaecological conditions, incidental endometrial polyps are diagnosed more frequently, which can pose a dilemma for women and for gynaecologists. The presence of endometrial polyps in postmenopausal women can lead to anxiety about malignancy, even though the malignant potential of endometrial polyps is low.

The aetiology of endometrial polyps is unknown, but their close relationship with the background endometrium is demonstrated by the similar way in which they proliferate and express apoptosis-regulating proteins during the menstrual cycle. However, in both pre- and postmenopausal women, endometrial polyps lose their apoptotic regulation and overexpress oestrogen and progesterone receptors, thus avoiding the usual control mechanisms.

Endometrial polyps are generally asymptomatic and may be an incidental finding during pelvic ultrasonography.

Incidental small endometrial polyps in premenopausal women may be amenable to conservative treatment due to their low malignant potential and chances of regression. However, endometrial polyps that lead to infertility, postmenopausal bleeding, menorrhagia and abnormal bleeding patterns and those in postmenopausal women warrant hysteroscopic removal under vision, which is superior to blind avulsion.

References Annan JJ, Aquilina J, Ball E. The management of endometrial polyps in the twenty-first century. Obstet Gynaecol. 2012;14:33–8.

GYN17

GYN17 Answer: B

Explanation There may be times when an obese woman requests a certain surgical treatment and alternatives are available. Such instances could include hysterectomy for menorrhagia or repair surgery for prolapse. Doctors should act in the best interests of their patients and that may mean refusing surgery when the risk is assessed as too high. The General Medical Council states that a doctor 'should provide effective care based on the best available evidence', and patients do not have an automatic right to treatments on demand. Most people will accept a specialist's advice, particularly when appropriate written information is provided. However, they do have a right to a second opinion and, similarly, doctors should 'consult and take advice from colleagues, where appropriate'.

References Biswas N, Hogston P. Surgical risk from obesity in gynaecology. Obstet Gynaecol. 2011;13:87–91.

GYN18

GYN18 Answer: C

Explanation The clinical history is very typical of endometriosis and blue nodules in vagina are characteristic of the same.

The vaginal discharge is most likely physiological, and irritability 'during' period can be explained due to severe physical discomfort as such.

References Essentials of obstetrics and gynaecology by Barry O'Reilly, Cecilia Bottomley, Janice Rymer, Chapter 6 Pelvic pain, Endometriosis and minimal access surgery. 2nd ed. Elsevier handbook series; 2012.

GYN19

GYN19 Answer: B

Explanation The urogenital system develops from the intermediate mesothelium of the peritoneal cavity and the endoderm of the urogenital sinus. The ovaries are derived from the mesodermal epithelium lining of the posterior abdominal wall, and primordial germ cells form by week 4, subsequently migrating into the developing ovary at week 6 and differentiating into oogonia. Both male and female fetuses initially have both a Wolffian (mesonephric) duct that lies medially and a Müllerian (paramesonephric) duct that lies laterally. The presence of a Y chromosome leads to male sex determination, and in its absence and in the presence of two X chromosomes, the Wolffian ducts regress due to a lack of testosterone and the Müllerian ducts persist due to the absence of Müllerian inhibitory factor. The paramesonephric duct develops into the uterus and fallopian tubes, while the vagina develops from the vaginal plate. The two Müllerian ducts fuse at the caudal end to form the body of the developing uterus and the unfused lateral arms form the fallopian tubes. The fused caudal portion extends cranially, eventually developing a central cavity, leading to development of the functional uterus.

References Edmonds DK. Normal and abnormal development of the genital tract. In: Edmonds DK, editor. Dewhurst's textbook of obstetrics and gynaecology. 8th ed. Oxford: Wiley; 2012. p. 421–4.

GYN20

GYN20 Answer: B

Explanation The presence of a chaperone is considered essential for every pelvic examination. Verbal consent should be obtained in the presence of the chaperone who is to be present during the examination and recorded in the notes.

If the patient declines the presence of a chaperone, the doctor should explain that a chaperone is also required to help in many cases and then attempt to arrange for the chaperone to be standing nearby within earshot. The reasons for declining a chaperone and alternative arrangements offered should be documented. Consent should also be specific to whether the intended examination is vaginal, rectal or both.

There is no evidence to support routine breast examination in the pregnant woman nor in the routine gynaecological patient. Should examination of the breast be considered necessary for clinical reasons, verbal consent should be obtained, again in the presence of a chaperone.

Communication skills are essential in conducting intimate examinations.

References https://www.rcog.org.uk/globalassets/documents/guidelines/clinical-governance-advice/cga6.pdf

GYN21

GYN21 Answer: D

Explanation Over 20 % of women attending gynaecology clinics have psychosexual dysfunction, yet there is little or no training in this area for medical students, obstetrics and gynaecology trainees and consultants. Sexual matters increasingly feature in the media and literature. Common problems include sexual pain disorders, protracted pelvic or vulval pain, hypoactive sexual desire disorder and repeated requests for gynaecological surgery where no pathology has been found.

References Cowan F, Frodsham L. Management of common disorders in psychosexual medicine. Obstet Gynaecol. 2015;17:47–53.

GYN22

GYN22 Answer: B

Explanation Women with premature ovarian insufficiency have an earlier onset of both CVD episodes and osteoporosis. They are also noted to have a reduced breast cancer risk compared with their menstruating peers. The risk of breast cancer with HRT use in these women is deemed to be no greater than the population risk for their age, while the benefits are greater by prevention of long-term morbidity. Hence, it is strongly advised that these women should consider taking HRT, at least until the age of 50.

References 1. Panay N, et al. The British menopause society & women's health concern recommendations on hormone replacement therapy. Menopause Int. 2013;19:59–68.

2. Maclaran K, Horner E, Panay N. Premature ovarian failure: long-term sequelae. Menopause Int. 2010;16:38–41.

GYN23

GYN23 Answer: E

Explanation Classical presentation of a cervical ectropion is seen commonly during puberty, pregnancy and the use of the oral contraceptive pill.

A cervical ectropion is defined as the presence of everted endocervical columnar epithelium on the ectocervix. It requires no treatment if asymptomatic, but 5 % of women with a cervical ectropion report postcoital bleeding. Ectopy and ectropion can produce significant mucoid discharge without being inflamed. Inflammation tends to give rise to postcoital bleeding.

Secondary infection of cervical ectopy or ectropion may involve both the epithelium and stroma, producing symptoms of cervicitis.

Symptomatic lesions may be treated by outpatient cryotherapy, but ablative treatment under local or general anaesthesia may be needed if symptoms persist after cryotherapy or where the lesion is inflamed. Prior to performing any treatment, it is essential to ensure that the woman has had a recent, normal cervical smear and that sexually transmitted infection has been excluded

References Connoley A, Esther Jones S. Nonmenstrual bleeding in women under 40 years of age. Obstet Gynaecol. 2004;6:153–8.

GYN24

GYN24 Answer: D

Explanation From an outflow tract perspective, the only uterine anomaly that may cause a problem is the presence of a rudimentary horn. In this circumstance, the caudal ends of the Müllerian duct fail to fuse, and a unicornuate uterus with an adjacent or attached uterine horn may result. This horn is functional and therefore at the time of the onset of menses, the endometrium within the horn will shed and therefore create a haematometra, with retrograde menstruation and severe dysmenorrhoea. In girls with dysmenorrhoea that is unresolved through normal medication, an ultrasound scan should be performed to identify whether or not there is a rudimentary horn present. When these are noncommunicating, the horn needs to be removed surgically and the uterus reconstructed. If this is carried out meticulously, reproductive performance is the same as with a unicornuate uterus. Occasionally, these horns may be communicating, in which case they are usually asymptomatic. However, if diagnosed prior to pregnancy, they should be removed because a pregnancy in a communicating horn can lead to uterine rupture and maternal fatality.

References Edmonds DK, Rose GL. Outflow tract disorders of the female genital tract. Obstet Gynaecol. 2013;15:11–7.

GYN25

GYN 25 Answer: B

Explanation All the clinical features strongly suggest Turner's syndrome. This is a chromosomal abnormality—monosomy X. Karyotyping will help in confirming the diagnosis in this case.

References Puberty and its disorders. In: Edmonds DK, editor. Dewhurst's textbook of obstetrics and gynaecology. 8th ed. Oxford: Wiley; 2012. p. 474.

GYN26

GYN26 Answer: D

Explanation DSR scores were better with luteal phase scoring, although the results were not statistically different. However, luteal phase dosing also helped control symptoms that persisted postmenstrually. Withdrawal of SSRI is not necessary when given only during the luteal phase. Although it may appear that SSRIs may have synergistic effects with hormonal suppression, there is no evidence to confirm this possibility.

References Management of premenstrual syndrome. RCOG Green-Top guideline No. 48. 2007.

GYN27

GYN 27 Answer: A

Explanation Occasionally, unexpected diseases, such as endometriosis or suspected cancer, may be discovered at the time of an operation, for which additional surgical procedures are indicated. If problems related to the woman's complaint, such as minor endometriosis or adhesions, are encountered during a diagnostic procedure, treatment can be performed if the woman has been made aware of the types of minor treatment that she could receive and has given her consent to the consequences of this treatment. If such a preoperative discussion has not occurred, then additional treatment should not take place. Where complications of the surgery occur, for example, trauma to a viscus that in itself is life-threatening, then corrective surgery must proceed and full explanation given as soon as practical during the woman's recovery. Generally, it is unwise to proceed with any additional surgical procedures without discussing them with the woman, even if this means a second operation, unless clear boundaries about additional procedures are documented by the carers prior to the procedure.

References Obtaining valid consent, clinical governance advice No. 6. 2015.
https://www.rcog.org.uk/globalassets/documents/guidelines/clinical-governance-advice/cga6.pdf

GYN28

GYN28 Answer: C

Explanation There is a number of complementary therapy options that are in use for the treatment of PMS. The use of St John's wort is fraught with possible significant interactions with conventional medicines especially SSRI. Although placebo-controlled RCTs do not show any benefit for evening primrose oil, it may be useful in the treatment of cyclical mastalgia. Vitamin A and other multivitamin combinations have unknown benefits, and it is unclear which one is the active ingredient. The use of *Ginkgo biloba*, although shown to have some benefit in placebo-controlled trials, requires further data. Apart from magnesium, the other options for which data exists are calcium/vitamin D and for *Vitex agnus-castus*.

References Management of premenstrual syndrome. RCOG Green-Top guideline No. 48. 2007.

GYN29

GYN 29 Answer: D

Explanation All reasonable steps should be taken to exclude pregnancy before embarking upon any surgical procedure.

A potentially viable pregnancy should not be terminated without the woman's consent and following the processes outlined in the 1967 Abortion Act. If a pregnancy is discovered at the start of a hysterectomy, including one for cancer, the operation should be rescheduled. An unexpected ectopic pregnancy should be removed. It is reasonable to presume that the woman would wish this and would wish the surgeon to act in favour of life-saving treatment.

References https://www.rcog.org.uk/globalassets/documents/guidelines/clinical-governance-advice/cga6.pdf

GYN30

GYN30 Answer: C

Explanation Atrophic vaginitis is treatable with topical oestrogen, resulting in cornification and regeneration of the vaginal epithelium. This improves lubrication and sexual function. Systemic absorption is insignificant with low-dose topical oestrogen. Additional systemic progestogen is not required. Vaginal oestrogen may reduce symptoms of urgency of micturition and recurrent urinary tract infections. Vaginal symptoms can persist even when on adequate systemic HRT; in such cases both topical and systemic are required. The safety of topical vaginal oestrogen has not been assessed in patients with breast cancer, where theoretically the risks are small. The benefits to the genitourinary tract along with improved sexual intimacy may outweigh the risk.

References Bakour SH, Williamson J. Latest evidence on using hormone replacement therapy in the menopause. Obstet Gynaecol. 2015;17:20–8.

Subfertility and Endocrinology: Answers and Explanations

22

SFE1

SFE1 Answer: B

Explanation Premature ovarian failure, categorised under WHO classification group III, is associated with high FSH and low oestrogen levels. Other causes of premature ovarian failure include microdeletions in the X chromosome, surgery and chemotherapy.

Kallmann's syndrome is a hypogonadotrophic hypogonadism and is associated with low FSH and low oestrogen levels. Other features include anosmia or hyposmia where the sense of smell is completely absent or diminished. Mutations in the *KAL1*, *FGFR1*, *PROKR2* and *PROK2* genes cause Kallmann's syndrome. Although some of their specific functions are unclear, these genes appear to be involved in the formation and migration of a group of nerve cells that are specialised to process smells (olfactory neurons). These nerve cells come together into a bundle forming the olfactory bulb, which is critical for the perception of odours. The *KAL1*, *FGFR1*, *PROKR2* and *PROK2* genes also play a role in the migration of neurons that produce gonadotrophin-releasing hormone (GnRH).

References Carol C, Bolarinde O. The subfertile couple. Obstet Gynaecol Reprod Med. 23:5;154–9.

SFE2

SFE2 Answer: B

© Springer India 2016
C. Ratha, J. Gupta, *SBAs and EMQs for MRCOG II*,
DOI 10.1007/978-81-322-2689-5_22

Explanation The strongest independent risk factors for having further miscarriages due to any aetiology are increasing maternal age and number of previous miscarriages. The risk of miscarriage doubles when maternal age doubles from 20 to 40 years. A 1997 longitudinal study found the rate of miscarriage in the next pregnancy to be 25 % in women under 30, 28 % in women aged 31–36 years, 33 % in women aged 36–39 years and 52 % in women over 40 years. Increased paternal age is also associated with miscarriage, with 1.6 times the risk when comparing a paternal age of 40 to that of a 25–29-year-old man. However, recurrent miscarriage has not been linked to any specific paternal health factors.

A poorer prognostic outcome with increasing numbers of miscarriages has been widely documented, with a 53 % chance of further miscarriage with six or more miscarriages versus 29 % with three pregnancy losses. Although, based on these data, 48 % of women over 40 years of age and 47 % of women with more than six previous miscarriages did achieve a live birth in the next pregnancy without having treatment.

References Morley L, Shillito J, Tang T. Preventing recurrent miscarriage of unknown aetiology. Obstet Gynaecol. 2013;15:99–105.

SFE3

SFE3 Answer: C

Explanation Heavy alcohol consumption, but not moderate consumption, may affect sexual and reproductive performance in a reversible fashion. Tobacco smoking and cannabis consumption have been shown to reduce semen parameters, although the relationship between male smoking habits and fertility remains uncertain. Although smokers in general may not experience reduced fertility, men with suboptimal semen quality may benefit from quitting smoking, and this should be strongly encouraged. Varicoceles, a collection of dilated refluxing veins in the spermatic cord, are found in 11.7 % of men with normal semen and 25.4 % of men with abnormal semen. The exact mechanism by which a varicocele can affect fertility is not well understood, but theories include increased scrotal heating and altered testicular steroidogenesis. The diagnostic significance, however, is debatable.

References Karavolos S, Stewart J, Evbuomwan I, McEleny K, Aird I. Assessment of the infertile male. Obstet Gynaecol. 2013;15:1–9.

SFE4

SFE4 Answer: D

Explanation Obstruction, excluding vasectomy, accounts for up to 41 % of causes of azoospermia. The diagnosis is based on normal serum FSH levels, normal testicular volume and evidence of complete spermatogenesis on biopsy. Causes include surgical trauma and vasectomy, infection (chlamydia, gonorrhoea, tuberculosis) and congenital bilateral absence of vas deferens (CBAVD). Treatment options include urological surgery when feasible as in vasectomy reversal or sperm retrieval from testes or epididymides. Techniques for sperm retrieval from the testes include testicular sperm aspiration (TESA), testicular sperm extraction (TESE) and microsurgical TESE (micro-TESE). Sperm from the epididymis can be retrieved by microsurgical (MESA) or percutaneous (PESA) epididymal sperm aspiration under local anaesthetic.

References Karavolos S, Stewart J, Evbuomwan I, McEleny K, Aird I. Assessment of the infertile male. Obstet Gynaecol. 2013;15:1–9.

SFE5

SFE5 Answer: C   *IUI alone - 6 cycles*

Explanation NICE currently recommends the use of up to six cycles of unstimulated IUI in mild cases of male factor infertility in order to reduce the rate of multiple pregnancies. IUI involves the placement of a washed pellet of ejaculated sperm within the uterine cavity, thus bypassing the cervical barrier. It may be performed with or without ovarian stimulation. Other indications include immunologic infertility and mechanical problems of sperm delivery such as erectile dysfunction or hypospadias. NICE recommends that IUI be used in mild forms of oligozoospermia; however, specific semen criteria for its use have not been standardised. Monthly conception rates of 8–16 % have been reported for IUI; however its efficacy has been questioned by recent studies.   *Cumulative = 40%*

References National Collaborating Centre for Women's and Children's Health. Fertility: assessment and treatment for people with fertility problems. London: RCOG Press; 2004.

SFE6

IVF Success = 28-32% (±30-40%)
rate
in
UK

SFE6 Answer: C

Explanation Average pregnancy rates of 33.0 % per embryo transfer have been reported after ICSI. Although IVF can be used to treat milder forms of sperm abnormalities, more severe forms require ICSI. ICSI was originally described in 1988 and has since revolutionised the treatment of male factor infertility. It involves the micromanipulation and injection of a single human sperm into the cytoplasm of the oocyte. ICSI requires ovarian stimulation, oocyte retrieval and sperm preparation as for IVF. It is used for uncorrectable severe forms of male factor infertility including oligospermia and asthenoteratozoospermia or following fertilisation failure in a previous IVF cycle.

References Karavolos S, Stewart J, Evbuomwan I, McEleny K, Aird I. Assessment of the infertile male. Obstet Gynaecol. 2013;15:1–9.

SFE7

SFE7 Answer: E

Explanation The most significant short-term complication associated with ovarian stimulation is ovarian hyperstimulation syndrome (OHSS), with moderate or severe OHSS reported in 3–8 % of IVF cycles. The characteristic feature of the pathophysiology of OHSS is increased vascular permeability. This is mediated by vasoactive substances derived from the hyperstimulated ovary following the action of human chorionic gonadotrophin (hCG) or luteinising hormone (LH). Vascular endothelial growth factor (VEGF) appears to play a critical role in the development of OHSS. In vitro studies have shown hCG to be a potent stimulator for granulosa cell VEGF production, which may explain the clinically observed link between hCG exposure and the development of OHSS. Increased vascular permeability is most marked in the peritoneal surfaces nearest to the ovary, leading to ascites, but may also affect pleural and pericardial cavities and the systemic circulation. Loss of fluid into the third space causes hypovolaemia and effusions.

References Prakash A, Mathur R. Ovarian hyperstimulation syndrome. Obstet Gynaecol. 2013;15:31–5.

SFE8

SFE8 Answer: B

Explanation Antiphospholipid antibodies are present in 15 % of women with recurrent miscarriage.

By comparison, the prevalence of antiphospholipid antibodies in women with a low-risk obstetric history is less than 2 %. In women with recurrent miscarriage associated with antiphospholipid antibodies, the live birth rate in pregnancies with no pharmacological intervention has been reported to be as low as 10 %. Adverse pregnancy outcomes associated with APLA include:

- Three or more consecutive miscarriages before 10 weeks of gestation
- One or more morphologically normal fetal losses after the tenth week of gestation
- One or more preterm births before the 34th week of gestation owing to placental disease

References http://www.rcog.org.uk/files/rcog-corp/GTG17recurrentmiscarriage.pdf

SFE9

SFE9 Answer: E

Explanation The main causes of infertility in the UK are:

- Unexplained infertility (no identified male or female cause) (25 %)
- Ovulatory disorders (25 %)
- Tubal damage (20 %)
- Factors in the male causing infertility (30 %)
- Uterine or peritoneal disorders (10 %).

In about 40 % of cases, disorders are found in both the man and the woman. Uterine or endometrial factors, gamete or embryo defects and pelvic conditions such as endometriosis may also play a role.

References NICE. Fertility: assessment and treatment for people with fertility problems. NICE clinical guideline 156. Manchester; 2013. http://www.nice.org.uk/nicemedia/live/14078/62769/62769.pdf

SFE10

SFE10 Answer: A

Explanation Polycystic ovarian syndrome is diagnosed when two of the three following criteria are met:

- Polycystic ovaries: either 12 or more peripheral follicles or increased ovarian volume (greater than 10 cm³)
- Oligo- or anovulation
- Clinical and/or biochemical signs of hyperandrogenism

A raised LH:FSH ratio is no longer a diagnostic criteria for PCOS owing to its inconsistency. The diagnosis of PCOS can only be made when other aetiologies have been excluded. The recommended baseline screening tests are thyroid function tests, a serum prolactin and a free androgen index (total testosterone divided by sex hormone-binding globulin (SHBG) × 100 to give a calculated free testosterone level). In cases of clinical evidence of hyperandrogenism and total testosterone greater than 5 nmol/l, 17-hydroxyprogesterone should be sampled and androgen-secreting tumours excluded. If there is a clinical suspicion of Cushing syndrome, this should be investigated according to local practice.

References Royal College of Obstetricians and Gynaecologists. Long term consequences of polycystic ovary syndrome. Green-Top guideline No. 33. London: RCOG Press; 2007. http://www.rcog.org.uk/files/rcog-corp/uploaded-files/GT33_LongTermPCOS.pdf

SFE11

SFE11 Answer: B

Explanation Women with regular menstrual cycles and more than 1 year's infertility can be offered a blood test to measure serum progesterone in the midluteal phase of their cycle (day 21 of a 28-day cycle) to confirm ovulation. Progesterone production from the corpus luteum peaks at this time if ovulation has occurred. There is a significant association between smoking and reduced fertility among female smokers. There is inconsistent evidence about the impact of alcohol intake and caffeine on female fertility. Alcohol in excess of 1 unit/day, maternal and paternal smoking and caffeine consumption all have adverse effects on the success rates of assisted reproduction procedures, including IVF. Women who are not known to have comorbidities (such as pelvic inflammatory disease, previous ectopic pregnancy or endometriosis) should be offered hysterosalpingography (HSG) to screen for tubal occlusion because this is a reliable test for ruling out tubal occlusion, and it is less invasive and makes more efficient use of resources than laparoscopy. Women who are thought to have comorbidities should be offered laparoscopy and dye so that tubal and other pelvic pathologies can be assessed at the same time. Women should not be offered an endometrial biopsy to evaluate the luteal phase as part of the investigation of fertility problems because there is no evidence that medical treatment of luteal phase defect improves pregnancy rates.

References National Collaborating Centre for Women's and Children's Health. Fertility assessment and treatment for people with fertility problems. London: RCOG Press; 2004. http://www.rcog.org.uk/files/rcog-corp/uploaded-files/NEBFertilityFull.pdf

SFE12

SFE12 Answer: D

Explanation Hydrosalpinx is dilatation of the fallopian tube in the presence of distal tubal obstruction, which may result from a number of causes. In women undergoing IVF, the presence of hydrosalpinx is associated with early pregnancy loss and poor implantation and pregnancy rates, probably due to alteration in endometrial receptivity. Women with hydrosalpinges should be offered salpingectomy, preferably by laparoscopy, before in vitro fertilisation treatment because this improves the chance of a live birth. Luteal support using human chorionic gonadotrophin or progesterone improves pregnancy rates in women who are undergoing IVF treatment using gonadotrophin-releasing hormone agonists for pituitary downregulation. The chance of a live birth following IVF treatment decreases with rising female age. The optimal female age range for IVF treatment is 23–39 years. Donor oocyte IVF success rates are reported to be similar in women with or without primary ovarian failure. Preimplantation genetic diagnosis (PGD) of the embryo is not a requirement prior to uterine transfer. It can be offered to couples with a family history of a serious genetic condition to avoid passing it on to their children.

References National Collaborating Centre for Women's and Children's Health. Fertility assessment and treatment for people with fertility problems. London: RCOG Press; 2004. http://www.rcog.org.uk/files/rcog-corp/uploaded-files/NEBFertilityFull.pdf

Human Fertilisation and Embryology Authority. Pre-implantation genetic diagnosis [online]. Available at http://www.hfea.gov.uk/preimplantation-genetic-diagnosis.html

SFE13

SFE13 Answer: E

Explanation Polycystic ovarian syndrome is diagnosed when two of the three following criteria are met:

- Polycystic ovaries: either 12 or more peripheral follicles or increased ovarian volume (greater than 10 cm^3)
- Oligo- or anovulation
- Clinical and/or biochemical signs of hyperandrogenism.

A raised LH:FSH ratio is no longer a diagnostic criteria for PCOS owing to its inconsistency. The diagnosis of PCOS can only be made when other aetiologies have been excluded. The recommended baseline screening tests are thyroid function tests, a serum prolactin and a free androgen index (total testosterone divided by sex hormone-binding globulin (SHBG)×100 to give a calculated free testosterone level). In cases of clinical evidence of hyperandrogenism and total testosterone greater than 5 nmol/l, 17-hydroxyprogesterone should be sampled and androgen-secreting tumours excluded. If there is a clinical suspicion of Cushing syndrome, this should be investigated according to local practice.

References Royal College of Obstetricians and Gynaecologists. Long term consequences of polycystic ovary syndrome. Green-Top guideline No. 33. London: RCOG Press; 2007. http://www.rcog.org.uk/files/rcog-corp/uploaded-files/GT33_LongTermPCOS.pdf

SFE14

SFE14 Answer: B

Explanation The NICE guidelines state that the following measures can be used to predict the likely ovarian response to gonadotrophin stimulation in IVF:

- Total antral follicle count of ≤4 for a low response and >16 for a high response
- Anti-Müllerian hormone of ≤5.4 pmol/l for a low response and ≥25.0 pmol/l for a high response
- Follicle-stimulating hormone >8.9 IU/l for a low response and <4 IU/l for a high response

The following tests should not be used individually to predict any outcome of fertility treatment:

- Ovarian volume
- Ovarian blood flow
- Inhibin B
- Oestradiol (E2)

References NICE. Fertility: assessment and treatment for people with fertility problems. NICE clinical guideline 156. Manchester; 2013. http://www.nice.org.uk/nicemedia/live/14078/62769/62769.pdf

SFE15

SFE15 Answer: B

Explanation Women with World Health Organization group II ovulation disorders (hypothalamic pituitary dysfunction) such as polycystic ovarian syndrome should be offered treatment with clomiphene citrate (or tamoxifen) as the first line of treatment for up to 12 months because it is likely to induce ovulation. Anovulatory women with polycystic ovarian syndrome who have not responded to clomiphene citrate and who have a body mass index of more than 25 should be offered metformin combined with clomiphene citrate because this increases ovulation and pregnancy rates. If there is no response to clomiphene citrate, women with PCOS should be offered laparoscopic ovarian drilling because it is as effective as gonadotrophin treatment and is not associated with an increased risk of multiple pregnancy. Treatment with gonadotrophins can be offered if ovulation does not occur with clomiphene citrate (or tamoxifen). Human menopausal gonadotrophin, urinary FSH and recombinant FSH are equally effective in achieving pregnancy, and consideration should be given to minimising cost when prescribing. Women with ovulatory disorders due to hyperprolactinaemia should be offered treatment with dopamine agonists such as bromocriptine. Consideration should be given to safety for use in pregnancy and minimising cost when prescribing.

References National Collaborating Centre for Women's and Children's Health. Fertility assessment and treatment for people with fertility problems. London: RCOG Press; 2004. http://www.rcog.org.uk/files/rcog-corp/uploaded-files/NEBFertilityFull.pdf

SFE16

SFE16 Answer: E

Explanation The World Health Organization classifies ovulation disorders into three groups. Group 1 is hypothalamic pituitary failure (hypothalamic amenorrhoea or hypogonadotrophic hypogonadism). This group of disorders is characterised by low gonadotrophins, normal prolactin and low oestrogen, and it accounts for about 10 % of ovulatory disorders. Failed ovarian follicular development results in hypo-oestrogenic amenorrhoea in this group of disorders. This group can improve their chance of regular ovulation, conception and an uncomplicated pregnancy by:

- Increasing their body weight if they have a BMI of less than 19
- Moderating their exercise levels if they undertake high levels of exercise

References National Collaborating Centre for Women's and Children's Health. Fertility assessment and treatment for people with fertility problems. London: RCOG Press; 2004. http://www.rcog.org.uk/files/rcog-corp/uploaded-files/NEBFertilityFull.pdf

NICE. Fertility: Assessment and treatment for people with fertility problems. NICE clinical guideline 156. Manchester, 2013. Available at http://www.nice.org.uk/nicemedia/live/14078/62769/62769.pdf

SFE17

SFE17 Answer: C

Explanation The World Health Organization classifies ovulation disorders into three groups. Group 3 is ovarian failure. This group, which is characterised by high gonadotrophins with hypogonadism and low oestrogen, accounts for about 4–5 % of ovulatory disorders.

References National Collaborating Centre for Women's and Children's Health. Fertility assessment and treatment for people with fertility problems. London: RCOG Press: 2004. http://www.rcog.org.uk/files/rcog-corp/uploaded-files/NEBFertilityFull.pdf

SFE18

SFE18 Answer: B

Explanation NICE recommends IVF as the treatment of choice in cases of unexplained infertility, mild male factor infertility and mild to moderate endometriosis if not conceived after 2 years of unprotected intercourse. Gonadotrophins/laparoscopic ovarian drilling/clomiphene + metformin can be offered as the second line of treatment for clomiphene-resistant PCOS cases for ovulation induction.

References NICE clinical guideline 156. Fertility – assessment and treatment for people with fertility problems.

SFE19

SFE19 Answer: B

Explanation Fertility may be reduced in transfusion-dependent individuals where chelation has been suboptimal and iron overload has occurred resulting in damage to the anterior pituitary. There is no contraindication to the use of hormonal methods of contraception such as the combined oral contraceptive pill, the progestogen-only pill, the Nexplanon® implant (Merck Sharp & Dohme Limited, Hoddesdon, Herts, UK) and the Mirena® intrauterine system (Bayer PLC, Newbury, Berks, UK) in women with thalassaemia. They may require ovulation induction using injectable gonadotrophins to conceive. Puberty is often delayed and incomplete. Aggressive chelation in the preconception stage can reduce and optimise body iron burden and reduce end-organ damage.

References Beta thalassemia in pregnancy – RCOG Green-Top guideline No. 66. 2014. http://www.rcog.org.uk/files/rcog-corp/GTG_66_Thalassaemia.pdf

SFE20

SFE20 Answer: A

Explanation The results of semen analysis conducted as part of an initial assessment should be compared with the following World Health Organization reference values:

- Semen volume: 1.5 ml or more
- pH: 7.2 or more
- Sperm concentration: 15 million spermatozoa per ml or more
- Total sperm number: 39 million spermatozoa per ejaculate or more
- Total motility (percentage of progressive motility and non-progressive motility): 40 % or more motile or 32 % or more with progressive motility
- Vitality: 58 % or more live spermatozoa
- Sperm morphology (percentage of normal forms): 4 % or more

References NICE. Fertility: assessment and treatment for people with fertility problems. NICE clinical guideline 156. Manchester; 2013. http://www.nice.org.uk/nicemedia/live/14078/62769/62769.pdf

SFE21

SFE21 Answer: C

Explanation *Chlamydia trachomatis* is the single largest cause of acquired tubal pathology, and evidence of both current and past infection can be easily measured using *C. trachomatis* antibody test (CAT). The sensitivity (21–90 %) and specificity (29–100 %) vary depending on the cut-off value used to define a positive result

References Suresh YN, Narvekar NN. The role of tubal patency tests and tubal surgery in the era of assisted reproductive techniques. Obstet Gynaecol. 2014;16:37–45.

SFE22

SFE22 Answer: A

Explanation With regard to the surgical therapy for cysts, a Cochrane review, based on four randomised trials involving 312 women, concluded that laparoscopic aspiration or cystectomy of endometrioma prior to ART does not show evidence of benefit over expectant management with regard to the clinical pregnancy rate.

References http://www.eshre.eu/~/media/Files/Guidelines/ESHRE%20guideline%20on%20endometriosis%202013.pdf

SFE23

SFE23 Answer: D

Explanation Unexplained infertility – NICE recommendations
   Do not offer oral ovarian stimulation agents (such as clomiphene citrate, anastrozole or letrozole) to women with unexplained infertility.

Inform women with unexplained infertility that clomiphene citrate as a stand-alone treatment does not increase the chances of pregnancy or a live birth.

Advise women with unexplained infertility who are having regular unprotected sexual intercourse to try to conceive for a total of 2 years (this can include up to 1 year before their fertility investigations) before IVF will be considered.

Offer IVF treatment to women with unexplained infertility who have not conceived after 2 years (this can include up to 1 year before their fertility investigations) of regular unprotected sexual intercourse.

References http://www.nice.org.uk/guidance/cg156/chapter/1-Recommen dations#unexplained-infertility-2

SFE24

SFE24 Answer: C

15% SIN = PTD – Resection c anast

85% PID = DTD.

Explanation Proximal tubal disease accounts for approximately 15 % of cases of tubal factor infertility; the most common cause is salpingitis isthmica nodosa (SIN), a tubal disease of inflammatory aetiology which is associated with other infective PID stigmata such as distal tubal disease and pelvic and perihepatic adhesions. The underlying histopathology reveals endosalpingeal diverticula encased in myosalpingeal hypertrophy and fibrosis resulting in a firm proximal tubular nodule which can be seen on laparoscopic examination. As the disease involves both endosalpingeal and myosalpingeal compartments, it is no surprise that tubal resection and anastomosis of the diseased inflammatory area result in higher success compared to tubal catheterisation or expectant management irrespective of tubal patency.

Distal tubal disease accounts for approximately 85 % of cases of tubal factor infertility. Hydrosalpinx is an end stage of distal tubal disease and is best managed by salpingectomy followed by IVF.

References Suresh YN, Narvekar NN. The role of tubal patency tests and tubal surgery in the era of assisted reproductive techniques. Obstet Gynaecol. 2014;16:37Narv

SFE25

SFE25 Answer: B

Explanation Evidence from a Swedish study suggests that not only does IVF double the risk of VTE compared to natural conception, but the risk in the first trimester was fourfold higher and the risk of PE during the first trimester was seven times higher. Women with ovarian hyperstimulation syndrome are particularly prone to VTE in the upper body.

References GTG 37a.

[handwritten notes: 1st trimester VTE = 4 fold ↑. PE 7x ↑. IVF double the risk of VTE > in upper body]

SFE26

SFE26 Answer: E

Explanation A womantion and the risk of PE during the first trimester was seven times higher. Women with ovarian hyperstimulation synIVF.

Use one of the following to predict the likely ovarian response to gonadotrophin stimulation in IVF:

– Total antral follicle count of ≤4 for low response and >16 for a high response
– Anti-Müllerian hormone ≤5.4 pmol/L for a low response and ≥25 pmol/L for a high response
– Follicle-stimulating hormone >8.9 IU/L for a low response and <4 IU/L for a high response

References Nice clinical guideline on Infertility. 2013.

SFE27

SFE27 Answer: C

Explanation Fertiloscopy is an outpatient technique that combines hysteroscopy, THL and salpingoscopy.

Salpingoscopy is the endoscopic visualisation of the endosalpinx of the tubal infundibulum and ampulla at laparoscopy and/or THL, whereas falloposcopy is the endoscopic visualisation of the whole endosalpinx at hysteroscopy.

Transvaginal hydrolaparoscopy (THL) involves insufflation of the pelvis with 0.4fund l of a fluid medium through an insufflating needle inserted into the posterior fornix, followed by the introduction of a small diameter rigid angled endoscope to visualise the pouch of Douglas (POD), pelvic side walls, adnexa and tubal patency (the dye injected transcervically).

References 1. Suresh YN, Narvekar NN. The role of tubal patency tests and tubal surgery in the era of assisted reproductive techniques. Obstet Gynaecol. 2014;16:37Narv

2. Watrelot A. Fertiloscopy. Gynecol Obstet Fertil. 2001;29:462Fer

SFE28

SFE28 Answer: B

Explanation In a couple where the man is HIV positive, the risk of HIV transmission to female partner is negligible through unprotected sexual intercourse (UPSI) when all the following criteria are met:

- The man is compliant with HAART.
- The man has had viral load <50 copies/ML for more than 6 months.
- There are no other infections present.
- Unprotected intercourse is limited to the time of ovulation.

If all the above criteria are met, sperm washing may not further reduce the risk of infection and may reduce the likelihood of pregnancy.

References NICE clinical guideline on Fertility. 2013.

SFE29

SFE29 Answer: A

Explanation Hypogonadotrophic hypogonadism is rare and accounts for <1 % of male factor fertility problems. It results from decreased production of FSH and LH secondary to hypothalamic or pituitary dysfunction, which leads to failure of spermatogenesis and testosterone secretion by the testes. It may be congenital or acquired. Causes include craniopharyngiomas, surgery for pituitary tumours, head trauma, haemochromatosis, Kallmann's syndrome and other congenital genetic syndromes of reduced gonadotrophin-releasing hormone (GnRH) secretion like Prader–Willi syndrome, Laurence–Moon–Biedl syndrome, etc.

References TOG. 2013;15(1).

SFE30

SFE30 Answer: C

Explanation Some androgen production occurs in all healthy women and is required for the synthesis of oestrogens. In hyperandrogenic states, there is either dysfunctional production of androgens or inadequate conversion to estrogens or both. This review focuses on the pathophysiology, biochemistry and differential diagnoses of hyperandrogenism in women.

In healthy women, 80 % of circulating testosterone is bound to sex hormone-binding globulin (SHBG), 19 % is bound to albumin, and 1 % circulates freely in the blood stream. Traditionally, only the unbound fraction is considered metabolically active, although this is now disputed. Of the circulating androgens, only testosterone and its active metabolite dihydrotestosterone (DHT) are able to activate androgen receptors. The remaining androgens, DHEA-S, DHEA and androstenedione, are almost entirely bound to albumin and can be converted to testosterone in peripheral tissue. Most of the circulating testosterone is metabolised in the liver into androsterone and etiocholanolone, which are conjugated with glucuronic acid or sulphuric acid and excreted in the urine as 17-ketosteroids.

References Meek CL, Bravis V, Don A, Kaplan F. Polycystic ovary syndrome and the differential diagnosis of hyperandrogenism. Obstet Gynaecol. 2013;15:171–6.

SFE31

SFE31 Answer: E

Explanation Despite the increasing numbers and the wide availability of ART, particularly IVF, the number of gynaecological cancers (ovarian and uterine) as well as breast and other cancers remains relatively small—as per expectation from various studies, including more recent and large ones, that corrected for confounding factors, namely, infertility and nulliparity.

There is some reliable evidence to suggest that CC when given in large doses and with multiple cycles increases the risks of the gynaecological cancers and probably breast cancer. However, guidelines for current practice recommend not to use CC for more than 12 cycles; furthermore, CC is only licensed for a maximum use of six cycles.

There is also some weak evidence to suggest that multiple IVF cycles might be associated with an increased risk of breast cancer. While pointing out that all the studies have methodological limitations, it will be sensible to ensure that women who have had multiple IVF cycles (regardless of the outcome) are informed of this possible risk as part of their counselling. The decision to proceed with IVF subsequently should be patient-centred and must respect the patient's informed choice.

The aetiology of malignant melanoma, and to a lesser extent that of thyroid cancer, is known to involve endogenous and exogenous hormones. It is also associated with parity and COCs. It was therefore hypothesised that the exogenous hormones administered for fertility treatment might be linked with both cancers. However, there is no strong evidence linking infertility treatment with non-gynaecological cancers.

One should remember that since the average age of IVF patients is 35 years and that the average age for ovarian and uterine cancer diagnosis is around 60 years, most of the treated patients have not yet reached that stage; therefore, vigilance is paramount to determine any future trends.

When counselling, patients in general should be reassured about the current data: that there is no significant increase in risk of cancer with IVF treatment for them or their offspring. We should also remember that infertile patients are at significantly higher risk of cancer due to their infertility and other confounding factors. Nevertheless, future data may indicate otherwise.

References Louis LS, Saso S, Ghaem-Maghami S, Abdalla H, Smith JR. The relationship between infertility treatment and cancer including gynaecological cancers. Obstet Gynaecol. 2013;15:177–83.

SFE32

SFE32 Answer: A

Explanation Surgical reversal of tubal sterilisation is just as successful as IVF; however, it is not funded on the NHS (nor is IVF for this patient group). Good prognostic factors include female age <35 years and residual tubal length of more than 4 cm. _– 75% successfull in 1yr after reversal. – IVF if no preg_

References Suresh YN, Narvekar NN. The role of tubal patency tests and tubal surgery in the era of assisted reproductive techniques. Obstet Gynaecol. 2014;16:37–45.

SFE33

SFE33 Answer: C

Explanation CAH is a group of autosomal recessive disorders, each of which involves a deficiency of one of five enzymes involved in the synthesis of cortisol in the adrenal cortex. In CAH, insufficient cortisol is produced, which stimulates hypothalamic CRH secretion, due to the absence of normal feedback inhibition. This leads to chronically elevated adrenocorticotrophic hormone (ACTH), which in turn stimulates the adrenal gland to become hyperplastic with excess androgen hormones and steroid precursors being produced and secreted from the normally functioning metabolic pathways. The most common form of CAH is due to a deficiency of 21-hydroxylase activity, which accounts for 90–95 % of cases of CAH. It is associated with a wide range of clinical effects and severity can vary depending on the mutation

References Speiser PW, White PC. Congenital adrenal hyperplasia. N Engl J Med. 2003;349:776–88.

SFE34

SFE34 Answer: E

Explanation Women with unexplained recurrent miscarriage have an excellent prognosis for future pregnancy outcome without pharmacological intervention if offered supportive care alone in the setting of a dedicated early pregnancy assessment unit.

References https://www.rcog.org.uk/globalassets/documents/guidelines/gtg_17.pdf

SFE35

SFE35 Answer: E

Explanation It is widely accepted that an elevated serum testosterone level provides biochemical evidence of hyperandrogenism. However, different analytical methods demonstrate significant differences in analytical specificity for testosterone—some methods have interference from non-testosterone androgens. Many practitioners believe that a serum total testosterone of <5.0 nmol/L, measured using an extraction immunoassay, makes serious pathology in a female unlikely. Mild hyperandrogenism with a serum total testosterone level of around 2–5 nmol/L is thought to be consistent with PCOS, while marked elevations (>5 nmol/L) should prompt investigation for other causes, such as an androgen-secreting tumour.

References Meek CL, Bravis V, Don A, Kaplan F. Polycystic ovary syndrome and the differential diagnosis of hyperandrogenism. Obstet Gynaecol. 2013;15:171–6.

Sexual and Reproductive Health: Answers and Explanations

23

SRH1

SRH1 Answer: E

Explanation Hot flushes begin as a sudden sensation of heat centred on the face and upper chest which rapidly becomes generalised. The sensation of heat lasts a few minutes, can be associated with profuse perspiration and can be followed by chills and shivering. Symptoms result from inappropriate peripheral vasodilatation leading to rapid heat loss and a decrease in core body temperature, and shivering then occurs to restore the core temperature to normal.

Approximately two-third of postmenopausal women will experience hot flushes, with 10–20 % experiencing severe symptoms. For most women, symptoms spontaneously resolve within a few years. However, one-third of postmenopausal women will experience symptoms for up to 5 years, and 20 % will have symptoms for up to 15 years. For women with surgically induced menopause, 90 % experience hot flushes during the first year.

References Tong IL. Nonpharmacological treatment of postmenopausal symptoms. Obstet Gynaecol. 2013;15:19–25.

SRH2

SRH2 Answer: E

Explanation Nexplanon® is a progestogen-only subdermal implant that has now replaced the contraceptive implant, Implanon. Nexplanon and Implanon are bioequivalent (i.e. they both contain 68 mg etonogestrel and they have the same release rate and 3-year duration of action). The progestogen-only implant is a long-acting reversible method of contraception (LARC). The primary mode of action is to prevent ovulation. Implants also prevent sperm penetration by altering the cervical mucus and possibly prevent implantation by thinning the endometrium. The implant is a highly effective contraceptive. The overall pregnancy rate reported in the National Institute of Health and Care Excellence (NICE) guideline on long-acting reversible contraception is <1 in 1000 over 3 years.

References http://www.fsrh.org/pdfs/CEUGuidanceProgestogenOnlyImplants.pdf

SRH3

SRH3 Answer: A

Explanation COC may be recommended for women who are not breastfeeding the baby. However, in breastfeeding women, it is recommended that COC not be used (WHO category 4, unacceptable health risk). Evidence suggested a reduction in milk volume (assessed by weight gain following morning feeds, weekly infant weight and supplements) associated with COC use from day 14 postpartum.

References http://www.fsrh.org/pdfs/archive/breastfeeding04.pdf

SRH4

SRH4 Answer: A

Explanation Treatment of BV is recommended for all women who are symptomatic of vaginal discharge. Up to 50 % of women with a clinical diagnosis of BV are asymptomatic. When present, however, the symptoms include a profuse, malodorous vaginal discharge. The offensive smell is due to the production of amines by anaerobic bacteria and is often worse after sex and during menses, when the higher pH causes further release of the amines. The discharge itself is usually white, thin and homogenous and not associated with any inflammation of the vulva or vagina. The diagnosis of a *Candida* infection can be made entirely clinically, based on the symptoms and signs. They include vulval itching or soreness, curdy white vaginal discharge without a smell, dysuria or superficial dyspareunia. Vulval itching is the most common symptom, and the discharge might be absent in 50 % of cases. The clinical signs include erythema of the vulva or vagina, vulval fissuring and oedema and satellite lesions.

References McCathie R. Vaginal discharge: common causes and management. Curr Obstet Gynaecol. 2006;16:211–7.

SRH5

SRH5 Answer: C

Explanation Missing pills or starting the pack late may make your pill less effective. The chance of pregnancy after missing pills depends on *when* pills are missed and *how many* pills are missed. A pill is late when you have forgotten to take it at the usual time. A pill has been missed when it is more than 24 h since the time you should have taken it.

If you miss one pill anywhere in your pack or start the new pack 1 day late, you will still have contraceptive cover.

However, missing *two or more pills* or starting the pack *two or more days late* (more than 48 h late) may affect your contraceptive cover. As soon as you realise you have missed any pills, take the last pill you missed immediately. In particular, during the 7-day pill-free break, your ovaries are not getting any effects from the pill. If you make this pill-free break longer by forgetting two or more pills, your ovaries might release an egg and there is a real risk of becoming pregnant.

References Faculty of Sexual and Reproductive Healthcare Clinical Effectiveness Unit CEU Statement. Missed pill recommendations; 2011.

SRH6

SRH6 Answer: E

Explanation The main feature of primary syphilis is one or more chancres. These macules develop within 90 days of inoculation and become papular, indurated and then ulcerate. They are usually painless. They are classically solitary and can appear anywhere on the body, although usually at the inoculation site. The ulcers resolve within 3 weeks, differentiating them from herpes ulcers, which resolve more quickly.

Secondary syphilis comprises multisystem involvement within 2 years. Features vary but classically include a generalised polymorphic rash often affecting the palms and soles. Alopecia, mucocutaneous lesions, uveitis, meningitis, cranial nerve palsies, hepatitis, splenomegaly, periostitis and glomerulonephritis might also occur.

References Kieran E, Hay DP. Sexually transmitted infections. Curr Obstet Gynaecol. 2006;16:218–25.

SRH7

SRH7 Answer: D

Explanation *N. gonorrhoeae* is a Gram-negative intracellular diplococcus. The primary sites of infection in women are the cervix (85–95 % of cases) and the urethra (65–75 % of cases).

Other sites that might be involved include the rectum (25–50 %), the oropharynx (5–15 %) and the conjunctiva. Gonorrhoea is the second most common pathogen causing PID and Fitz–Hugh–Curtis syndrome, with the attendant risk of long-term sequelae, as with *Chlamydia*. Gonorrhoea has been associated with miscarriage, premature labour and neonatal infection. In about 1 % of cases infection can spread haematogenously to the distant site, resulting in disseminated gonococcal infection with manifestations ranging from tendon/joint pain to meningitis or endocarditis.

References Kieran E, Hay DP. Sexually transmitted infections. Curr Obstet Gynaecol. 2006;16:218–25.

SRH8

SRH8 Answer: C

Explanation It is the most common STI in the UK. Between 3 % and 5 % of sexually active women attending UK general practices test positive for *Chlamydia*. Most women (80 %) are asymptomatic. If symptoms occur, this will generally be within 3 weeks of infection and comprise postcoital or intermenstrual bleeding, dysuria, lower abdominal pain and/or purulent vaginal discharge. The severity of the symptoms is variable. Approximately one-third of women will progress to ascending infection, presenting with PID. Even short delays in treatment of PID will markedly increase the risk of subsequent complications, which include infertility, ectopic pregnancy and chronic pelvic pain.

References Kieran E, Hay DP. Sexually transmitted infections. Curr Obstet Gynaecol. 2006;16:218–25.

SRH9

SRH9 Answer: E

Explanation A diagnosis of PID, and empirical antibiotic treatment, should be considered and usually offered in any young (under 25) sexually active woman who has recent onset, bilateral lower abdominal pain associated with local tenderness on bimanual vaginal examination, in whom pregnancy has been excluded. PID may be symptomatic or asymptomatic. Even when present, clinical symptoms and signs lack sensitivity and specificity (the positive predictive value of a clinical diagnosis is 65–90 % compared to laparoscopic diagnosis).

- Testing for gonorrhoea and *Chlamydia* in the lower genital tract is recommended since a positive result supports the diagnosis of PID. The absence of infection at this site does not exclude PID however.
- An elevated ESR or C-reactive protein also supports the diagnosis but is non-specific.
- The absence of endocervical or vaginal pus cells has a good negative predictive value (95 %) for a diagnosis of PID, but their presence is non-specific (poor positive predictive value—17 %).

References http://www.bashh.org/documents/3572.pdf

SRH10

SRH10 Answer: D

Explanation Rifampicin-like drugs (e.g. rifampicin, rifabutin) are the only antibiotics that are enzyme inducers and that have consistently been shown to reduce serum levels of ethinyl estradiol. Pregnancies have also been reported following concomitant use of COC and a wide range of antimicrobial agents, including penicillins, tetracyclines, macrolides, fluoroquinolones and imidazole antifungal drugs, which are not enzyme inducers.

Women who do not wish to change from a combined method while on short-term treatment with an enzyme-inducing drug (and for 28 days after stopping treatment) may opt to continue using a COC containing at least 30 μg EE, the patch or ring together with additional contraception. An extended or tricycling regimen should be used with a hormone-free interval of 4 days. Additional contraception should be continued for 28 days after stopping the enzyme-inducing drug.

With the exception of the very potent enzyme inducers rifampicin and rifabutin, women who are on an enzyme-inducing drug and who do not wish to change from COC may increase the dose of COC to at least 50 µg EE (maximum 70 µg) and use an extended or tricycling regimen with a pill-free interval of 4 days.

References http://www.fsrh.org/pdfs/CEUGuidanceDrugInteractionsHormonal. pdf

SRH11

SRH11 Answer: A

Explanation Progestogen-only injectable contraception containing DMPA works primarily by inhibiting ovulation. There is thickening of cervical mucus inhibiting sperm penetration into the upper reproductive tract. In addition, changes to the endometrium make it an unfavourable environment for implantation. Repeat injections of DMPA should be planned at 12-week intervals. The SPC suggests that DMPA can be given up to 12 weeks and 5 days since the last injection

References http://www.fsrh.org/pdfs/CEUGuidanceProgestogen OnlyInjectables09.pdf

SRH12

SRH12 Answer: C

Explanation A collaborative reanalysis of 45 epidemiological studies demonstrated that with every 5 years of use, there is approximately a 20 % reduction in the risk of ovarian cancer. A woman's risk after 15 years of use was around half of those who had never used COC. Risk reductions of at least 50 % have also been noted for endometrial cancer. The protective effect increases with increasing duration of use, and while it decreases over time after stopping, it has been shown to last up to several decades after use.

Among BRCA mutation carriers, COC use has been shown to provide a protective effect against ovarian cancer. Data also suggest a reduction in the incidence of ovarian cysts and benign ovarian tumours among women using COCs. COC use is not associated with an increased risk of mortality from endometrial or ovarian cancer.

References http://www.fsrh.org/pdfs/CEUGuidanceCombinedHormonal Contraception.pdf

SRH13

SRH13 Answer: E

Explanation Altered bleeding patterns is the most common reason given by women for stopping POPs. Indeed almost half of POP users experience prolonged bleeding, and up to 70 % report breakthrough bleeding or spotting in one or more cycles. Bleeding patterns associated with POPs may depend upon the progestogen used, the dose at which it is given and the circulating endogenous estradiol concentrations. Ovulation and subsequent endogenous progestogen concentrations may also influence bleeding patterns. Women should be advised about the likelihood and types of bleeding patterns expected with POP use. As a general guide:

- 20 % of women will be amenorrhoeic.
- 40 % will bleed regularly.
- 40 % will have erratic bleeding.

Between 10 % and 25 % of women using a POP will discontinue this method within 1 year as a result of these bleeding patterns.

References http://www.fsrh.org/pdfs/CEUGuidanceProgestogenOnlyPill09.pdf

SRH14

SRH14 Answer: A

Explanation All eligible women presenting between 0 and 120 h of UPSI or within 5 days of expected ovulation should be offered a Cu-IUD because of the low-documented failure rate.

The efficacy of ulipristal acetate (UPA) has been demonstrated up to 120 h and can be offered to all eligible women requesting EC during this time period. It is the only oral EC licensed for use between 72 and 120 h. The efficacy of levonorgestrel (LNG) has been demonstrated up to 96 h; between 96 and 120 h efficacy is unknown. Use of LNG beyond 72 h is outside the product licence.

References http://www.fsrh.org/pdfs/CEUguidanceEmergencyContraception11.pdf

SRH15

SRH15 Answer: B

Explanation The majority of studies show no adverse effects of POPs or DMPA on breastfeeding, milk volume, infant growth or development. In the first 6 weeks postpartum, WHOMEC recommends that the risks for breastfeeding women of using progestogen-only contraception (pills, injectables, implants or the LNG-IUS) outweigh any benefits. COC if used in the first 6 weeks postpartum may have an adverse effect on breast milk volume (grade B). Breastfeeding women should be advised to avoid COC in the first 6 weeks postpartum (grade B).

LAM is over 98 % effective in preventing pregnancy in breastfeeding women if they are <6 months postpartum, amenorrhoeic and fully breastfeeding (grade B). In women using LAM, it should be advised that the risk of pregnancy is increased if breastfeeding decreases (particularly stopping night feeds), when menstruation recurs or when >6 months postpartum.

References http://www.fsrh.org/pdfs/archive/breastfeeding04.pdf

SRH16

SRH16 Answer: E

Explanation Doctors are able to provide contraception, sexual and reproductive health advice and treatment, without parental knowledge or consent, to a young person aged under 16, provided that he/she understands the advice provided and its implications, and her/his physical or mental health would otherwise be likely to suffer, and so provision of advice or treatment is in their best interest.

An under 16 is deemed to be Gillick competent if they can understand the nature of the advice being given and have a sufficient maturity to understand what is involved.

Fraser guidelines state that:

- The young person understands the health professional's advice.
- The health professional cannot persuade the young person to inform his or her parents or allow the doctor to inform the parents that he or she is seeking contraceptive advice.

- The young person is very likely to begin or continue having intercourse with or without contraceptive treatment.
- Unless he/she receives contraceptive advice or treatment, the young person's physical or mental health or both are likely to suffer.
- The young person's best interests require the health professional to give contraceptive advice, treatment or both without parental consent.

Sexual activity with a child under 13 is a criminal offence and should always result in a child protection referral.

The Sexual Offences Act 2003 does not affect the ability of health professionals and others working with young people to provide confidential advice or treatment on contraception and sexual and reproductive health to young people under 16.

Under the Sexual Offences Act 2003, a person aged 18 or over commits an offence if they have sexual intercourse/any form of sexual touching with a person under 16.

References Department of Health. Best practice guidance for doctors and other health professionals on the provision of advice and treatment to young people under 16 on contraception, sexual and reproductive health; 2004. http://www.bashh.org/documents/1993.pdf

Sexual Offences Act 2003. http://www.legislation.gov.uk/ukpga/2003/42/section/9

SRH17

SRH17 Answer: D

Explanation Women with minimal or mild endometriosis who undergo laparoscopy should be offered surgical ablation or resection of endometriosis plus laparoscopic adhesiolysis because this improves the chance of pregnancy. Treatment with ovulation-suppression agents (medroxyprogesterone, gestrinone, combined oral contraceptives and GnRHa) or with danazol is ineffective in the treatment of endometriosis-associated infertility. Commonly used ovulation-suppression agents have been known to cause significant adverse effects such as weight gain, hot flushes and bone loss. Medical treatment of minimal and mild endometriosis does not enhance fertility in subfertile women and should not be offered.

References National Collaborating Centre for Women's and Children's Health. Fertility assessment and treatment for people with fertility problems. London: RCOG Press; 2004. http://www.rcog.org.uk/files/rcog-corp/uploaded-files/NEBFertilityFull.pdf

SRH18

SRH18 Answer: C

Explanation Prophylactic antibiotic use and bacterial screening for lower genital tract infection reduces this risk of infection after surgical abortion. Incidence rates among the control groups in trials of prophylactic antibiotics for abortion suggest that infective complications occur in up to 10 % of cases.

Vacuum aspiration under 7 weeks of gestation should be performed with appropriate safeguards to ensure complete abortion, including inspection of aspirated tissue. Prostaglandin analogues and osmotic cervical dilators are used for cervical preparation. The risk of uterine perforation is in the order of 1–4 in 1000 and is lower for early abortions and those performed by experienced clinicians.

References Royal College of Obstetricians and Gynaecologists. The care of women requesting induced abortion. Evidence-based clinical guideline number 7. London: RCOG Press; 2011. http://www.rcog.org.uk/files/rcog-corp/Abortion%20 guideline_web_1.pdf

SRH19

SRH19 Answer: E

Explanation Services should offer antibiotic prophylaxis effective against *Chlamydia trachomatis* and anaerobes for both surgical abortion (evidence grade, A) and medical abortion (evidence grade, C).

The following regimens are suitable for peri-abortion antibiotic prophylaxis:

- Azithromycin 1 g orally on the day of abortion, *plus* metronidazole 1 g rectally or 800 mg orally prior to or at the time of abortion
  OR
- Doxycycline 100 mg orally twice daily for 7 days, starting on the day of the abortion, *plus* metronidazole 1 g rectally or 800 mg orally prior to or at the time of the abortion
  OR
- Metronidazole 1 g rectally or 800 mg orally prior to or at the time of abortion for women who have tested negative for *C. trachomatis* infection

References RCOG Evidence based clinical guideline. Care of women requesting induced abortion. 2011.

SRH20

SRH20 Answer: A

Explanation Women with GTD should be advised to use barrier methods of contraception until hCG levels revert to normal. Once hCG level have normalised, the combined oral contraceptive pill may be used. There is no evidence as to whether single-agent progestogens have any effect on GTN. If oral contraception has been started before the diagnosis of GTD was made, the woman can be advised to remain on oral contraception, but she should be advised that there is a potential but low increased risk of developing GTN. Intrauterine contraceptive devices should not be used until hCG levels are normal to reduce the risk of uterine perforation.

References https://www.rcog.org.uk/globalassets/documents/guidelines/gtg_38.pdf

SRH21

SRH21 Answer: A

Explanation Cytogenetic analysis should be performed on products of conception of the third and subsequent consecutive miscarriage(s).

Parental peripheral blood karyotyping of both partners should be performed in couples with recurrent miscarriage where testing of products of conception reports an unbalanced structural chromosomal abnormality.

References https://www.rcog.org.uk/globalassets/documents/guidelines/gtg_17.pdf

SRH22

SRH22 Answer: E

Explanation The copper-bearing intrauterine device (Cu-IUD) can be inserted up to 120 h after the first episode of unprotected sexual intercourse (UPSI) or within 5 days of the earliest expected date of ovulation.

All eligible women presenting between 0 and 120 h of UPSI or within 5 days of expected ovulation should be offered a Cu-IUD because of the low-documented failure rate. The efficacy of ulipristal acetate (UPA) has been demonstrated up to

120 h and can be offered to all eligible women requesting EC during this time period. It is the only oral EC licensed for use between 72 and 120 h.

References http://www.fsrh.org/pdfs/CEUguidanceEmergencyContraception11.pdf

---

SRH23

SRH23 Answer: B

Explanation Qlaira is a new contraceptive pill which contains natural oestrogen, i.e. oestradiol valerate. It has continuous 28 days' cycle with 26 active pills with decreasing oestrogen and increasing progesterone dose to match the natural cycle followed by 2 placebos. There are no clinically significant benefits over the pills containing synthetic oestrogen. Missed pills rule vary, and the second method of contraception needs to be taken for 9 days if Qlaira is missed.

References FSRH publication. Qlaira; 2009.

SRH24

SRH24 Answer: B

Explanation Women with GTD should be advised to use barrier methods of contraception until hCG levels revert to normal.

Once hCG level have normalised, the combined oral contraceptive pill may be used. There is no evidence as to whether single-agent progestogens have any effect on GTN.

If oral contraception has been started before the diagnosis of GTD was made, the woman can be advised to remain on oral contraception but she should be advised that there is a potential but low increased risk of developing GTN.

Intrauterine contraceptive devices should not be used until hCG levels are normal to reduce the risk of uterine perforation.

It is true that barrier methods help protect against sexually transmitted diseases.

References Green-Top guideline – gestational trophoblastic disease.

SRH25

SRH25 Answer: C

Explanation Gonorrhoea is an STI caused by *Neisseria gonorrhoeae* which are Gram-negative cocci (not bacilli). Up to 50 % of women will be asymptomatic. Common symptoms may include increased or altered vaginal discharge and lower abdominal pain. It can also be a rare cause of heavy menstrual, postcoital or intermenstrual bleeding due to cervicitis or endometritis.

References British Association for Sexual Health and HIV Clinical Effectiveness Group. UK National guideline for the management of gonorrhoea in adults. 2011. http://www.bashh.org/documents/3611

SRH26

SRH26 Answer: B

Explanation Apart from infections, other causes of vaginal discharge include foreign bodies (e.g. retained tampons or condoms), cervical ectopy or polyps, genital tract malignancy, fistulae and allergic reactions.

Exclusion of infective and other causes can help confirm that a vaginal discharge is physiological.

There is some association between methods of contraception and vaginal discharge. Women complaining of vaginal discharge should be asked about current and past contraception.

Douching is the process of intravaginal cleaning with a liquid solution. Some women use the practice of douching as part of their general hygiene or cultural practice. Data suggest that douching changes vaginal flora and may predispose women to BV, although not all studies have reported this finding. Overall, the evidence suggests that douching should be discouraged as there are no proven health benefits.

Women with cervical ectopy may complain of increased physiological discharge. Ectopy is a normal finding in women of reproductive age, but treatments such as acidic gel, silver nitrate cauterisation, laser or cold coagulation are occasionally used in a gynaecology setting for symptomatic relief of vaginal discharge or postcoital bleeding. There is a lack of robust evidence for the effectiveness of these treatments in reducing vaginal discharge. Cervical pathology must be excluded prior to treatment, and women should be informed of potential risks of treatment and the fact that discharge symptoms may initially worsen before there is any improvement.

References   http://www.fsrh.org/pdfs/CEUGuidanceVaginalDischarge.pdf

SRH27

SRH27 Answer: C

Explanation   Women with cardiac diseases may be offered an intrauterine contraceptive device for contraception after considering all the clinical factors.

For women with cardiac disease, the decision to use an IUCD should involve a cardiologist.

The intrauterine method should be inserted in a hospital setting if vasovagal reaction presents a particularly high risk, e.g. women with a single ventricular physiology, Eisenmenger syndrome, tachycardia or pre-existing bradycardia.

Prophylactic antibiotics are not routinely required for insertion or removal of intrauterine contraceptive devices in women at high risk of infective endocarditis

References   http://www.fsrh.org/pdfs/CEUGuidanceContraceptiveChoices WomenCardiacDisease.pdf

SRH28

SRH28 Answer: D

Explanation   Women can be informed that a causal association between combined oral contraception (COC) use and onset or exacerbation of IBD is unsubstantiated.

Women should be advised that the efficacy of oral contraception is unlikely to be reduced by large bowel disease but may be reduced in women with Crohn's disease who have small bowel disease and malabsorption.

Health professionals should consider the impact of IBD-associated conditions such as venous thromboembolism, primary sclerosing cholangitis and osteoporosis and other medical conditions when prescribing contraception to women with IBD.

Women using combined hormonal contraception should use additional contraception while taking antibiotic courses of less than 3 weeks and for 7 days after the antibiotic has been discontinued.

Health professionals should check whether any prescribed medications for rectal or genital administration contain products that may reduce the efficacy of condoms.

Women with IBD should stop COC at least 4 weeks before major elective surgery and alternative contraception should be provided. An advice regarding recommencing COC should be given individually.

Laparoscopic sterilisation is an inappropriate method of contraception for women with IBD who have had previous pelvic or abdominal surgery.

Women with IBD considering sterilisation, and their partners, should be counselled about alternative methods of contraception including long-acting reversible contraception (LARC) and vasectomy.

References http://www.fsrh.org/pdfs/CEUGuidanceIBD09.pdf

SRH29

SRH29 Answer: B

Explanation The following regimens are recommended for early medical abortion:

- At ≤63 days of gestation, mifepristone 200 mg orally followed 24–48 h later by misoprostol 800 micrograms given by the vaginal, buccal or sublingual route
- At ≤49 days of gestation, 200 mg oral mifepristone followed 24–48 h later by 400 μ grams of oral misoprostol

For women at 50–63 days of gestation, if abortion has not occurred 4 h after administration of misoprostol, a second dose of misoprostol 400 micrograms may be administered vaginally or orally (depending upon preference and amount of bleeding).

References https://www.rcog.org.uk/globalassets/documents/guidelines/abortion-guideline_web_1.pdf

SRH30

SRH30 Answer: C

Explanations High vaginal swabs (HVS) are often used to diagnose causes of vaginal discharge but they are of limited value.

BV may be underdiagnosed if no other diagnostic criteria are used. Reporting of commensal bacteria can cause anxiety and lead to overtreatment.

HVS may be used to aid the diagnosis of BV, VVC, TV or other genital tract infections (e.g. streptococcal organisms), but their use should generally be reserved for the following situations:

1. When symptoms, signs and/or pH are inconsistent with a specific diagnosis
2. Pregnancy, postpartum, postabortion or post-instrumentation

3. Recurrent symptoms
4. Failed treatment

If TV (*Trichomonas vaginalis*) is suspected, an HVS can be taken from the posterior fornix but sensitivity may be low because motility reduces with transit time. Therefore, referral to GUM is recommended for confirmation by wet microscopy +/− culture and also for partner notification.

References   http://www.fsrh.org/pdfs/CEUGuidanceVaginalDischarge.pdf

Gynaecologic Oncology: Answers and Explanations

24

GYNONCO1

GYNONCO1 Answer: C

Explanation Epithelial ovarian cancers (EOCs) are the most common cause of death from gynaecological malignancy in the developed world. EOCs comprise a heterogeneous group of neoplasms including serous (68 %), clear cell (13 %), endometrioid (9 %) and mucinous (3 %) pathological subtypes.

References https://www.rcog.org.uk/globalassets/documents/guidelines/scientific-impact-papers/sip44hgscs.pdf

GYNONCO2

GYNONCO2 Answer: D

Explanation The risk of endometrial cancer in a low-risk woman in the UK is 2.7 %. However, it may be increased in certain high-risk groups. The hereditary non-polyposis colon cancer syndrome (HNPCC—Lynch syndrome) is a predominantly colorectal cancer syndrome with an increased risk for cancer of the endometrium, ovary, stomach, urothelium and pancreas. Two genes account for the majority of the families with HNPCC – *MLH1* and *MSH2*. Germline *MSH6* mutations, which are rare in HNPCC, have been reported in several families with multiple members affected with endometrial carcinoma. These genes show highly penetrant autosomal dominant inheritance. In males the lifetime risk of colorectal cancer by 70 is 70 %. In females it is 50 % by 70, with an equally high risk for endometrial cancer and a lifetime risk for ovarian cancer of 12 %.

© Springer India 2016
C. Ratha, J. Gupta, *SBAs and EMQs for MRCOG II*,
DOI 10.1007/978-81-322-2689-5_24

HNPCC families are usually identified clinically by their family history of colorectal cancer rather than endometrial or ovarian cancer. Families most likely to have HNPCC fulfil all the Amsterdam criteria:

- Colorectal cancer in at least three first-degree relatives of each other and where familial adenomatous polyposis coli has been excluded
- Colorectal cancer in at least two successive generations
- Colorectal cancer diagnosed under the age of 50 years in one relative

The appropriate surveillance method for endometrial cancer is still disputed, and some would argue that, given the relatively early presentation with symptoms and the relatively good prognosis, active surveillance is not warranted. Surveillance methods have included transvaginal ultrasound scans, pipelle aspiration and hysteroscopy. The detection rates for endometrial cancer using the pipelle were 97 % and 91 % in post- and premenopausal women, respectively.

References   Gardiner C. Family history of gynaecological cancers. Obstet Gynaecol Reprod Med. 17(12):356–61.

GYNONCO3

GYNONCO3 Answer: D

Explanation Use of the combined oral contraceptive pill has been shown to decrease the risk of endometrial cancer. This effect is likely to be due to the suppression of endometrial proliferation by the progestagen component of the oral contraceptive pill. Duration of use is important as patients with 12–23 months of use have a 40 % reduction in risk, and women with 10 years use have a 60 % reduction. There is an ongoing research study to identify whether intrauterine progestagens, delivered using the MIRENA intrauterine contraceptive device, can reduce the risk of endometrial cancer in women with HNPCC mutations.

References   Gardiner C. Family history of gynaecological cancers. Obstet Gynaecol Reprod Med. 17(12):356–61.

GYNONCO4

GYNONCO4 Answer: C

Explanation It is not uncommon to find foci of malignant tumours in the ovaries of women who have undergone prophylactic oophorectomy for a high risk of ovarian cancer. A recent study found 12 % of women who underwent an oophorectomy because of a *BRCA1* or *BRCA2* mutation had occult ovarian tumours, which had not been identified by surveillance. A small number of women who undergo prophylactic oophorectomy subsequently go on to develop intra-abdominal carcinomatosis that is indistinguishable from ovarian cancer. These tumours are thought to be papillary serous carcinomas of the peritoneum, which shares a common embryological origin with the ovarian epithelium.

References Gardiner C. Family history of gynaecological cancers. Obstet Gynaecol Reprod Med. 17(12):349–55. Subject – Gynaecology.

GYNONCO5

GYNONCO5 Answer: B

Explanation Increasing use of laparoscopy in oncology has led to a change in the surgical approach for borderline tumours, but there are concerns regarding the possibilities of cyst rupture, development of port-site metastases and understaging of disease; higher risk of recurrence and worsened survival have been documented. In the absence of clear evidence to the contrary, staging and treatment of borderline ovarian tumours should ideally be performed by midline laparotomy.

No role for *adjuvant* chemotherapy has been demonstrated for borderline ovarian tumours and there are no relevant clinical trials. Consideration may be given to chemotherapy in the setting of recurrent borderline ovarian tumour that is not amenable to surgical resection, particularly as undiagnosed invasive disease cannot be excluded in this situation.

The risk of recurrence varies between 0 and 58 %, depending upon the histological type of borderline ovarian tumour and extent of primary surgery. Published evidence suggests that the incidence of invasive disease at recurrence varies from 8 to 73 %. For women treated with conservative surgery, clinical examination and vaginal ultrasound have been shown to benefit the detection of recurrent disease. Currently, we follow up every 3 months for the first 2 years, every 6 months for the next 2 years and annually thereafter.

References Bagade P, Edmondson R, Nayar A. Management of borderline ovarian tumours. Obstet Gynaecol. 2012;14:115–20.

GYNONCO6

GYNONCO6 Answer: A

Explanation Borderline tumours represent a disease that is distinct from invasive ovarian cancer. It is now clear from molecular studies that there are at least two distinct forms of ovarian cancer.

High-grade serous cancers, which are associated with very high rates of p53 mutation, are the most common form of invasive neoplasm. Low-grade tumours, which include borderline ovarian tumours, are characterised by mutations of the BRAF/KRAS pathway. It is thus clear that there is no progression from one type to the other and that, although borderline ovarian tumours can progress to invasive disease, this tends to be the low-grade invasive phenotype rather than the high grade. There is no evidence that women with mutations of the BRCA genes, which clearly predispose to invasive cancers, are at increased risk for the development of borderline ovarian tumours.

References Bagade P, Edmondson R, Nayar A. Management of borderline ovarian tumours. Obstet Gynaecol. 2012;14:115–20.

GYNONCO7

GYNONCO7 Answer: E

Explanation Ultrapotent steroids are important in the management of women diagnosed with lichen sclerosus. Corticosteroids have anti-inflammatory and immunosuppressive properties by altering lymphocyte differentiation and function and inhibiting cytokine production. Clobetasol propionate is the most potent topical corticosteroid available. Response rates reported from large-case series of women diagnosed with lichen sclerosus are high, with either complete or partial resolution of symptoms in 54–96 % of women. Approximately 4–10 % of women with anogenital lichen sclerosus will have symptoms that do not improve with topical ultrapotent steroids (steroid-resistant disease). The recommended second-line treatment is topical tacrolimus under the supervision of a specialist clinic.

Tacrolimus and pimecrolimus belong to the class of immunosuppressant drugs known as calcineurin inhibitors. Their mode of action differs from that of corticosteroids, mainly reducing inflammation by suppressing T-lymphocyte responses. Tacrolimus and pimecrolimus have both been shown to be effective at controlling a number of vulval dermatoses including lichen sclerosus and lichen planus.

References RCOG Green-Top guideline No. 58 – The management of vulval skin disorders.

GYNONCO8

GYNONCO8 Answer: B

Explanation Anogenital lichen sclerosus can present at any age but is more commonly seen in postmenopausal women. It causes severe pruritus, which may be worse at night. The whole vulval perianal area may be affected in a figure-of-eight distribution. Uncontrollable scratching may cause trauma with bleeding and skin splitting and symptoms of discomfort, pain and dyspareunia. Lichen sclerosus is not linked to female hormone changes, contraceptives, hormone replacement therapy or the menopause. Evidence suggests that it is an autoimmune condition, with around 40 % of women with lichen sclerosus having or going on to develop another autoimmune condition.

References RCOG Green-Top guideline No. 58 – The management of vulval skin disorders.

GYNONCO9

GYNONCO9 Answer: B

Explanation Lichen planus is a common skin disease which may affect the skin anywhere on the body. It usually affects mucosal surfaces and is more commonly seen in the oral mucosa. Lichen planus presents with polygonal flat-topped violaceous purpuric plaques and papules with a fine white reticular pattern (Wickham striae). However, in the mouth and genital region, it can be erosive and is more commonly associated with pain than with pruritus. Erosive lichen planus appears as a well-demarcated, glazed erythema around the introitus. The aetiology is unknown, but it may be an autoimmune condition. It can affect all ages and is not linked to hormonal status.

References RCOG Green-Top guideline No. 58 – The management of vulval skin disorders.

GYNONCO10

GYNONCO10 Answer: A

Explanation Long-term follow-up of randomised clinical trials have reported similar survival rates for women treated by mastectomy or breast conservation surgery. However. all of these studies had selection criteria and indeed the vast majority of patients in these studies presented with tumours < 2.5 cm. Accurate preoperative assessment of the size and extent of the tumour is essential for deciding whether breast conservation surgery is an alternative option to mastectomy. Routine methods for assessing the extent of disease in the breast are clinical examination, mammography and ultrasound. In a significant number of cases, the true extent of disease is underestimated, particularly with invasive lobular cancer.

While many women may be suitable for breast conservation surgery, various factors (e.g. biological, patient choice) may lead to some women being advised or choosing to have a mastectomy for their disease.

References Surgical guidelines for the management of breast cancer, association of breast surgery at BASO 2009. Eur J Surg Oncol. 2009. doi:10.1016/j.ejso.2009.01.008

GYNONCO11

GYNONCO11 Answer: D

Explanation Some patients with invasive breast cancer may be diagnosed with axillary disease prior to definitive surgery. The use of preoperative axillary assessment with ultrasound and appropriate fine-needle aspiration (or core biopsy if feasible) can yield a diagnosis of involved nodes in some cases. If a positive diagnosis of axillary nodal metastasis is made in a patient with early breast cancer, that patient should normally proceed to an axillary clearance. If an axillary clearance is carried out, all axillary lymph nodes should be removed unless there are specific reasons or unit policies not to do this. In the latter cases the anatomical level of dissection should be specified in the operation note. The number of nodes retrieved from axillary node clearance histology specimens will be both surgeon and pathologist dependent. However, for a full axillary clearance, at least 10 nodes should be retrieved in >90 % of cases.

References Surgical guidelines for the management of breast cancer, Association of Breast Surgery at BASO 2009. Eur J Surg Oncol. 2009. doi:10.1016/j.ejso.2009.01.008

GYNONCO12

GYNONCO12 Answer: D

Explanation The NHS Breast Screening Programme provides free breast screening every three years for all women aged between 50 and 70 years. Once women reach the upper age limit for routine invitations for breast screening, they are encouraged to make their own appointment.

Women under 50 are not currently offered routine screening. Research has shown that routine screening in the 40–50 age group is less effective. As a woman goes through menopause, the glandular tissue in her breast 'involutes', that is to say, the proportion of fat in her breast increases. This makes the mammogram easier to interpret.

However, the DMIST study has shown that digital mammography is better for screening younger women and women with denser breasts and is equally effective as film mammography in older women. So the programme is now being gradually extended to women aged 47–49, as well as to those aged 71–73.

References http://www.cancerscreening.nhs.uk/breastscreen

GYNONCO13

GYNONCO13 Answer: E

Explanation A lump in the breast is a cause of great concern. High-frequency, high-resolution USG helps in its evaluation. This is exemplified in women with dense breast tissue where USG is useful in detecting small breast cancers that are not seen on mammography.

Several studies have described the sonographic characteristics commonly seen in benign lesions of the breast:

1. Smooth and well circumscribed
2. Hyperechoic, isoechoic or mildly hypoechoic
3. Thin echogenic capsule
4. Ellipsoid shape, with the maximum diameter being in the transverse plane
5. Three or fewer gentle lobulations
6. Absence of any malignant findings

The following are the common benign causes of breast lump and their ultrasound characteristics:

Breast cysts—the commonest cause of breast lumps in women between 35 and 50 years of age. A cyst occurs when fluid accumulates due to obstruction of the extralobular terminal ducts, either due to fibrosis or because of intraductal epithelial proliferation. A cyst is seen on USG as a well-defined, round or oval, anechoic structure with a thin wall.

Fibroadenosis—the USG appearance of the breast in this condition is extremely variable since it depends on the stage and extent of morphological changes. In the early stages, the USG appearance may be normal, even though lumps may be palpable on clinical examination. There may be focal areas of thickening of the parenchyma, with or without patchy increase in echogenicity. Discrete single cysts or clusters of small cysts may be seen in some. Focal fibrocystic changes may appear as solid masses or thin-walled cysts. About half of these solid masses are usually classified as indeterminate and will eventually require a biopsy

Duct ectasia—this lesion has a variable appearance. Typically, duct ectasia may appear as a single tubular structure filled with fluid or sometimes may show multiple such structures as well. Old cellular debris may appear as echogenic content. If the debris fills the lumen, it can be sometimes mistaken for a solid mass, unless the tubular shape is picked up.

Fibroadenoma—on USG, it appears as a well-defined lesion. A capsule can usually be identified. The echotexture is usually homogenous and hypoechoic as compared to the breast parenchyma, and there may be low-level internal echoes. Typically, the transverse diameter is greater than the anteroposterior diameter. In a small number of patients, the mass may appear complex, hyperechoic or isoechoic. A similar USG appearance may be seen with medullary, mucinous or papillary carcinoma.

References Gokhale S. Ultrasound characterization of breast masses. Indian J Radiol Imaging. 2009;19(3):242–7.

GYNONCO14

GYNONCO14 Answer: C

Explanation Community-based surveys indicate that one fifth of women have significant vulval symptoms. The common conditions with which women present are dermatitis, vulval candidiasis, lichen simplex, Lichen sclerosus and Lichen planus. Anogenital lichen sclerosus can present at any age but is more commonly seen in postmenopausal women. It causes severe pruritus, which may be worse at night. The whole vulval perianal area may be affected in a figure-of-eight distribution. Uncontrollable scratching may cause trauma with bleeding and skin splitting and symptoms of discomfort, pain and dyspareunia. Lichen sclerosus is not linked to female hormone changes, contraceptives, hormone replacement therapy or menopause. Evidence suggests that it is an autoimmune condition, with around 40 % of women with lichen sclerosus having or going on to develop another autoimmune condition. Pruritus is related to active inflammation with erythema and keratinisation of the vulval skin. Hyperkeratosis can be marked with thickened white skin. The skin is often atrophic, classically demonstrating subepithelial haemorrhages (ecchymoses), and it may split easily. Continuing inflammation results in inflammatory adhesions. Often there is lateral fusion of the labia minora, which become adherent and eventually are completely reabsorbed. The hood of the clitoris and its lateral margins may fuse, burying the clitoris. Midline fusion can produce skin bridges at the fourchette and narrowing of the introitus. Occasionally, the labia minora fuse together medially, which also restricts the vaginal opening and can cause difficulty with micturition and even urinary retention.

References RCOG Green-Top guideline No. 58. The management of vulval skin disorders. 2011.

GYNONCO15

GYNONCO15 Answer: B

Explanation Vulval intraepithelial neoplasia (VIN) is commonly associated with HPV 16 and has a varied clinical presentation. Symptoms include irritation, mild discomfort, pain or ulceration.

It can however be asymptomatic, and a change in texture and/or appearance is noted. On examination, VIN presents as an area of glazed erythema, thickened, macerated skin, an area of brown pigmentation or a combination of these features. VIN patients are more likely to develop cervical intraepithelial neoplasia (CIN) and anal intraepithelial neoplasia (AIN) and should be examined to exclude this. There are two main histological subtypes of VIN—well differentiated and basaloid. The latter is more common, particularly in premenopausal women. Untreated VIN may progress to invasive squamous cell carcinoma (SCC) in approximately 5 % of cases.

References Hussain SH, Sterling J. Skin diseases affecting the vulva. Obstet Gynaecol Reprod Med. 24(5):141–7.

GYNONCO16

GYNONCO16 Answer: C

Explanation The proportion of vulval carcinomas associated with HPV infection varies from 15 % to 79 %. HPV16 is by far the most common type identified in both vulval carcinomas and VINs, although other HPV types, such as 18, 31, 33 and 45, have also been reported. Low-risk HPV types, especially HPV6 and HPV11, have been found in a small percentage of vulval lesions, but their role is not clear. HPV is detected in most cases of undifferentiated VIN (usual type) and only in few cases of differentiated VIN. Prophylactic HPV vaccines, which cover HPV16 and HPV18, have been associated with a significant reduction in the incidence of VIN in young women

References Gajjar K, Shafi M. Invasive vulval cancer. Obstet Gynaecol Reprod Med. 24(6):177–85.

GYNONCO17

GYNONCO17 Answer: D

Explanation Groin node dissection should not be underestimated, as it allows adequate staging and, therefore, remains an important factor in reducing the mortality from vulval cancer. The incidence of lymph node metastasis is related to the clinical stage of the disease and depth of invasion. A recurrence in the groin carries a very high mortality. Systematic inguinofemoral lymphadenectomy comprises resection of superficial inguinal lymph nodes as well as deep femoral nodes. Patient selection is important due to the significant morbidity associated with lymphadenectomy. Lymphadenectomy is not required in early stage 1A vulval cancer due to the very low risk of metastasis. Therefore, majority of the patients with early stage disease may undergo an unnecessary lymph node resection and the associated complications. Complications include wound dehiscence, infection, lymphocysts and lymphoedema.

References Gajjar K, Shafi M. Invasive vulval cancer. Obstet Gynaecol Reprod Med. 24(6):177–85.

GYNONCO18

GYNONCO18 Answer: D

Explanation Histologically and biologically, endometrial cancers are broadly classified into two main categories: type 1 and type 2 cancers. The vast majority (80 %) of endometrial carcinomas are type 1, i.e. endometrioid adenocarcinoma, and arise from the glandular epithelium, usually on a background of atypical hyperplasia. Endometrial adenocarcinoma is found in up to 50 % of cases of severe atypical hyperplasia. They are associated with obesity, nulliparity, insulin resistance and a hyper-oestrogenic environment, e.g. the use of unopposed oestrogens or ovarian granulosa cell tumour. These tumours often exhibit mutations in the PTEN tumour suppressor gene, KRAS oncogene and mismatch repair genes and frequently stain positively for oestrogen and progesterone receptors.

Type 2 tumours, i.e. serous, clear cell, squamous and undifferentiated carcinomas, carcinosarcoma (previously called malignant mixed Müllerian tumour) and endometrial stromal sarcomas (ESS), are less common, more aggressive and have a poorer prognosis. They are not associated with the risk factors for type 1 cancers. Often these tumours occur in older women. At a molecular level, mutations of the p53 tumour suppressor gene are common.

References Kay J, Mehasseb MK. Endometrial cancer. Obstet Gynaecol Reprod Med. 24(6):177–85.

GYNONCO19

GYNONCO19 Answer: A

Explanation Endometrial cancer is one of the extra-colonic cancers caused by hereditary non-polyposis colon cancer syndrome (HNPCC) or Lynch II syndrome. This is an autosomal dominant cancer susceptibility syndrome resulting of a germ cell line mutation in one of the DNA mismatch repair genes (MSH2, MLH1 or MSH6). Despite the name of the syndrome, 50 % of affected women will develop endometrial carcinoma as their index cancer (rather than bowel cancer). Women with confirmed HNPCC have a 40–60 % lifetime risk of developing endometrial cancer and a 10 % risk of developing a number of other cancers. Strict criteria have been developed to identify these women at risk (the Amsterdam criteria). There is no uniform screening strategy, and risk-reducing hysterectomy and bilateral salpingo-oophorectomy are recommended for those women who have completed their family. Endometrial surveillance with annual endometrial imaging and biopsy is offered to women with HNPCC who wish to retain their uterus, although this is not proven to be effective in prevention

References Kay J, Mehasseb MK. Endometrial cancer. Obstet Gynaecol Reprod Med. 24(6):177–85.

GYNONCO20

nGYNONCO20 Answer: C

Explanation Vulval SCC is staged surgically and the International Federation of Gynaecology and Obstetrics (FIGO) classification system is used. Mortality is directly related to the stage of disease at presentation.

FIGO stage	Description
I	Tumour confined to the vulva
IA	Lesions 2 cm in size, confined to the vulva or perineum and with stromal invasion of 1.0 mm, no nodal metastasis
IB	Lesions >2 cm in size or with stromal invasion >1.0 mm, confined to the vulva
	Or perineum, with negative nodes
II	Tumour of any size with extension to adjacent perineal structures (lower third of urethra, lower third of vagina, anus) with negative nodes
III	Tumour of any size, with or without extension to adjacent perineal structures, with positive inguinofemoral nodes
IIIA	(i) With 1 lymph node metastasis ($\geq$5 mm)
	(ii) With 1–2 lymph node metastasis(es) (<5 mm)

FIGO stage	Description
IIIB	(i) With 2 or more lymph node metastases ($\geq$5 mm)
	(ii) With 3 or more lymph node metastases (<5 mm)
IIIC	With positive nodes with extra-capsular spread
IV	Tumour invading other regional (upper 2/3 urethra, upper 2/3 vagina) or distant structures
IVA	Tumour invades any of the following: (i) upper urethral and/or vaginal mucosa, bladder mucosa, rectal mucosa or fixed to the pelvic bone or (ii) fixed or ulcerated inguinofemoral lymph nodes
IVB	Any distant metastasis including pelvic lymph nodes

References Gajjar K, Shafi M. Invasive vulval cancer. Obstet Gynaecol Reprod Med. 24(6):177–85.

GYNONCO21

GYNONCO21 Answer: B

Explanation Obesity accounts for about 40 % of endometrial cancer cases in the developed world. Endometrial carcinoma was the first malignancy to be recognised as being linked to obesity. A linear increase in the risk of type 1 endometrial cancer with increasing weight and BMI has been observed. Overweight and obese women have two to four times greater risk of developing endometrial cancer than women of a healthy weight, regardless of their menopausal status. Obesity affects the production of peptides (e.g. insulin and IGFe1, SHBG) and steroid hormones (i.e. oestrogen, progesterone and androgens). It is likely that prolonged exposure to high levels of oestrogen and insulin associated with obesity may contribute to the development of endometrial cancer.

References Kay J, Mehasseb MK. Endometrial cancer. Obstet Gynaecol Reprod Med. 24(6):177–85.

GYNONCO22

GYNONCO22 Answer: A

Explanation Cancer is the second most common cause of death within reproductive years of life; however, its association with pregnancy is a rare circumstance, complicating approximately 1 in 1000 pregnancies. The most commonly encountered malignancies within pregnancy include breast, cervix, thyroid, ovary, colon, leukaemias, melanomas and lymphomas. Breast cancer is the commonest cancer affecting women with a lifetime risk of 11 % in the UK. It also accounts for the most prevalent cancer complicating pregnancy and the puerperium, occurring in about 1 in 3000 women. Physiological changes within the breast hinder the detection of discrete lumps in pregnancy, and therefore prognosis is worse where pregnancy coexists due to delays in diagnosis and treatment.

References Cooke L, Shafi MI. Cancer in pregnancy. Obstet Gynaecol Reprod Med. 23(10):317–9.

GYNONCO23

GYNONCO23 Answer: E

Explanation Cervical cancer is still staged clinically using the International Federation of Gynaecology and Obstetrics (FIGO) system. Traditionally, this included procedures such as pathology review, examination under anaesthesia with combined rectovaginal examination, cystoscopy, proctoscopy, chest radiography and perhaps intravenous urography. In practice, currently, all women undergo ultrasound scan, MRI, CT and possibly PET in some developed countries. Although the imaging results cannot change the clinical FIGO staging, they are often used to plan management.

References Kyrgiou M, Shafi MI. Invasive cancer of the cervix. Obstet Gynaecol Reprod Med. 23(11):343–51.

GYNONCO24

GYNONCO24 Answer: E

Explanation The majority of cervical cancers are squamous in origin, but adenocarcinomas appear to be increasingly common, accounting for approximately 20 % of all primary cervical cancers. This increase partly reflects an increased awareness of the disease. Adenocarcinoma is more likely to be diagnosed in younger women and has largely poorer prognosis in comparison to cervical squamous carcinoma, which partly reflects the delay in diagnosis. Cytology screening programmes were designed to detect squamous lesions and, as a result, the endocervical distribution of glandular abnormalities reduces their accuracy. Specific oncogenic HPV types, and in particular HPV 18, have been related to adenocarcinoma.

References Kyrgiou M, Shafi MI. Invasive cancer of the cervix. Obstet Gynaecol Reprod Med. 23(11):343–51.

GYNONCO25

GYNONCO25 Answer: E

Explanation Hysteroscopy and endometrial sampling can be performed safely in the outpatient setting in >80 % of women, providing prompt reassurance and a diagnosis in those cases where an endometrial abnormality is suggested on ultrasound scan. The pipelle is the best endometrial sampling device, with detection rates for endometrial cancer in postmenopausal and premenopausal women of 99.6 % and 91 %, respectively. The sensitivity for the detection of endometrial hyperplasia is 81 %, with a specificity of 98 %.

References Kay J, Mehasseb MK. Endometrial cancer. Obstet Gynaecol Reprod Med. 24(6):177–85.

GYNONCO26

GYNONCO26 Answer: C

Explanation The staging system used for endometrial carcinoma is the International Federation of Gynaecology and Obstetrics (FIGO) classification, revised in 2009. The staging is based upon findings at surgery and histological assessment of the surgical specimen, providing prognostic information. After omission from the 2009 FIGO staging for endometrial carcinoma, the need for and the significance of a positive peritoneal cytology result became controversial. In women with stage I and II disease, positive peritoneal cytology results do not influence survival. Poor prognosis associated with positive washings is most common in women with other adverse prognostic factors, i.e. grade 3 histologic types, metastases to the adnexa, deep myometrial invasion or positive pelvic or para-aortic nodes. Positive peritoneal cytology may thus carry a prognostic significance only when the endometrial carcinoma has spread beyond the uterus. It does not carry any therapeutic significance as yet.

References Kay J, Mehasseb MK. Endometrial cancer. Obstet Gynaecol Reprod Med. 24(6):177–85.

GYNONCO27

GYNONCO27 Answer: C

Explanation Lymphatic spread occurs to the external iliac, internal iliac and obturator lymph nodes in the pelvis and to the para-aortic nodes. Involvement of para-aortic nodes is less common if the pelvic nodes are not involved, although direct spread via lymphatic channels draining the upper uterus can occur.

References Kay J, Mehasseb MK. Endometrial cancer. Obstet Gynaecol Reprod Med. 24(6):177–85.

GYNONCO28

GYNONCO28 Answer: D

Explanation The overall prognosis for endometrial cancer is generally good and reflects early presentation of the disease in most cases. The 5-year survival rate for all stages is approximately 80 % but varies with tumour grade and depth of myometrial invasion. Survival in stage 1 disease is 85–90 % but approximately 70–75 % for stage II, 45 % for stage III and <30 % for stage IV disease. Other factors that adversely affect prognosis include non-endometrioid histological subtype and lymphovascular space invasion.

References Kay J, Mehasseb MK. Endometrial cancer. Obstet Gynaecol Reprod Med. 24(6):177–85.

GYNONCO29

GYNONCO29 Answer: B

Explanation Call–Exner bodies are small eosinophilic fluid-filled spaces between granulosa cells. They are usually associated with granulosa cell tumour. The microfollicular variant, the most easily recognised, is characterised by multiple small rounded spaces formed by cystic degeneration in small aggregates of granulosa cells, containing eosinophilic PAS-positive material (chondroitin 6-sulphate) and often fragments of nuclear debris or pyknotic nuclei. These spaces, known as Call–Exner bodies, are found in only 30–50 % of tumours.

References Gynecologic pathology by Nucci and Oliva. Elsevier Churchill Livingstone 2009. Chapter 12, Sex cord stromal tumours of the ovary. p. 463.

GYNONCO30

GYNONCO30 Answer: E

Explanation Calculating the risk of malignancy index (RMI), these are modifications of the original RMI using modified scores: RMI = UxMxCA125.

U = 0 (for ultrasound score of 0); U = 1 (for ultrasound score of 1); U = 3 (for ultrasound score of 2–5). Ultrasound scans are scored one point for each of the following characteristics: multilocular cyst, evidence of solid areas, evidence of metastases, presence of ascites and bilateral lesions.

M = 3 for all postmenopausal women dealt with by this guideline: CA125 is serum and CA125 measurement in u/ml.

References https://www.rcog.org.uk/globalassets/documents/guidelines/gtg34ovariancysts.pdf

GYNONCO31

GYNONCO31 Answer: C

Explanation All ovarian cysts that are suspicious of malignancy in a postmenopausal woman, as indicated by a high risk of malignancy index, clinical suspicion or findings at laparoscopy, are likely to require a full laparotomy and staging procedure. This should be performed by an appropriate surgeon, working as part of a multidisciplinary team in a cancer centre, through an extended midline incision, and should include:

- Cytology: ascites or washings
- Laparotomy with clear documentation
- Biopsies from adhesions and suspicious areas
- TAH, BSO and infracolic omentectomy

The laparotomy and staging procedure may include bilateral selective pelvic and para-aortic lymphadenectomy.

References https://www.rcog.org.uk/globalassets/documents/guidelines/gtg34ovariancysts.pdf

GYNONCO32

GYNONCO32 Answer: C

Explanation Simple, unilateral, unilocular ovarian cysts, less than 5 cm in diameter, have a low risk of malignancy. It is recommended that, in the presence of a normal serum CA125 levels, they be managed conservatively.

Numerous studies have looked at the risk of malignancy in ovarian cysts, comparing ultrasound morphology with either histology at subsequent surgery or by close follow-up of those women managed conservatively. The risk of malignancy in these studies of cysts that are less than 5 cm, unilateral, unilocular and echo-free with no solid parts or papillary formations is less than 1 %.

In addition, more than 50 % of these cysts will resolve spontaneously within three months.

Thus, it is reasonable to manage these cysts conservatively, with a follow-up ultrasound scan for cysts of 2–5 cm, a reasonable interval being four months. This, of course, depends upon the views and symptoms of the woman and on the gynaecologist's clinical assessment.

References https://www.rcog.org.uk/globalassets/documents/guidelines/gtg34ovariancysts.pdf

---

GYNONCO33

GYNONCO33 Answer: D

Explanation Recommendations for follow-up protocols are currently determined by an expert consensus opinion.

- Women treated for high-grade disease (CIN 2, CIN 3, cGIN) require six- and 12-month follow-up cytology and annual cytology for the subsequent 9 years at least before returning to screening at the routine interval (high-risk follow-up).
- Women treated for low-grade disease require 6-, 12- and 24-month follow-up cytology. If all results are negative, then women may be returned to screening at the routine interval (low-risk follow-up).

If a woman has not attended for all the specified cytology for her high-risk follow-up, she should be allowed to return to routine screening provided her samples are normal at least 10 years after treatment

References http://www.cancerscreening.nhs.uk/cervical/publications/nhscsp20.pdf

GYNONCO34

GYNONCO34 Answer: D

Explanation Women with suspected PE should be advised that, compared with CTPA, V/Q scanning may carry a slightly increased risk of childhood cancer but is associated with a lower risk of maternal breast cancer; in both situations, the absolute risk is very small. Lifetime risk is increased by 13.6 % with CTPA.

References RCOG GTG No. 37b. 2015.

GYNONCO35

GYNONCO35 Answer: D

Explanation Borderline ovarian tumours are a heterogeneous group of tumours often seen in younger women. They are a distinct pathological group of neoplasms that demonstrate higher proliferative activity when compared with benign neoplasms but which do not show stromal invasion. Younger women are more likely to have borderline tumours compared with older women. Parous women have a reduced risk of developing borderline ovarian tumours compared with nulliparous women. Lactation is found to be protective. These risk factors are similar to those recognised for invasive ovarian cancer.

However, unlike invasive ovarian cancer, oral contraceptive use is not protective against the development of borderline ovarian tumours. It has been suggested that this finding may support the concept that borderline tumours represent a disease that is distinct from invasive ovarian cancer. Furthermore, there is no evidence that women with mutations of the *BRCA* genes, which clearly predispose to invasive cancers, are at increased risk for the development of borderline ovarian tumours.

Many are only diagnosed after primary surgery has already taken place for a presumed benign lesion. The subsequent management often causes confusion. Complete surgical staging is the cornerstone of management, but conservative surgery is an acceptable alternative in those keen to retain their fertility. The role of long-term follow-up is controversial.

References Bagade P, Edmondson R, Nayar A. Management of borderline ovarian tumours. Obstet Gynaecol. 2012;14:115–20.

GYNONCO36

GYNONCO36 Answer: C

Explanation Cervical screening in pregnancy

- If a woman has been called for routine screening and she is pregnant, the test should be deferred.
- If a previous test was abnormal and in the interim the woman becomes pregnant, then the test should not be delayed but should be taken in mid-trimester unless there is a clinical contraindication.

References http://www.cancerscreening.nhs.uk/cervical/publications/nhscsp20.pdf

GYNONCO37

GYNONCO37 Answer: E

Explanation Women who have had a hysterectomy with CIN present are potentially at risk of developing vaginal intraepithelial neoplasia (VaIN) and invasive vaginal disease. There is no clear evidence that colposcopy increases the detection of disease on follow-up. Expert consensus opinion recommends that for women who undergo hysterectomy and have incompletely excised CIN (or uncertain excision), follow-up should be as if their cervix remained in situ.

- CIN 1: vault cytology at six, 12 and 24 months
- CIN 2/3: vault cytology at 6 and 12 months, followed by nine annual vault cytology samples – follow-up for incompletely excised CIN, continues to 65 years or until 10 years after surgery (whichever is later).
- As women who have undergone hysterectomy have no cervix and so are no longer eligible for recall within the NHSCSP, their vault cytology following treatment of CIN must be managed outside the programme.

References http://www.cancerscreening.nhs.uk/cervical/publications/nhscsp20.pdf

GYNONCO38

GYNONCO38 Answer: A

Explanation In a median tumour location (lower commissure, periurethral, periclitoris) and stage 1B cancer, bilateral inguinofemoral lymphadenectomy should be carried out. For the lateral tumours, an ipsilateral lymphadenectomy is sufficient since the risk of contralateral lymph node involvement is less than 1 %. In the case of ipsilateral positive lymph nodes, the other side has to be removed.

References Gajjar K, Shafi M. Invasive vulval cancer. Obstet Gynaecol Reprod Med. 24(6):177–85.

GYNONCO39

GYNONCO39 Answer: E

Explanation If the frozen section is reported as borderline, for the older woman with no fertility concerns, a complete staging should be undertaken, which should include:

- Exploration of the entire abdominal cavity with peritoneal washings
- Total abdominal hysterectomy
- Bilateral salpingo-oophorectomy and infracolic omentectomy
- Appendicectomy in the case of mucinous tumours

Conservative surgery is defined as surgery with complete staging but with preservation of the uterus and at least a part of one ovary to preserve fertility. The two common options are cystectomy and unilateral salpingo-oophorectomy, with/without infracolic omentectomy and peritoneal washings. Systematic biopsies of a macroscopically normal contralateral ovary are not recommended because they do not exclude recurrent disease, they yield no abnormal histological findings and they interfere with fertility further as a result of adhesions. Morbidity may also be reduced by less radical surgery, but clearly this must not be at the expense of safety with regard to cancer prognosis.

Approximately one-third of cases reported as borderline at frozen section are later reclassified as invasive tumours. Although no survival benefit has been shown with lymphadenectomy in borderline ovarian tumours, to ensure that such cases of invasive disease are fully staged, lymphadenectomy should be considered.

References Bagade P, Edmondson R, Nayar A. Management of borderline ovarian tumours. Obstet Gynaecol. 2012;14:115–20.

GYNONCO40

GYNONCO40 Answer: E

Explanation Sentinel node detection has been investigated as a safe, accurate method of ascertaining the status of clinically non-suspicious groin nodes preoperatively to allow inguinofemoral lymphadenectomy, with all its attendant morbidity, to be restricted to patients who need it.

Sentinel node detection involves injection of intradermal isosulfan blue dye around the primary vulval lesion, either alone or commonly with a 99mTc radioactive sulphur colloid. The sentinel node is the node that receives the primary lymphatic flow from the tumour and is detected positive by uptake of radioactive colloids and blue dye. Central tumours may have bilateral sentinel nodes. The negative predictive value for dual technique of sentinel node detection is quoted between 89 and 100 %. The finding of a positive node with metastasis would lead to full systematic lymphadenectomy, but those with negative node would be spared the significant morbidity associated with procedure. Sentinel node detection should only be performed by appropriately trained gynaecological oncologist within a skilled multidisciplinary team.

Sentinel lymphadenectomy is associated with a lower rate of lymphoedema compared to complete groin lymphadenectomy. Nevertheless, the procedure has a small but definite false-negative rate (2–5 %); therefore, appropriate counselling of risks and benefits and close surveillance are paramount as groin recurrence in vulval cancer carries a very poor prognosis.

References Gajjar K, Shafi M. Invasive vulval cancer. Obstet Gynaecol Reprod Med. 24(6):177–85.

Urogynecology and Pelvic Floor: Answers and Explanations

25

UGN1

UGN1 Answer: D

Explanation The pudendal nerve (S2–S4) exits the pelvis initially through the greater sciatic foramen below the piriformis. Importantly, it runs behind the lateral third of the sacrospinous ligament and ischial spine alongside the internal pudendal artery and immediately re-enters the pelvis through the lesser sciatic foramen to the pudendal canal (Alcock's canal). This nerve is susceptible to entrapment injuries during sacrospinous ligament fixation as it runs behind the lateral aspect of the sacrospinous ligament.

The anterior branches of L2–L4 give rise to the obturator nerve and converge behind the psoas muscle. The obturator nerve then passes over the pelvic brim in front of the sacroiliac joint and behind the common iliac vessels to enter the thigh via the obturator foramen. This nerve is most frequently injured during retroperitoneal surgery, excision of endometriosis, the passage of a trocar through the obturator foramen, insertion of transobturator tapes and during paravaginal defect repairs.

The sciatic nerve arises from the L4–S3 nerve roots. It emerges from the pelvis below the piriformis muscle, curving laterally and downward through the gluteal region. Initially it lies midway between the posterior superior iliac spine and ischial tuberosity. Lower down in the thigh, it courses midway between the ischial tuberosity and greater trochanter.

The common peroneal nerve and tibial nerve are its two derivatives at the mid-thigh. The common peroneal nerve importantly winds forward around the neck of the fibula.

The genitofemoral nerve originates from the upper L1–2 segments. It passes downwards and emerges from the anterior surface of the psoas muscle.

C. Ratha, J. Gupta, *SBAs and EMQs for MRCOG II*,
DOI 10.1007/978-81-322-2689-5_25

References Kuponiyi O, Alleemudder DI, Latunde-Dada A, Eedarapalli P. Nerve injuries associated with gynaecological surgery. Obstet & Gynaecol. 2014; 16:29–36.

UGN2

UGN2 Answer: C

A major issue with the use of synthetic meshes in the repair of prolapse is mesh erosion. This has been reported to be as high as 12 % in vaginal procedures and can be difficult to manage. If the repair is carried out laparoscopically without opening the vaginal vault and a macroporous mesh is used, the erosion rate can be reduced to 1–2 %. The laparoscopic route also has the additional benefit of not shortening or narrowing the vagina.

References Morrion J, MacKenzie I. Avoiding and managing complications during gynaecological surgery. Obstet, Gynaecol Reprod Med. 17(4):105–11.

UGN3

UGN 3 Answer: D

Explanation Painful bladder syndrome (PBS) is categorised by suprapubic pain related to bladder filling, accompanied by other symptoms such as increased daytime and night-time frequency in the absence of proven urinary tract infection or other pathology. There is considerable overlap between the overactive bladder syndrome, the urethral pain syndrome and PBS. Whereas the principal complaint of women with OAB is urgency, in women with PBS, it is predominantly pain related to bladder filling. Women with urethral pain syndrome, on the other hand, complain of pain on voiding.

References Jha S, Parsons M, Toozs-Hobson P. Painful bladder syndrome and interstitial cystitis. Obstet Gynaecol. 2007;9:34–41.

UGN4

UGN 4 Answer: E

Explanation The ureters are muscular tubes whose peristaltic contractions convey urine from the kidneys to the urinary bladder. Each descends slightly medially anterior to psoas major and enters the pelvic cavity where it curves laterally and then medially, as it runs down to open into the base of the urinary bladder. In the female pelvis, it forms an important relation to the ovarian fossa and comes to lie posterior to the ovaries. It is closely related to the uterine artery lateral to the uterine cervix and runs under it—best remembered as 'water under the bridge'.

Ureteric tunnel is the Mackenrodt's or the cardinal ligaments through which the ureter passes before entering the bladder. 'Unroofing of the ureter' and freeing it from the ligaments is necessary to excise a portion of the parametria during radical hysterectomy for cervical cancer. It ends by piercing the posterior aspect of the bladder after emerging from the ureteric tunnel.

References Gray's anatomy – Chapter – Kidneys and ureter.

UGN5

UGN 5 Answer: D

Explanation Postpartum voiding dysfunction is failure to pass urine within 6 h of vaginal delivery. Epidural anaesthesia decreases sensation as hence is a recognised risk factor. Other risk factors are primigravida, instrumental delivery, prolonged labour and perineal trauma. Postpartum measuring residual urine volume in asymptomatic women is not helpful.

References Post partum voiding dysfunction. TOG. 2008;10:71–4.

UGN6

UGN 6 Answer: C

Explanation Obliterating the uterosacrals by continuous sutures and the peritoneum of the posterior cul de sac as high as possible (high uterosacral suspension) helps to prevent vault prolapse during vaginal hysterectomy. Moschowitz-type operation involves a purse-string technique, incorporating the distal ends of the uterosacral and cardinal ligaments and thereby drawing these structures to the midline. Simple closure of the peritoneum is done with a purse-string suture, with none of the uterosacral-cardinal ligaments incorporated into the repair. Cruikshank and Kovac performed the only prospective, randomised comparison of procedures used at the time of hysterectomy to prevent enterocele. In their study, 100 patients undergoing vaginal hysterectomy for various indications (excluding prolapse of the posterior superior segment of the vagina) were randomised to 1 of 3 surgical methods to prevent enterocele. The McCall repair was significantly more effective than the other 2 types of repair, with a 6.1 % risk of subsequent prolapse, versus 30.3 % in women who had a Moschcowitz-type closure and 39.4 % in those who underwent simple closure of the peritoneum.

References Cruikshank SH, Kovac SR. Randomized comparison of three surgical methods used at the time of vaginal hysterectomy to prevent posterior enterocele. Am J Obstet Gynecol. 1999;180:859–65.

   RCOG Green-Top guideline No. 46. The management of pot hysterectomy vaginal vault prolapse. 2007.

UGN7

UGN7 Answer: C

Explanation Offer a trial of supervised pelvic floor muscle training of at least 3 months' duration as first-line treatment to women with stress or mixed UI. Pelvic floor muscle training programmes should comprise at least 8 contractions performed 3 times per day.

References http://www.nice.org.uk/guidance/cg171

UGN8

UGN 8 Answer: A

Explanation Use bladder diaries in the initial assessment of women with UI or OAB. Encourage women to complete a minimum of 3 days of the diary covering variations in their usual activities, such as both working and leisure days.

References http://www.nice.org.uk/guidance/cg171

UGN9

UGN 9 Answer: C

Explanation Start treatment with botulinum toxin A only if women:

• Have been trained in clean intermittent catheterisation and have performed the technique successfully and

- are able and willing to perform clean intermittent catheterisation on a regular basis for as long as needed.

Use 200 units when offering botulinum toxin A.

Consider 100 units of botulinum toxin A for women who would prefer a dose with a lower chance of catheterisation and accept a reduced chance of success.

References Sinha Dd, Arunkalaivanan AS. Botulinum toxin type A: applications in urogynaecology. Obstet Gynaecol. 2006;8:177–80. doi:10.1576/toag.8.3.177.27254

UGN10

UGN10 Answer: C

Explanation

Point	Description	Range of Values
Aa	Anterior vaginal wall 3 cm proximal to the hymen	-3 cm to +3 cm
Ba	Most distal position of the remaining upper anterior vaginal wall	-3 cm to +tvl
C	Most distal edge of cervix or vaginal cuff scar	
D	Posterior fomix (N/A if post-hysterectomy)	
Ap	Posterior vaginal wall 3 cm proximal to the hymen	-3 cm to +3 cm
Bp	Most distal position of the remaining upper posterior vaginal wall	-3 cm to + tvl
Genital hiatus (gh) – Measured from middle of external urethral meatus to posterior midline hymen **Perineal body (pb)** – Measured from posterior margin of gh to middle of anal opening **Total vaginal length (tvl)** – Depth of vagina when point D or C is reduced to normal position		

References http://www.lasvegasurogynecology.com/POPstix%20insert_opt.pdf

UGN11

UGN11 Answer: D

Explanation

Point	Description	Range of Values
Aa	Anterior vaginal wall 3 cm proximal to the hymen	-3 cm to +3 cm
Ba	Most distal position of the remaining upper anterior vaginal wall	-3 cm to +tvl
C	Most distal edge of cervix or vaginal cuff scar	
D	Posterior fomix (N/A if post-hysterectomy)	
Ap	Posterior vaginal wall 3 cm proximal to the hymen	-3 cm to +3 cm
Bp	Most distal position of the remaining upper posterior vaginal wall	-3 cm to + tvl

Genital hiatus (gh) – Measured from middle of external urethral meatus to posterior midline hymen
Perineal body (pb) – Measured from posterior margin of gh to middle of anal opening
Total vaginal length (tvl) – Depth of vagina when point D or C is reduced to normal position

References http://www.lasvegasurogynecology.com/POPstix%20insert_opt.pdf

UGN12

UGN 12 Answer: E

Explanation Duloxetine is a serotonin and noradrenaline (norepinephrine) reuptake inhibitor which has been approved for the treatment of stress incontinence. Viktrup and Yalcin reviewed the impact of pre-existing risk factors, including BMI, on the efficacy of duloxetine in the management of stress incontinence. Significant improvements in all outcome measures (incontinence quality of life, incontinence episode frequency and patient global impression of improvement) were observed for the duloxetine group compared with placebo, independent of BMI strata. Overweight women tended to have a greater increase in incontinence quality-of-life score than women with a BMI <28.

It has clinically important interactions with other drugs including warfarin and antidepressants. Duloxetine is believed to act by increasing sphincter activity in the storage phase of the micturition cycle.

References 1. Jain P, Parsons M. The effects of obesity on the pelvic floor. Obstet Gynaecol. 2011;13:133–42.

2. Orme S, Ramsay I. Duloxetine: the long awaited drug treatment for stress urinary incontinence. Obstet Gynaecol. 2005;7:117–9. doi:10.1576/toag.7.2.117.27070

UGN13

UGN13 Answer: E

Explanation Urinary tract catheterisation is commonly employed in routine gynaecological practice. A sound knowledge of catheter types, indications and complications is an important part of gynaecological training.

Common indications and contraindications[10] are shown in Box 3.

Box 3. *Indications and contraindications of suprapubic catheterisation*

Indications

- **Short term:**
  - urogynaecological/gynaecological operations
  - urological (urethral stricture/trauma)
  - anorectal surgery
  - acute retention
  - severe pelvic trauma
- **Long term:**
  - neurogenic bladder
  - chronic retention
  - inability to self-catheterise
  - persistent expulsion of IUC (spasm/deliberate)
  - mobility problems
  - intractable incontinence (last resort)

Contraindications

- **Absolute:**
  - unexplained haematuria due to risk of placing the catheter through a bladder tumour
- **Relative:**
  - extensive abdominal adhesions from previous surgeries, especially closed insertion
  - extensive intraoperative bladder reconstruction
  - anticoagulation therapy/blood clotting disorders
  - inability to fill the bladder to a minimum of 300 ml
  - ascites
  - suspicion of ovarian cyst
  - very obese patients

References Aslam N, Moran PA. Catheter use in gynaecological practice. Obstet Gynaecol. 2014;16:161–8.

UGN14

UGN14 Answer: B

Explanation Anterior repair should be used to describe the procedure that provides support along the whole length of the anterior vaginal wall, thereby supporting both the urethra and the bladder base. Anterior repair is performed for symptomatic anterior vaginal wall prolapse. A woman who is found to have a prolapse on routine examination for cervical screening is not well served by being encouraged to have surgery. While troublesome urinary symptoms may be improved by anterior repair, a significant proportion of women develop new urinary symptoms following surgery, which will be particularly unwelcome if they were symptom free before

There is no consensus on whether interrupted or continuous sutures produce a more robust repair.

There is much debate about the optimal technique for performing anterior repair and whether fascial repair should be augmented by insertion of absorbable or non-absorbable graft material. The limited evidence available suggests that use of a non-absorbable graft reduces the risk of operative failure or recurrence but is associated with a risk of graft erosion and bladder injury.

References Reid F, Smith T. Anterior vaginal repair. Obstet Gynaecol. 2012;14:137–41.

UGN15

UGN 15 Answer: B

Explanation Pelvic floor disorders encompass a wide range of problems which include urinary incontinence, pelvic organ prolapse, faecal incontinence and sexual dysfunction. They are extremely prevalent, affecting up to 40 % of women attending gynaecology clinics. These disorders rarely result in serious morbidity or mortality, but they often impair quality of life severely. The multifaceted and taboo nature of pelvic floor disorders means that clinical interview data are prone to inaccuracy and non-disclosure. It is generally acknowledged that only women themselves can report objectively on their symptoms and health-related quality of life (HRQoL), hence the potential value of practical and reliable tools allowing the identification, prioritisation, appropriate management and monitoring of these intimate and often complex problems.

References Radley S, Dua A. Quality of life measurement and electronic assessment in urogynaecology. Obstet Gynaecol. 2011;13:219–23.

UGN16

UGN 16 Answer: D

Explanation The duration for which a medium- or long-term catheter can stay in place depends on the bonding or coating used. The coating used for medium-term latex catheters is PTFE or Teflon which makes the latex more inert and gives it a smooth surface. This reduces the incidence of urethritis and encrustation. A PTFE-coated catheter can stay in place for up to 28 days. Bard Urology (UK) recommends that the PTFE latex catheters can stay between 7 and 21 days.

The coating used for long-term latex and 100 % silicone catheters is a hydrophilic polymer. The catheter surface absorbs a small amount of bodily fluid which lubricates its surface and reduces the friction between the catheter and urethral wall. This helps to reduce the risk of bacterial colonisation and encrustation.

References Aslam N, Moran PA. Catheter use in gynaecological practice. Obstet Gynaecol. 2014;16:161–8.

UGN17

UGN17 Answer: D

Explanation The woman's age, postmenopausal status, multiple child births remain risk factors for pelvic floor dysfunction. In posterior wall prolapse, the patient has difficulty in defecation, while in anterior wall prolapse, there are more urinary symptoms.

References Hughe and Jackson. The scientific basis of prolapse. Obstet Gynecol. 2000;3(2):10–5.

UGN18

UGN 18 Answer: B

Explanation The aetiology of UD remains largely unknown, but it is thought it may be congenital or acquired in origin. Congenital cases may occur from remnants of Gartner's duct or abnormal union of primordial folds or persisting cell rests, especially Müllerian, but they are rarely found in children. It is three times higher in Black American compared with White American women, suggesting a genetic susceptibility in this population. Most cases are acquired and result from repeated infections and obstruction of the periurethral glands. These rupture into the urethral lumen and the cyst epithelialises and persists. Traumatic childbirth, especially with assisted delivery, has been suggested as a cause of UD development, but it may equally develop in nulliparous patients. UD has also been reported following transurethral collagen injection for stress urinary incontinence. The UD usually dissects within the urethral pelvic ligament with the orifice/neck just off centre at 4 and 8 o'clock. Occasionally it may extend proximally beneath the bladder neck and trigonal area. Most UD have a single connection to the urethra and vary in size and shape. Complex patterns may occur with multiple ostia; UD may be multiple and loculated and may extend partially ('saddlebag' or 'horseshoe') or circumferentially around the urethra and thereby compromise urethral sphincter function. They are usually lined by urothelium, but squamous and glandular metaplasia can occur and even leiomyoma.

UD may present with multiple symptoms. The historical classical triad of dysuria, post-void dribbling and dyspareunia is only seen in a minority of patients. Lower urinary tract symptoms (LUTS), namely, frequency and urgency, are present in 40–100 % of cases.

References Archer R, Blackman J, Stott M, Barrington J. Urethral diverticulum. Obstet Gynaecol. 2015;17:125–9.

UGN19

UGN 19 Answer: C

Explanation As per NICE offer one of the following choices first to women with OAB or mixed UI:

- Oxybutynin (immediate release)
- Tolterodine (immediate release)
- Darifenacin (once daily preparation)

References https://www.nice.org.uk/guidance/CG171/chapter/1-Recommendations

UGN20

UGN 20 Answer: D

Explanation A third-degree perineal tear is defined as a partial or complete disruption of the anal sphincter muscles, which may involve either or both the external (EAS) and internal anal sphincter (IAS) muscles. A fourth-degree tear is defined as a disruption of the anal sphincter muscles with a breach of the rectal mucosa. Obstetric anal sphincter injury encompasses both third- and fourth-degree perineal tears.

References GTG third and fourth degree perineal tears.

Core Surgical Skills and Postoperative Care: Answers and Explanations

26

CSPO1

CSPO1 Answer: B

Explanation Though popularly used, evidence has proved that steroids are not useful for prevention of adhesions in fertility-conserving surgeries. Dextran can cause anaphylaxis, and its use is not preferred.

Adept has found to be useful as adhesion prevention agent. Interceed is oxidised regenerated cellulose. Evidence shows no definite benefit of using adhesion prevention agents in caesarean section.

References Scientific Impact Paper No 39. The use of adhesion prevention agents. Obstetr Gynaecol. 2013.

CSPO2

CSPO2 Answer: B

Explanation The advantages that transverse incisions offer are that they are less painful, have better cosmetic results, interfere less with postoperative respiration and have greater strength. The disadvantages being that there is greater blood loss and injury to nerves and muscle which can result in potential spaces with haematoma or seroma. Also, there is compromised view of upper abdominal cavity.

Skin preparation is done before all surgical procedures. Preoperative showering with antiseptics reduces the infection rate in clean wound (1.3 % versus 2.3 %). Wound infection rate of 0.6 % is seen with depilatory preparation, as with procedure done with no hair removal. Hair removal is done to prevent interference with wound

© Springer India 2016
C. Ratha, J. Gupta, *SBAs and EMQs for MRCOG II*,
DOI 10.1007/978-81-322-2689-5_26

approximation in certain incisions. Same scalpel can be safely used for both superficial and deep incisions.

References   Raghavan R, Arya P, Arya P, China S. Abdominal incisions and sutures in obstetrics and gynaecology. Obstet Gynaecol. 2014;16:13–8.

CSPO3

CSPO 3 Answer: C

Explanation   Injury occurs most frequently in the lower third of the ureter (51 %), followed by the upper third (30 %) and the middle third (19 %).
   The most common sites of injury are:

- Lateral to the uterine vessels
- The area of the ureterovesical junction close to the cardinal ligaments
- The base of the infundibulopelvic ligament as the ureters cross the pelvic brim at the ovarian fossa
- at the level of the uterosacral ligament

   Most studies show the most common site of injury to be lateral to the uterine vessels, but Daly et al. report this to be at the ovarian fossa. During laparoscopy, the ureter is injured most frequently adjacent to the uterosacral ligaments.

References   Jha S, Coomarasamy A, Chan KK. Ureteric injury in obstetric and gynaecological surgery. Obstet Gynaecol. 2004;6:203–8. doi:10.1576/toag.6.4.203.27016

CSPO4

CSPO4 Answer: E

Explanation   Three main types of suture include the nonabsorbable, slowly absorbable and the rapidly absorbable. These can be further divided into monofilament or braided sutures. The incidence of wound infection is low with monofilament sutures. Silk and polyester are examples of braided non-reabsorbable sutures. Silk has higher tissue reaction, lower tensile strength as compared to nylon. Polypropylene has the least tissue reaction ability.
   The incidence of wound dehiscence and hernia is similar for nonabsorbable and slowly absorbable sutures. The incidence of prolonged wound pain and suture sinus is significantly higher with a nonabsorbable suture.

References   Raghavan R, Arya P, Arya P, China S. Abdominal incisions and sutures in obstetrics and gynaecology. Obstet Gynaecol. 2014;16:13–8.

CSPO5

CSPO5 Answer: A

Explanation Self-retaining abdominal retractors can cause a femoral neuropathy—either by direct pressure on the nerve or exaggerated extension of the retractor blades. The diagnosis is made some days after the surgery with a complaint of numbness over the skin on the anterior surface of the upper thigh. Specific action is not indicated, as there are no serious sequelae and symptoms will usually spontaneously resolve over a few months. Obturator nerve injury causes numbness in the inner thigh and difficulty in adduction of hip joint causing gait difficulties and posture instability. Pudendal nerve entrapment also known as Alcock canal syndrome can cause pain in genital area and urinary and faecal incontinence sometimes.

Sciatic nerve and peroneal nerve are usually not encountered in gynaec surgeries.

References Morrion J, MacKenzie I. Avoiding and managing complications during gynaecological surgery. Obstet Gynaecol Reprod Med. 17;4:105–11.

CSPO6

CSPO6 Answer: E

Explanation There are two types of staple: nonabsorbable and absorbable. The nonabsorbable staple (Proximate; Ethicon Endo-Surgery, Inc., Blue Ash, OH, USA) is made of stainless steel and has the highest tensile strength of any wound closure material. Staples have a low tissue reactivity. Prior to stapling, it is useful to grasp the wound edges with forceps to evert the tissue so as to prevent inverted skin edges.

Additionally, contaminated wounds closed with staples have a lower incidence of infection compared with those closed with sutures. Disadvantages of staples include the potential for staple track formation, bacterial migration into the wound bed and discomfort during staple removal. The absorbable staple (Insorb; Incisive Surgical, Inc., Minneapolis, MN, USA) is a novel device which deploys U-shaped absorbable staples into the dermal layer of tissue.

These staples contain an absorbable copolymer of predominantly polylactide and a lesser component of polyglycolide. They maintain 40 % of their strength at 14 days and are completely absorbed over a period of months (tissue half-life of 10 weeks). The Insorb staples are associated with a significantly lower infection rate.

References Raghavan R, Arya P, Arya P, China S. Abdominal incisions and sutures in obstetrics and gynaecology. Obstet Gynaecol. 2014;16:13–8.

CSPO7

CSPO 7 Answer: D

Explanation FFP at a dose of 12–15 ml/kg should be administered for every 6 units of red cells during major obstetric haemorrhage. Subsequent FFP transfusion should be guided by the results of clotting tests if they are available in a timely manner, aiming to maintain prothrombin time (PT) and activated partial thromboplastin time (APTT) ratios at less than 1.5 x normal.

References Green to guideline blood transfusion in Obstetrics. 2015.

CSPO8

CSPO8 Answer: B

Explanation Iatrogenic nerve injury following gynaecological surgery occurs more commonly than is recognised and is a significant cause of postoperative neuropathy.

Neuropathy results when there is a disruption to the blood supply of the nerve caused by injury. Three types of microvascular changes occur with nerve injury. Neuropraxia is the result of external nerve compression leading to a disruption of conduction across a small portion of the axon. Nerve recovery takes weeks or months once remyelination occurs.

Axonotmesis is caused by profound nerve compression or traction. Damage occurs to the axon only, with preservation of the supporting Schwann cells. Regeneration is possible because supporting Schwann cells remain intact. Recovery time is longer than neuropraxia.

The most severe form of injury is termed neurotmesis, and it results from complete nerve transection or ligation, where both the axon and Schwann cells are disrupted. Regeneration is rendered impossible, and without restorative surgery, prognosis is usually poor

References Kuponiyi O, Alleemudder DI, Latunde-Dada A, Eedarapalli P. Nerve injuries associated with gynaecological surgery. Obstet Gynaecol. 2014;16:29–36.

CSPO9

CSPO9 Answer: C

Explanation Because of the high risk of bowel being densely adherent to the underside of a midline incision, using closed entry techniques (i.e. with a Veress needle) in women with a midline scar is absolutely contraindicated. Most gynaecologists feel comfortable using closed entry techniques in women with a previous transverse suprapubic incision, but, in view of the known 20 % chance of periumbilical adhesions, perhaps we should be considering alternative entry techniques more often. Not only is there an increased risk of periumbilical adhesions, but adherence of the greater omentum to the underside of a Pfannenstiel incision can pull the transverse colon down, making it more at risk from the Veress needle and primary trocar.

Hasson first described his open entry technique in 1974. Although it is the preferred entry method for most general surgeons, the technique has never really been embraced with much enthusiasm by gynaecologists. It is certainly the entry technique that should be used in all thin women, as it will avoid accidental injury to the great vessels on the posterior abdominal wall.

Palmer's point is situated in the left midclavicular line, 2–3 cm below the costal margin. We know that the left upper quadrant is the area where adhesions are least likely to be found following previous surgery, except, of course, where the surgery was performed in this area, for example, splenectomy.

In the presence of a midline laparotomy scar, the open entry incision can be placed well lateral to the midline and beyond the lateral border of the rectus muscle. This minimises the risk of encountering bowel adherent to the midline scar and avoids having to cut through the bulk of the rectus muscle and potentially damaging the epigastric blood vessels. It is certainly an option worth considering where there are concerns about using the closed entry technique at Palmer's point.

References Frappell J. Laparoscopic entry after previous surgery. Obstet Gynaecol. 2012;14:207–9. doi: 10.1111/j.1744-4667.2012.00119.x

---

CSPO10

CSPO10 Answer: A

Explanation Retractors are used to hold back the abdominal wall and/or the viscus and can be hand-held or self-retaining. The commonly used ones are Doyens, Deaver, Langenbeck, Morris and the self-retaining Balfour retractor.

References Monaghan J, Lopes T, Naik R, Spirtos N. Instruments, operative materials and basic surgical techniques. In: Bonney's gynaecology surgery. 11th ed. Chichester: Wiley-Blackwell; 2011.

CSPO11

CSPO11 Answer: D

Explanation LMWH should not be given for 4 h after the use of spinal anaesthesia or after the epidural catheter has been removed, and the epidural catheter should not be removed within 12 h of the most recent injection.

References https://www.rcog.org.uk/globalassets/documents/guidelines/gtg-37b.pdf

CSPO12

CSPO12 Answer: A

Explanation

References http://www.nrls.npsa.nhs.uk/resources/?entryid45=59860

CSPO13

CSPO 13 Answer: B

Explanation Lloyd Davies position is also known as Trendelenburg position with legs apart or head-down lithotomy. It is defined as supine position of the body with hips flexed at 15° as the basic angle and with a 30° head-down tilt. Lloyd Davies position is used in pelvic and rectal surgery where access is required from both abdominal and perineal aspects.

The key difference between lithotomy and Lloyd Davies is the degree of hip and knee flexion.

References Strat OG module on technical skills https://stratog.rcog.org.uk/uploads/File/elearn/BPS

CSPO14

CSPO14 Answer: D

Explanation An intra-abdominal pressure of 20–25 mmHg should be used for gas insufflation before inserting the primary trocar.

The distension pressure should be reduced to 12–15 mmHg once the insertion of the trocars is complete. This gives adequate distension for operative laparoscopy and allows the anaesthetist to ventilate the patient safely and effectively.

It is necessary to achieve a pressure of 20–25 mmHg before inserting the trocar, as this results in increased splinting and allows the trocar to be more easily inserted through the layers of the abdominal wall.

References http://bsge.org.uk/userfiles/file/GtG%20no%2049%20 Laparoscopic%20Injury%202008.pdf

---

CSPO15

CSPO15 Answer: E

Explanation Intraoperative cell salvage is a strategy to reduce the use of banked blood. Where IOCS is used during caesarean section in RhD-negative, previously nonsensitised women and where cord blood group is confirmed as RhD positive (or unknown), a minimum dose of 1500 iu anti-D immunoglobulin should be administered following the reinfusion of salvaged red cells. A maternal blood sample should be taken for estimation of fetomaternal haemorrhage 30sly min after reinfusion in case more anti-D is indicated.

References Green Top guideline blood transfusion in Obstetrics.

CSPO16

CSPO16 Answer: E

Explanation Needles are designed to carry suture material through tissue with the minimal trauma. Surgical needles have 3 basic components—he attachment point, the body and the point.

The body is the section of the needle grasped by the needle holder. The diameter should be as close as possible to that of the suture material being used. The curvature varies depending on the job and is expressed as eighths of a circle. In general the deeper the plane, the more curved the needle should be. Straight is useful for skin, there is also ½ curve (half circle), 3/8 or a J needle that is used to close the rectus sheath after laparoscopy. Some needles are eyed, allowing the surgeon to choose the needle and suture material to suit the job. However, they are rarely used. The point extends from the extreme point of the needle to the maximum diameter of the body. The different points are designed to give the required amount of cutting for different tissues. The needles used in gynaecology surgery include:

Blunt point—for blunt dissection and suturing friable tissue. It is also used in patients with blood-borne viruses such as hepatitis B.

Tapered point—for soft, easily penetrated tissue, shown by a circle with a dot inside.

Tapercutting—used to cut through most tissues with minimum trauma; this is shown on the bottom left.

Cutting—used to cut through tougher tissues.

References Strat OG module on technical skills. https://stratog.rcog.org.uk/tutorial/general-principles/preliminary-reading-6759

CSPO17

CSPO 17 Answer: C

Explanation Tissue adhesives are a valuable alternative for mechanical tissue fixation by sutures or staples. Types:

1. Biological: include fibrin-based glues, gelatin-based hydrogels and composite glues
2. Synthetic: cyanoacrylates and polymeric sealants
   - Non-resorbable: limited to surface applications
   - Resorbable (biodegradable): deployed for both surface applications and internal use

3. Genetically engineered protein glues

Advantages:

- Faster, no need for suture removal.
- Cyanoacrylates have been shown to have antimicrobial properties (especially against Gram-positive organisms).

The synthetic adhesive 2-octylcyanoacrylate (Dermabond, Ethicon) is US Food and Drug Administration-approved surgical adhesive. The cyanoacrylates polymerise upon contact with blood, forming a solid film that bridges the wounds and holds the apposed wound edges together.

References Raghavan R, Arya P, Arya P, China S. Abdominal incisions and sutures in obstetrics and gynaecology. Obstet Gynaecol. 2014;16:13 8.

CSPO18

CSPO18 Answer: B

Explanation The Gridiron incision is a downward and inward incision from the McBurney point. The incision is carried through the skin and subcutaneous fat to the abdominal wall muscles, which is split along the direction of the fibres. The peritoneum may then be reflected away from the abdominal wall inferiorly. This allows extraperitoneal drainage of abscess, avoiding peritoneal contamination. The Gridiron incision can be performed on the left lower quadrant to drain abscess on the left side of the pelvis and can be varied for appendicectomy in pregnant women.

Rockeyidiron incision (or Elliot) is a transverse incision made at the junction of the middle and lower thirds of the line joining the anterior superior iliac spine to the umbilicus.

The Keustner incision, sometimes incorrectly referred to as modified Pfannenstiel incision, involves a slightly curved skin incision beginning below the level of the anterior superior iliac spine and extending just below the pubic hairline. The Mouchel incision is a transverse abdominal incision that runs at the upper limit of the pubic hair and is thus lower than the Maylard incision.

References Raghavan R, Arya P, Arya P, China S. Abdominal incisions and sutures in obstetrics and gynaecology. Obstet Gynaecol. 2014;16:13 8.

CSPO19

CSO19 Answer: A

Explanation The T12tionr:rya P, Arya P, China S. Abdominal incisions and sutures in obstetrics and gynaecology. a slightly curved skin incision beginning below the level of the anterior superior iliac spine and extending just below the pubic hairline. The Mouchel inneurosis above the superficial inguinal ring, while the ilioinguinal nerve emerges through it.

Both nerves have a sensory function only. While the Iliohypogastric provides sensation to the skin of the gluteal and hypogastric regions, the ilioinguinal nerve provides sensory innervation to the skin overlying the groin, inner thigh and labia majora.

Injury to these nerves is typically caused by suture entrapment at the lateral borders of low transverse or Pfannenstiel incisions that extend beyond the lateral border of the rectus abdominus muscle. The reported incidence of ilioinguinal or iliohypogastric neuropathy following a Pfannenstiel incision is 3.7 %. Laparoscopic and retropubic mid-urethral tape procedures may also injure this nerve.

The diagnostic triad for ilioinguinal/iliohypogastric nerve entrapment syndrome consists of:

1. Sharp burning pain radiating from the incision site to the mons pubis, labia and thigh
2. Paraesthesia over the nerve distribution areas
3. Pain relief following administration of local anaesthetic

References 1. Kuponiyi O, Alleemudder DI, Latunde-Dada A, Eedarapalli P. Nerve injuries associated with gynaecological surgery. Obstet Gynaecol. 2014;16:29 All

2. Miyazaki F, Shook G. Ilioinguinal nerve entrapment during needle suspension for stress incontinence. Obstet Gynecol. 1992;80:246Sho

CSPO20

CSPO20 Answer: E

Explanation Studies have shown that patients who have a thin body habitus, ill-developed abdominal wall muscles or a narrow pelvis are more at risk of retractor blade-associated nerve injury. Such patients are at further risk if the operating time exceeds 4 h.

A large number of iatrogenic lumbosacral nerve injuries during gynaecological surgery can be attributed to the incorrect positioning of self-retaining retractor blades. The gold standard of correct positioning is for the self-retractor blades to cradle the rectus muscle without compressing the psoas muscle underneath.

When positioning the retractors, the surgeon must check visually and by direct palpation that the psoas muscle is not entrapped between the blades and the pelvic side wall.

References 1. Kuponiyi O, Alleemudder DI, Latunde-Dada A, Eedarapalli P. Nerve injuries associated with gynaecological surgery. Obstet Gynaecol. 2014;16:29 All

2. Winfree CJ, Kline DG. Intraoperative positioning nerve injuries. Surg Neurol. 2005;63:5, Kl

CSPO21

CSKPO 21 Answer: B

Explanation The inferior epigastric artery originates from the external iliac artery posterior to the inguinal ligament. Its accompanying veins, usually two, drain into the external iliac vein. It divides into numerous branches, which anastomose with those of the superior epigastric and lower six posterior intercostal arteries. The artery is an important inferomedial relation of the deep inguinal ring and may be damaged during extensive medial dissection of the deep ring during hernia repair, particularly when this is performed in the preperitoneal plane. It may also be injured during placement of secondary trocars in the iliac fossae during laparoscopic procedures.

Sometimes the inferior epigastric artery arises from the femoral artery. It then ascends anterior to the femoral vein, into the abdomen to follow its course as above. It occasionally arises from the external iliac artery, in common with an aberrant obturator artery and, rarely, from the obturator artery.

The superior and inferior epigastric arteries are an important source for a potential collateral circulation between the internal thoracic artery and the external iliac artery in situations in which flow in the thoracic or abdominal aorta is compromised. Small tributaries of the inferior epigastric vein drain the skin around the umbilicus and anastomose with the terminal branches of the umbilical vein, draining the inner surface of the umbilicus via the falciform ligament. These anastomoses may open widely in cases of portal hypertension, with portal venous blood draining into the systemic circulation via the inferior epigastric vessels. The radiating dilated veins seen under the umbilical skin are referred to as the 'caput medusae'.

References Gray's Anatomy 39th edition.

CSPO22

CSPO22 Answer: B

Explanation Diagnosis of AMI in pregnancy may be difficult because of its low prevalence and consequent low index of suspicion. Also as the presenting symptoms and signs can be attributed to normal manifestations of pregnancy or be masked during labour, it can lead to a delay in diagnosis. The diagnostic criteria of AMI are the same as for the nonpregnant patient. In addition to chest pain, typical features of pregnancy such as epigastric pain, vomiting or dizziness, particularly in the presence of known AMI risk factors, should be investigated further. A low index of suspicion is important, as two consecutive CMACE reports have shown a consistent failure to consider AMI as a cause of chest pain in women with risk factors.

Electrocardiograms (ECGs) are classically the first-line test in making a diagnosis of AMI in any patient presenting with chest pain. The most sensitive and specific ECG marker is ST elevation, which normally appears within a few minutes of onset of symptoms. Serial ECGs are fundamental as the initial ECG can be normal with changes evolving over time. The sensitivity of 12-lead ECGs has been reported to be as low as 50 % to identify ischaemia.

Cardiac-specific troponin I and troponin T are the biomarkers of choice for diagnosing myocardial infarction. Different hospitals will use either troponin I or troponin T, and recommended sampling times vary depending on the assay, so clinicians should check their local hospital guidelines. A negative troponin at presentation does not exclude cardiac damage as it can take 12 h for the level to peak. Troponin is never increased above the upper limit of normal in healthy pregnant women and is not affected by anaesthesia, a prolonged labour or caesarean section, and therefore is the investigation of choice.

In contrast, other cardiac markers—myoglobin, creatinine kinase, creatinine kinase isoenzyme MB—can be increased significantly in labour. The troponin levels can be raised in pre-eclampsia, gestational hypertension and pulmonary embolism in the absence of significant coronary disease. It is important to note that in pre-eclampsia the troponin level is never above standard threshold set for MI.

References Wuntakal R, Shetty N, Ioannou E, Sharma S, Kurian J. Myocardial infarction and pregnancy. Obstet Gynaecol. 2013;15:247She.

CSPO23

CSPO23 Answer: A

Explanation Common peroneal nerve injury is avoided when there is padding in place between the lateral fibular heads and the stirrup, thus preventing nerve compression against a hard surface. As with abdominal surgery, the length of operative time during lithotomy has been cited as a significant risk factor for increasing the risk of nerve injury, especially if operating time exceeds 2 h.

CSPO24

CSPO24 Answer: C

Explanation Where the torn IAS can be identified, it is advisable to repair this separately with interrupted or mattress sutures without any attempt to overlap the IAS.

References https://www.rcog.org.uk/globalassets/documents/guidelines/gtg-29.pdf

CSPO25

CSPO25 Answer: A

Explanation Third-degree tear: Injury to perineum involving the anal sphincter complex:
Grade 3a tear: Less than 50 % of external anal sphincter (EAS) thickness torn.
    Grade 3b tear: More than 50 % of EAS thickness torn.
Grade 3c tear: Both EAS and internal anal sphincter (IAS) torn.
Fourth-degree tear: Injury to perineum involving the anal sphincter complex (EAS and IAS) and anorectal mucosa.

References https://www.rcog.org.uk/globalassets/documents/guidelines/gtg-29.pdf

Surgical Procedures: Answers and Explanations

27

SP1

Answer: B

Explanation There are four causes of inadvertent laparoscopic electrosurgical injuries, namely, inadvertent tissue contact, insulation failure, direct coupling and capacitive coupling. The above apply to all visceral injuries that may occur during laparoscopic surgery.

Such injuries may be difficult to identify, as they can occur at a site distant to the surgeon's view and/or present as delayed tissue breakdown several days following the primary insult. Safety measures to prevent laparoscopic electrosurgical complications include:

- Inspect insulation carefully before use
- Use the *lowest* possible effective power setting.
- Use available technology; newer tissue response generators and active electrode monitoring technology eliminate concerns about insulation failure and capacitive coupling.
- Use a low-voltage waveform for monopolar diathermy (cut).
- Use bipolar electrosurgery when appropriate.
- Use brief intermittent activation.
- Do not activate in close proximity or direct contact with another instrument.
- Ensure that both the heel and the tips of the bipolar forceps are kept under direct view when activating.

References 1. Shirk GJ, et al. Complications of laparoscopic surgery: how to avoid them and how to repair them. J Minim Invasive Gynecol. 2006;13:352–9.
2. Alkatout I, et al. Principles and safety measures of electrosurgery in laparoscopy. JSLS. 2012;16:130–9.

© Springer India 2016
C. Ratha, J. Gupta, *SBAs and EMQs for MRCOG II*,
DOI 10.1007/978-81-322-2689-5_27

SP2

Answer: C

Explanation The two types of current used in hysteroscopic surgery are monopolar and bipolar. The energy is transmitted through the hysteroscope at the tip of a loop, rollerball or disc. Monopolar energy needs the patient to be part of the electrical circuit; hence, a return electrode is attached to the patient. In bipolar devices, the circuit is formed within the instrument itself, avoiding the risk of burn injury to patient. Bipolar energy is used with electrolytic solutions and produces a vapour at the end of the operating instrument leading to the tissue vaporization or desiccation needed to dissect the tissue. Monopolar current need non-electrolytic solutions as they do not conduct electricity.

References Stocker L, et al. An overview of hysteroscopy and hysteroscopic surgery. Obstet Gynaecol Rep Med. 23:5;146–53.

SP3

Answer: B

Explanation Pre-op counselling for procedures needs a clear explanation of risks. There is no need to discuss every conceivable risk posed by the surgery, but the main risks must be covered: both those that occur frequently and those less frequent but more severe. Vague terms such as 'low' and 'high' risk should be avoided, as should complicated statistical terms. Use of phrases such as 'a risk of 1 in 100 women' is more appropriate.

The serious risks that need to be mentioned for a diagnostic hysteroscopy are uterine perforation, pelvic infection and failure to visualise uterine cavity, pelvic or shoulder pain. Frequent risks are vaginal bleeding and discharge. Extra procedures that may become necessary are laparotomy to repair a uterine perforation and blood transfusion.

References Lebus CS, Shafi MI. Pre and post op care in gynaecology. Curr Obstet Gynaecol. 2006;16:84–92.

SP4

Answer: D

Explanation In a review by the Council of the Association of Surgeons, it was suggested that, after two failed attempts to insert the Veress needle, either the open Hasson technique or Palmer's point entry should be used.

References http://bsge.org.uk/userfiles/file/GtG%20no%2049%20 Laparoscopic%20Injury%202008.pdf

---

SP5

Answer: E

Explanation Trocars can either be inserted blind, after a pneumoperitoneum has been established with a Veress needle, or open, through a mini-laparotomy incision. Patients should be in a supine position with an empty bladder; the Trendelenburg position (head down) should not be used during primary trocar insertion, as this alters the angles, increasing the risk of vascular injury, and brings the bowel up out of the pelvis and towards the umbilicus. During the operative procedure, intra-abdominal pressures of 10–15 mmHg are normally used, although a pressure of 25 mmHg for trocar insertion may reduce the risk of injury. At this pressure, it is unlikely that the anterior abdominal wall can be compressed onto the aorta. If a Veress needle is used, its position can be checked by allowing saline to run into the abdominal cavity or by ensuring that gas readily passes in through the needle while the pressure is low. Higher pressures or lack of saline drainage would suggest that the needle was still extra-peritoneal. Another option is to insert the primary port sheath using an open technique; a small incision is made below or within the umbilicus. In published series, rates of bowel damage are similar to the closed technique, but as the open technique is often reserved for high risk patients, the comparison may not be valid. Vascular damage is, however, much reduced.

References Morrion J, MacKenzie I. Avoiding and managing complications during gynaecological surgery. Obstet Gynaecol Rep Med. 17(4):105–11.

SP6

Answer: E

Explanation Cochrane review concluded that the best route for performing hysterectomy was the vaginal route. In patients for whom the vaginal route is contraindicated or not technically possible, laparoscopic hysterectomy had benefits over the abdominal route and should be the default approach. The benefits of laparoscopic hysterectomy versus abdominal hysterectomy were lower intraoperative blood, a smaller drop in haemoglobin level, shorter duration of hospital stay, speedier return to normal activities, fewer wound or abdominal wall infections and fewer unspecified infections or febrile episodes, at the cost of longer operating time and more urinary tract injuries. There was no benefit in performing a total laparoscopic hysterectomy over a laparoscopically assisted vaginal hysterectomy.

References Slack A, McVeigh E. Laparascopy and laparascopic surgery. Obstet Gynaecol Rep Med. 17(4):112–8.

SP7

Answer: D

Explanation Before defibulation, identification of the urethra should be attempted and a catheter passed. Incision should be made along the vulval excision scar. Cutting diathermy reduces the amount of bleeding. The use of fine absorbable suture material such as polyglactin 910 (Vicryl® Rapide, Ethicon) is recommended.

Prophylactic antibiotic therapy should be considered. Defibulation can be carried out in the antenatal period or intrapartum. The decision should be made by a senior obstetrician with adequate experience in this field. If necessary, guidance should be sought from a centre that has developed expertise in the assessment and management of affected women. The technique for defibulation is described in the WHO document, management of pregnancy, childbirth and the postpartum period in the presence of female genital mutilation, which includes diagrams and photographs. Antenatal surgical correction should ideally be performed around 20 weeks of gestation to reduce the risk of miscarriage and allow time for healing before the birth.

Women should be recommended to undergo defibulation before conception, especially if difficult surgery is anticipated. Gynaecology and maternity units with little experience of genital mutilation should consult with a centre that has developed expertise in the assessment and management of affected women. It must be remembered that defibulation does not restore physical or emotional normality.

Urine should be screened for bacteriuria before surgery. Blood should be sent for group and serum save because of the risk of haemorrhage. Defibulation may be carried out in any suitable outpatient room equipped for minor procedures or in an operating theatre.

Ideally, the surgeon or midwife should have personal experience of defibulation. In emergency situations, senior obstetric help must be called.

References 1. Green-Top guideline FGM.

2. World Health Organization. Management of pregnancy, childbirth and postpartum period in the presence of female genital mutilation. Geneva: WHO; 2001. www.who.int/reproductivehealth/publications/mngt_pregnancy_childbirth_fgm/text.pdf

SP8

Answer: D

Explanation McCall culdoplasty at the time of vaginal hysterectomy is a recommended measure to prevent enterocele formation. A small randomised trial compared vaginal Moschowitz-type operation, McCall's culdoplasty and peritoneal closure of the cul-de-sac as preventive measures against the development of enterocele. It included 100 women and showed that McCall's culdoplasty was more effective than vaginal Moschowitz or simple closure of the peritoneum in preventing enterocele at 3 years' follow-up. The technique involves approximating the uterosacral ligaments using continuous sutures, so as to obliterate the peritoneum of the posterior cul-de-sac as high as possible

Suturing the cardinal and uterosacral ligaments to the vaginal cuff at the time of hysterectomy is a recommended measure to avoid vault prolapse. Attaching the uterosacral and cardinal ligaments to the vaginal cuff and high circumferential obliteration of the pouch of Douglas has been suggested to prevent vault prolapse and enterocele formation. No cases of vault prolapse or enterocele were recorded among 112 patients over a follow-up period extending from 7 to 42 months.

References 1. Green Top guideline – post hysterectomy vault prolapse.

2. Cruikshank SH, Kovac SR. Randomized comparison of three surgical methods used at the time of vaginal hysterectomy to prevent posterior enterocele. Am J Obstet Gynecol. 1999;180:859–65.

SP9

Answer: A

Explanation A lower segment caesarean section is unlikely to cause an anal sphincter injury. The other complications are rather well established in association with LSCS.

Immediate	Postpartum haemorrhage
	Wound haematoma
	Intra-abdominal haemorrhage
	Bladder/bowel trauma
	Neonatal—transient tachypnoea of the newborn
Intermediate	Infection
	Urinary tract infection if urinary symptoms
	Endometritis if excessive vaginal bleeding
	Respiratory (especially if general anaesthetic was used)
	Venous thromboembolism
	Spinal headache

(continued)

Late	Urinary tract trauma fistula
	Subfertility
	Regret and other negative psychological sequelae
	Rupture/dehiscence of scar
	Placenta praevia/accreta

References Strat OG Labour and Delivery. https://stratog.rcog.org.uk/tutorial/caesarean-section---teaching-resource/complications---model-answer-7439

SP10

Answer: C

Explanation The sign in needs to be completed before induction of anaesthesia and the time out needs to be completed before skin incision or surgical procedure. There is no time in as a part of the checklist.

References http://www.nrls.npsa.nhs.uk/resources/?entryid45=59860

Clinical Governance: Answers and Explanations

28

CG1

CG1 Answer: C

Explanation Respect for autonomy is the most important principle, and we cannot justify forcing patients to undergo treatment they choose 'autonomously' to refuse. In a woman refusing a caesarean section, undertaking such a procedure without her consent would be classed as assault.

Beneficence and non-maleficence are also considered here. The unborn fetus has no rights, and giving treatment against the patient's will constitute battery.

CG2

CG2 Answer: B

Explanation Ethics aims to understand the problem, and practical ethics helps with decision-making. The principles of ethics include beneficence, maleficence, autonomy and justice. The **four principles approach** provides a way of thinking about ethical issues/problems in a simple and accessible way that should cut across cultural differences. In current UK practice, care is delivered under the clinical governance framework using protocols, cost-effectiveness and NICE guidelines and underpinned by a risk management framework.

The 'four principles' approach may need to be used in exceptional circumstances where they may need to have recourse to a legal framework:

1. Respect for autonomy—obligation to respect the decision-making capacities of the autonomous person

© Springer India 2016
C. Ratha, J. Gupta, *SBAs and EMQs for MRCOG II*,
DOI 10.1007/978-81-322-2689-5_28

2. Beneficence—obligation to provide benefits and to balance benefits against risks
3. Non-maleficence—obligation to avoid causing harm
4. Justice—obligation of fairness in the distribution of benefits and risks

References Strat OG tutorial on clinical governance.

CG3

CG3 Answer: B

Explanation The contemporary teacher must be able to use knowledge and different methods of teaching, assess the needs and level of knowledge of the learners and conduct teaching in accordance with the curriculum.

The main roles of a clinical teacher are:

1. The information provider in the lecture and in the clinical context
2. The role model on the job and in more formal teaching settings
3. The facilitator as a mentor and learning facilitator
4. The student assessor and curriculum evaluator
5. The curriculum and course planner
6. The resource material creator and study guide provider

References Duthie SJ, Garden AS. The teacher, the learner and the method. Obstet Gynaecol. 2010;12:273–80.

CG4

CG4 Answer: A

Explanation FGM is illegal unless it is a surgical operation on a girl or woman irrespective of her age:

a. Which is necessary for her physical or mental health.
b. She is in any stage of labour, or has just given birth, for purposes connected with the labour or birth.

It is illegal to arrange, or assist in arranging, for a UK national or UK resident to be taken overseas for the purpose of FGM.

It is an offence for those with parental responsibility to fail to protect a girl from the risk of FGM.

If FGM is confirmed in a girl under 18 years of age (either on examination or because the patient or parent says it has been done), reporting to the police is mandatory, and this must be within 1 month of confirmation [New 2015].

CG5

CG5 Answer: D

Explanation Patients will expect hospitals to hold information about them in confidence by their doctors. You must treat information about them as confidential. It is essential to remember that the doctor's duty of care is always to the patient (the woman) and not to her relatives or her unborn child. It is especially important to be mindful of this duty when confronted by the relatives away from the patient.

This also applies where the patient is a child or young person, as well as when the patient is an adult. Without the trust that confidentiality brings, children and young people might not seek medical care and advice. The same duties of confidentiality apply when using, sharing or disclosing information about children and young people as about young children.

References GMC guidance document on confidentiality: www.gmc-uk.org/guidance

---

CG6

CG6 Answer: C

Explanation Consent is when a competent patient:

- Makes it clear that they are able to understand what a procedure involves
- Has been made aware of and been able to discuss the benefits and the risks of a procedure
- Has received appropriate written information

Thus, when taking consent, a patient must be able to understand the procedure, be able to retain that information, can make a decision based on that information and be able to communicate that decision to the carer by signing the consent form (see Mental Capacity Act.) The four elements are therefore:

1. Understanding
2. Retaining
3. Deciding
4. Communicating

References http://www.nhs.uk/Conditions/social-care-and-support-guide/Pages/mental-capacity.aspx

CG7

CG7 Answer: C

Explanation   The Mental Capacity Act (MCA) is designed to protect and empower individuals who may lack the mental capacity to make their own decisions about their care and treatment. It is a law that applies to individuals aged 16 and over. Examples of people who may lack capacity include those with:

Dementia
A severe learning disability
A brain injury
A mental health condition
A stroke

Unconsciousness caused by an anaesthetic or sudden accident
   However, just because a person has one of these conditions does not necessarily mean they lack the capacity to make a specific decision.

References   http://www.nhs.uk/Conditions/social-care-and-support-guide/Pages/mental-capacity.aspx

CG8

CG 8 Answer: C

   The 1-min preceptor **is a five-step process that can be carried out in minutes with the purpose of structuring teaching opportunities that arise in the clinical environment. This is an example of a teaching method that demands a good rapport between the teacher and the learner(s). The teacher must make the learner feel secure and allow the voicing of opinions, whether they are correct or incorrect. The five steps are:**

1. Commitment
2. Justification
3. Application
4. Positive reinforcement
5. Correction of mistakes

References   Duthie SJ, Garden AS. The teacher, the learner and the method. Obstet Gynaecol. 2010;12:273–80.

CG9

CG9 Answer: C

Explanation Medical negligence is part of the Tort Law and is part of civil as opposed to criminal law. It should be considered a legal term where 'a breach of a legal duty to take care results in damage to the claimant'. The law of negligence allows the Plaintiff i.e. the patient (A) to sue the Defendant i.e. the Doctor (B) (or in some circumstances B's employers) on the basis of vicarious responsibility, for compensation where A suffers harm as a result of B's carelessness.

A has to establish:

- B owed A a duty of care.
- B breached that duty of care (fell below the required standard, i.e. B did not act in accordance to that followed by a 'reasonable', 'respectable' or 'responsible' body of practitioners at the same level (Bolam test (1957))). Likewise it is important to also apply the Bolitho test (1997), which is a modification of the Bolam test, i.e. although a defence argument may be 'reasonable', 'respectable' or 'responsible', was that opinion based on 'logical' analysis?
- 'A' suffered harm as a result of that breach.

Once A has shown that there was a duty of care and proved that it has been breached, then A has to prove that the defendant's negligence actually caused the damage. The onus is on the claimant (A) to prove the causal link on a balance of probabilities. Causation is of crucial importance in medical negligence especially when related to informed consent. This may be a factual causation or a 'but for' test that the defendant's (B) negligent act or omission did in fact cause the claimants damage. The other way would be that the damage is still sufficiently proximate in law to hold the defendant liable.

CG10

CG10 Answer: D

Explanation The Caldicott guardian is a senior person (usually the medical director) who is responsible for protecting confidentiality of patient and service user information and enabling appropriate information sharing. Every planned use or transfer of patient identifiable information from or within an organisation should be clearly defined and analysed, with regular reviews, by the Caldicott guardian.

References http://webarchive.nationalarchives.gov.uk/20130502102046/http://connectingforhealth.nhs.uk/systemsandservices/infogov/caldicott

British Medical Association. *Confidentiality and disclosure of health information toolkit.* London: BMA; 2009.

Extended Matching Questions

29

Options for Questions 1–4

A. Amniocentesis
B. Fetal blood sampling
C. Chorionic villus sampling (CVS)
D. Maternal Doppler study
E. Fetal blood sampling
F. Fetal fibronectin
G. NT scan
H. Cervical length by TVS
I. Fetal ultrasound study

Instruction Select the most appropriate investigation for the given clinical scenario *(each option could be used once, more than once or not at all)*.

1. Consanguineous couple, now 11 weeks pregnant. G4 P2L1 A1 with one live child with thalassaemia minor, one previous child who died of thalassaemia major and one termination of pregnancy following fetal diagnosis.
2. Mrs. X, 34 years of age at 17 weeks' gestation has a 1 in 16 risk of Down syndrome on the quadruple test and wants to confirm fetal karyotype.
3. Mrs. Y, G3A2 previous two preterm births of AGA fetuses at 22–24 weeks' gestation due to cervical incompetence. Now 11 weeks pregnant.
4. Mrs.Z, 32 years of age, 29 weeks pregnant, has an SGA fetus with reduced amniotic fluid. She is perceiving reduced fetal movements since a day.

Options for Questions 5–8

A. Maternal IV antibiotics

© Springer India 2016
C. Ratha, J. Gupta, *SBAs and EMQs for MRCOG II*,
DOI 10.1007/978-81-322-2689-5_29

B. Fetal antibiotic therapy
C. Selective feticide
D. Fetoscopic laser coagulation of placental anastomotic vessels
E. Amniodrainage
F. Vesicoamniotic shunt
G. Fetal blood transfusion
H. LASER septostomy
I. Immediate delivery by LSCS

Instruction Select the most appropriate treatment for the given clinical scenario
(each option could be used once, more than once or not at all).

5. Mrs. A, a primary school teacher, 27 years of age, is 34 weeks pregnant. She
    contracted parvovirus infection following an outbreak at her school 2 weeks
    back. Now the ultrasound scan shows fetal hydrops.
6. Mrs. B has monochorionic diamniotic twins and is now 24 weeks pregnant. The
    fetal scan shows excessive amniotic fluid with a large fetal urinary bladder in one
    sac with almost no liquor and non-visualisation of fetal urinary bladder in the
    other with a growth discrepancy of 35 % between the twins.
7. Mrs. C has dichorionic diamniotic twins with one anencephalic fetus and a struc-
    turally normal co-twin. She is 22 weeks pregnant, and there is polyhydramnios
    in the sac of the anencephalic fetus. The mother understands that anencephaly is
    a lethal anomaly and wants to minimise the perinatal risks for the normal
    co-twin.
8. Mrs. D has a singleton fetus diagnosed with an omphalocele. Fetal karyotyping
    was normal and after conferring with the paediatric surgeon, she is planning for
    postnatal surgical correction of the abdominal wall defect. She is now 29 weeks
    pregnant and has developed severe polyhydramnios causing maternal respiratory
    discomfort.

Options for Questions 9–12

A. Lichen sclerosus
B. Seborrhoeic dermatitis
C. Atopic vulvitis
D. Lichen simplex
E. Psoriasis
F. Herpes simplex
G. Behcet's disease
H. Hidradenitis suppurativa
I. Paget's disease
J. Tinea cruris

For each of the following patients with vulval symptoms, please select the most
likely diagnosis from the list. Each option may be used once, more than once or not
at all.

9. A 5-year-old girl presents with burning on micturition and vulva I scratching. On examination the vulva is noted to have a well-demarcated white area around the introitus. The overlying skin appears thin with extensive fissuring. The perianal area is not involved.

10. A 70-year-old postmenopausal woman presents with vulval itching. On examination, she has a narrow introitus. The skin over the labia, the perineal area and the genitocrural folds is thin and dry, with white discoloration and superficial excoriations. A skin biopsy reveals atrophic epidermis with hyperkeratosis and superficial dermal hyalinisation with lymphocytic infiltrates.

11. A 23-year-old woman presents with vulval itching. On examination there is a well-demarcated symmetrical lesion involving the labia major and minor and extending to the genitocrural folds. The lesions appear beefy red with scaling. A biopsy shows papillomatosis, parakeratosis and neutrophil exocytosis.

12. A 34-year-old woman presents with a burning sensation in the vulval region. On examination the vulva is erythematous with marked oedema and numerous small superficial ulcerations. The inguinal lymph nodes are enlarged and tender.

Options for Questions 13–15

A. Average
B. Historical controlled observational study
C. Intention to treat analysis
D. Meta-analysis
E. Narrative review
F. Power calculation
G. Randomised controlled trial
H. Relative risk
 I. Secondary analysis
J. Systematic review

For each of the questions below, choose the most appropriate answer from the list of options above. Each option may be used once, more than once or not at all.

13. The sample size of a study is assessed by which calculation?
14. Reliable evidence of clinical practice should be derived from which type of evidence?
15. A chemotherapy trial that includes all the patients who started the trial is described as what type of analysis?

Options for Questions 16–18

A. Combined oral contraceptive pill
B. Copper intrauterine contraception device (IUCD)

C. Depo-Provera
D. GyneFix IUCD
E. Nexplanon implant
F. Laparoscopic sterilisation
G. Levonelle
H. Levonorgestrel intrauterine system
 I. Male contraception
 J. Mini-laparotomy and sterilisation
K. Progestogen-only pill
 L. Sheath/condom
M. Withdrawal

For each of the scenarios described below, choose the most appropriate contraceptive advice from the list of options above. Each option may be used once, more than once or not at all.

16. A 16-year-old with Eisenmenger's complex consults you for contraceptive advice.
17. A 42-year-old multiparous single woman with a BMI of 35 consults you for advice regarding contraception. She had a termination 6 months ago while on the combined oral contraceptive pill.
18. A 27-year-old nulliparous student is requesting contraception. She refuses any form of hormonal preparation.

Options for Questions 19–21

A. Ca-125
B. Cervical smear
C. Computed tomography (CT) scan
D. Diagnostic laparoscopy
E. Endometrial outpatient biopsy
F. Follicle-stimulating hormone (FSH), luteinising hormone (LH) and oestradiol
G. Full blood count
H. Inpatient hysteroscopy
 I. Magnetic resonance imaging (MRI)
 J. Outpatient hysteroscopy
K. Routine ultrasound scan
 L. Thyroid function tests
M. Triple swabs
N. Urgent ultrasound
O. Urodynamics

For each of the scenarios described below, choose the single most useful investigation from the list of options above. Each option may be used once, more than once or not at all.

19. A 55-year-old woman presents with postmenopausal bleeding. An ultrasound scan shows a normal uterus and ovaries with an endometrial thickness of 5 mm.
20. A 42-year-old woman presents with an irregular cycle. Her last cervical smear 1 year ago was normal and she has no menorrhagia.
21. A 45-year-old woman with human immunodeficiency virus (HIV) infection presents to the gynaecology clinic with intermenstrual bleeding and occasional postcoital bleeding.

Options for Questions 22–23

A. 0.05 %
B. 0.5 %
C. 5 %
D. 10 %
E. 20 %
F. 35 %
G. 50 %
H. 80 %
 I. Reduces incidence of bowel and vascular trauma only
 J. Reduces incidence of vascular trauma only
K. Reduces incidence of bowel trauma only

Lead in: for each of the questions below, choose the most appropriate answer from the list of options above. Each option may be used once, more than once or not at all.

22. Bowel adhesions to the anterior abdominal wall are found in what percentage of patients without prior surgery?
23. What is the advantage of open laparoscopy?

Options for Questions 24–28

Management of labour

A. Amniotomy (artificial rupture of membranes).
B. Caesarean section.
C. Change maternal labour position.
D. Commence continuous electronic fetal monitoring (CTG).
E. Commence intermittent fetal heart rate auscultation.
F. Episiotomy.
G. Intravaginal prostaglandin.
H. Intravenous antibiotics.
 I. Intravenous fluids.
 J. Instrumental (forceps or ventouse) delivery.

K. Fetal blood sampling.
L. Intravenous oxytocin.
M. Repeat vaginal examination at suitable time interval.
N. Subcutaneous terbutaline.

Instructions: for each clinical scenario listed, select the NEXT MOST appropriate clinical management. Unless stated otherwise, all scenarios refer to a 25-year-old woman who is 40 weeks pregnant and is in spontaneous-onset labour. Abbreviations: Cx = cervical dilatation; FHR = fetal heart rate.

24. CTG variable decelerations for 20 min at Cx 4 cm. CTG normal prior to decelerations. Currently, FHR baseline is 140 bpm. Membranes intact. Uterine contractions are 3–4 every 10 min. Epidural analgesia top-up was given 20 min prior. The woman is in left lateral supine position. Maternal BP 100/60 mmHg.

25. Progressed from Cx 5 cm to Cx 6 cm in 4 h. Membranes artificially ruptured 8 h ago. Uterine contractions are 2–3 every 10 min. The fetus has severe IUGR at 38 weeks. Continuous fetal CTG monitoring in progress; CTG is normal with normal FHR.

26. In the second stage of labour. Active pushing for 2 h. CTG shows deep decelerations. Fetal head just visible when labia are parted at peak of maternal expulsive effort. Epidural top-up 1 h ago. Uterine contractions are 4 every 10 min.

27. Appearance of meconium-stained liquor following amniotomy at Cx 5 cm labour. Spontaneous-onset labour. Low-risk pregnancy. Intermittent FHR monitoring prior to amniotomy showed normal FHR.

28. Progressed from Cx 5 cm to Cx 9 cm in 4 h. Spontaneous-onset labour with intact membranes. Uterine contractions are 2–3 every 10 min. Low-risk pregnancy. Intermittent FHR monitoring shows normal FHR. No urge to push.

Options for Questions 29–33

Management of Labour

A. Amniotomy (artificial rupture of membranes).
B. Caesarean section.
C. Change maternal labour position.
D. Commence continuous electronic fetal monitoring (CTG).
E. Commence intermittent fetal heart rate auscultation.
F. Episiotomy.
G. Intravaginal prostaglandin.
H. Intravenous antibiotics.
 I. Intravenous fluids.
 J. Instrumental (forceps or ventouse) delivery.
K. Fetal blood sampling.
L. Intravenous oxytocin.
M. Repeat vaginal examination at suitable time interval.

N. Subcutaneous terbutaline.

Instructions For each clinical scenario listed, select the NEXT MOST appropriate clinical management. Unless stated otherwise, all scenarios refer to a 25-year-old woman who is 40 weeks pregnant and is in spontaneous-onset labour. Abbreviations: Cx = cervical dilatation; FHR = fetal heart rate.

29. CTG decelerations for 40 min then a prolonged deceleration for 4 min without recovery of the FHR. Currently, FHR is 80 bpm. CTG was normal prior to decelerations. Cx is 5 cm. Membranes ruptured 3 h prior. The woman in left lateral supine position. No epidural analgesia. No oxytocin augmentation. Contractions 2 in 10 min.

30. Ruptured membranes for 24 h with no onset of uterine contractions. FHR is 150 bpm. Maternal temperature is 37.1° and maternal pulse 100 bpm. Maternal IV antibiotics commenced. Cervix <1 cm dilated, uneffaced and firm consistency.

31. Quick recovery variable decelerations on CTG for 40 min. Baseline FHR 165 bpm. Contracting 5–6 every 10 min. Vaginal prostaglandin inserted 1 h earlier and just removed. Cervix 5 cm dilated with ruptured membranes. No vaginal bleeding or uterine tenderness.

32. Appearance of meconium-stained liquor following amniotomy at Cx 5 cm labour. Spontaneous-onset labour. Low-risk pregnancy. Intermittent FHR monitoring prior to amniotomy showed normal FHR.

33. Progressed from Cx 3 cm to Cx 7 cm in 4 h. Spontaneous-onset labour with intact membranes. Uterine contractions are 2–3 every 10 min. Low-risk pregnancy. Intermittent FHR monitoring shows normal FHR. No urge to push.

Options for Questions 34–38

Postpartum problems

A. Pulmonary embolism
B. Pneumonia
C. Breast mastitis
D. Uterine endometritis
E. Infected perineum
F. Superficial leg vein thrombophlebitis
G. Leg deep-vein thrombosis
H. Wound infection
I. Infected pelvic haematoma
J. Urinary tract infection
K. Appendicitis
L. Glandular fever
M. Ruptured uterus

N. Secondary postpartum haemorrhage
O. Uterine involution

Instructions The options listed are recognised causes of puerperal pyrexia. For each of the clinical scenarios listed, select the SINGLE most likely diagnosis.

34. Pelvic pain, fever and malodorous vaginal discharge that persists 3 days post-delivery. History of 36 h of membrane rupture prior to delivery.
35. Low-grade pyrexia. Localised superficial lower abdominal pain and erythema around skin incision day 4 post-caesarean delivery. No pelvic pain, vaginal bleeding. Mobilising well.
36. Low-grade fever five days following uncomplicated spontaneous vaginal delivery without perineal trauma with epidural analgesia. Foley catheter reinserted 48 h postdelivery for 24 h due to inability to sense a full bladder and void.
37. Pyrexia day 1 postdelivery. General anaesthetic emergency caesarean with difficult intubation. Saturations 92 % on air. Known smoker. Bibasal crepitations on chest auscultation.
38. Low-grade fever, pleuritic chest discomfort 9 days postdelivery. No productive cough. Had emergency caesarean delivery for abruption. Required 4 unit transfusion. Obesity (BMI 36). Normal wound on inspection. No clinical leg pain or swelling. Saturations 94 % air, RR 24. No added breath sounds on auscultation.

Options for Questions 39–43

Postpartum problems

A. Atonic uterus
B. Broad ligament haematoma
C. Cervical trauma
D. Disseminated intravascular coagulation
E. Endometritis
F. Extrauterine pelvic haematoma
G. Perineal tear
H. Retained placental tissue
 I. Uterine inversion
J. Uterine rupture

Instructions The options listed are recognised causes of postpartum haemorrhage. For each of the clinical scenarios listed, select the most likely diagnosis.

39. Maternal collapse 4 h following ventouse instrumental delivery for fetal distress (CTG decelerations). Moderate vaginal bleeding. Placenta checked to be complete. She had undergone a caesarean section delivery 2 years earlier.

Abdominal examination reveals a tender moderately contracted uterus. Urinary catheter has shown new-onset haematuria.

40. Heavy vaginal bleeding 12 days following elective caesarean section for twin pregnancy. Abdominal examination reveals tender slightly enlarged uterus. She has a low-grade pyrexia and malodorous vaginal discharge.

41. Intrapartum haemorrhage just prior to delivery that appears watery. She presented with a history of antepartum haemorrhage, abdominal pain and stillbirth at 36 weeks' gestation. She also has bleeding from nostrils and IV cannulation sites.

42. Profound hypotension and maternal collapse one minute after delivering the placenta. Difficult placental delivery requiring considerable cord traction force. Moderate vaginal bleeding. Abdominal palpation reveals an indented uterine fundus. Vaginal examination reveals a bulging pulsating mass that does not feel like a remnant placenta.

43. Heavy vaginal bleeding immediately following spontaneous term delivery of diabetic mother. Baby birth weight 4.8 kg. Known to have polyhydramnios before delivery. Labour augmented with oxytocin. Abdominal examination reveals a boggy noncontracted enlarged uterus extending well above the umbilicus, which contracts down on manual uterine massage. No perineal tear occurred at delivery. The placenta was checked to be complete and intact.

Options for Questions 44–48

Antenatal care: congenital and perinatal infection

A. *Cytomegalovirus* (CMV)
B. Group B streptococcus
C. Hepatitis B
D. Herpes simplex virus (HSV)
E. Human immunodeficiency virus (HIV)
F. Human papilloma virus (HPV)
G. *Listeria monocytogenes*
H. Parvovirus B19
 I. *Toxoplasma gondii*
 J. *Treponema pallidum* (syphilis)
K. *Rubella*
L. *Varicella zoster* virus (VZV)

Instructions For each of the characteristics and fetal sequelae listed, select the SINGLE most likely causative infective organism from the options provided.

44. Uncooked meat; chorioretinitis, sensitive to spiramycin.
45. Vaccination of infant at birth, combined with specific immunoglobulin, will reduce vertical transmission.

46. Unpasteurised milk, soft cheese; IUFD, neonatal sepsis, neonatal abscesses.
47. Segmental skin scarring, mental retardation, limb hypoplasia, cataracts, microcephaly, chorioretinitis, hydrocephalus, and low birth weight.
48. Deafness and mental retardation is more common if the fetus is symptomatic at birth (hepatosplenomegaly, purpura, anaemia, IUGR).

Options for Questions 49–53

Antenatal care: screening tests

A. Preimplantation genetic diagnosis
B. 11+2 to 14+ 1
C. 14+2 to 20+0
D. 18+0 to 20+6
E. 28w
F. 32w
G. 36w
H. 41w

Instructions For each of the clinical scenarios listed, select the SINGLE most appropriate gestation when the screening test should be performed.

49. Optimal gestational age to accurately determine chorionicity of multiple pregnancies
50. Quadruple test or integrated (combined and quadruple test) screening tests for Down syndrome
51. Optimal time to commence ultrasonographic measurement of cervical length in women with a history of one or more spontaneous mid-trimester pregnancy loss
52. Screening that prevents the risk of single gene defect disorders such as Huntington disease
53. Testing for gestational diabetes

Options for Questions 54–58

Antenatal care: screening tests

A. Preimplantation genetic diagnosis
B. 11+2 to 14+ 1
C. 14+2 to 20+0
D. 18+0 to 20+6
E. 28w
F. 32w

G. 36w
H. 41w

Instructions For each of the clinical scenarios listed, select the SINGLE most appropriate gestation when the screening test should be performed.

54. Detailed fetal structural anomaly screening
55. Quadruple test or integrated (combined and quadruple test) screening tests for Down syndrome
56. Optimal time to commence ultrasonographic measurement of cervical length in women with a history of one or more spontaneous mid-trimester pregnancy loss
57. Screening that prevents the risk of single gene defect disorders such as Huntington disease
58. 'Preferred time to rescan a woman who has been identified to have a low-lying placenta'

Options for Questions 59–63

Subject: breast

A. Axillary mammary tissue
B. Breast abscess
C. Breast cyst
D. Breast lumpiness
E. Early breast cancer
F. Enlarged axillary lymph node
G. Fat necrosis
H. Fibroadenoma
 I. Galactocoele
J. Locally advanced breast cancer

Instructions For each of the clinical scenarios below, choose the single most likely diagnosis from the list above. Each diagnosis above may be used once, more than once or not at all.

59. A 25-year-old woman presents to the breast clinic with a 2-year history of a breast lump. She had breast ultrasound and fine-needle aspiration cytology and was discharged with no follow-up.
60. A 28-year-old woman who is 4 months' postnatal who was concerned about a mass in her left axilla which developed 2 months prior to delivery. Clinical examination revealed no breast abnormality.
61. A 31-year-old woman presents with a 2-month history of a painful right-sided breast lump. She was examined, no further investigations were arranged, and she was discharged.

62. A 75-year-old woman presented with pain in her left breast associated with skin oedema and redness. Examination revealed enlarged lymph nodes in the right axilla.

63. A 46-year-old woman presented with a 2-month history of a lump in her left breast. She had menopause 1 year ago and was started on HRT 6 months later. A mammogram 4 months ago was negative. On examination there is a single breast lump.

Options for Questions 64–68

Subject: early pregnancy care

A. Admission to hospital ward for observation
B. Diagnostic laparoscopy and proceed as necessary according to pathology identified
C. Intramuscular methotrexate
D. Intravenous fluid resuscitation
E. Intravenous antibiotics
F. Measure serum βhCG and serum progesterone
G. Measure FBC and determine blood group type
H. Oral mifepristone followed 24–48 h later by vaginal misoprostol
 I. Pelvic ultrasound
 J. Speculum and vaginal/cervical infection screening swab tests
K. Speculum and cervical smear test
L. Surgical evacuation of the uterus

Instructions For each of the following clinical scenarios involving early pregnancy, select the SINGLE most appropriate management action that should be undertaken next.

64. 28-year-old G1P0 is 12 weeks pregnant. She complains of PV bleeding after intercourse. Her last cervical smear, 6 months ago, was reported as normal.

65. A 19-year-old has undergone a medical termination of pregnancy at 9 weeks. She presents 2 weeks later with heavy vaginal bleeding

66. A 34-year-old is diagnosed by ultrasound to have probable complete molar pregnancy at 10 weeks' gestation.

67. A 17-year-old is bought in by ambulance after collapsing in a shop. Her BP is 100/70, HR 115 bpm and sats 98 % air. She complains of severe abdominal pain and shoulder pain and feels faint.

68. A 22-year-old is diagnosed with a 1.5 cm left tubal ectopic pregnancy (described as gestational sac-like structure) on ultrasound. Her βhCG is 1500 IU/L and has increased to 1600 IU/L in 48 h. She is asymptomatic (no pain or bleeding) and has no evidence of pelvic haemoperitoneum on ultrasound.

Options for Questions 69–73

Subject: early pregnancy care

A. Complete miscarriage
B. Early fetal demise
C. Intrauterine pregnancy of uncertain viability
D. Inevitable miscarriage
E. Incomplete miscarriage
F. Late miscarriage
G. Ongoing intrauterine pregnancy
H. Pregnancy of unknown location
 I. Recurrent miscarriage
 J. Ruptured tubal ectopic pregnancy
K. Stillbirth
L. Threatened miscarriage
M. Unruptured tubal ectopic pregnancy

Instructions For each of the following clinical scenarios involving early pregnancy, select the SINGLE most likely diagnosis.

69. 5w pregnant. βhCG 600 IU/L. Intrauterine gestation sac with mean diameter measuring 20 mm. A yolk sac was identified within the gestation sac, but there is no evidence of a fetal pole

70. 6w pregnant. βhCG 1000 IU/L. Intrauterine sac measuring 50 mm containing a fetal pole of crown-rump length 10 mm. No fetal heart activity is identified.

71. 6w pregnant. HCG 1800 IU/L. No evidence of an intrauterine or extrauterine pregnancy. No pelvic free fluid.

72. 10w pregnant with cramping pelvic pain and vaginal bleeding. Ultrasound shows fetus with CRL 25 mm and fetal heart activity. Speculum examination shows 3–4 cm dilated cervical os with evidence of active bleeding.

73. 9w pregnant. βhCG 2500 IU/L. left pelvic tenderness. Ultrasound shows an empty uterus, free fluid in the pelvis (40 mm by 60 mm) and a left adnexal mass containing a sac-like structure measuring 2.5 cm.

Options for Questions 74–78

Maternal medicine

A. Chronic hypertension
B. Chronic hypertension and superimposed pre-eclampsia
C. Chronic renal disease
D. Cushing's syndrome
E. Gestational hypertension

F. Hyperthyroidism
G. Pheochromocytoma
H. Pre-eclampsia

Instructions For each of the clinical scenarios involving pregnancy, select the most likely diagnosis from the list of options.

74. 20 weeks pregnant. Episodic headaches, palpitations, sweating and tremor. Examination shows BP 160/110 mmHg. BP tends to be highly labile.
75. 13 weeks pregnant with BP 160/100 mmHg. History of childhood glomerulonephritis. Urine dipstix shows +++ proteinuria. Similar BP recorded at prepregnancy counselling review 6 months earlier.
76. 32 weeks pregnant with proteinuria (0.2 g/24 h) and BP of 150/100 mmHg. Booking BP at 12 weeks was 90/60 mmHg and BP at 20 weeks 95/60 mmHg. No urine proteinuria detected antenatally until 32w. Normal fetal growth. Mild peripheral oedema.
77. 40 weeks pregnant. Admitted with headache, hypertension 150/105 mmHg and +++proteinuria on urine dipstix. Obstetric ultrasound shows fetal IUGR. At pregnancy booking, her BP was 100/60 mmHg and her urinalysis showed no abnormality.
78. 34 weeks pregnant. Worsening hypertension and proteinuria over 4 weeks. Booking BP was 160/100 mmHg with 3 g proteinuria/24 h quantified. Oral labetalol therapy commenced at booking. Now BP 180/100 mmHg and 9 g proteinuria/24 h.

Options for Questions 79–83

Maternal medicine

A. Acute fatty liver of pregnancy
B. Antiphospholipid syndrome
C. Beta-thalassaemia major
D. Disseminated intravascular coagulation (DIC)
E. Gestational thrombocytopenia
F. Immune thrombocytopenic purpura
G. Pernicious anaemia
H. Pre-eclampsia/HELLP syndrome
 I. Sickle cell disease
J. Systemic lupus erythematosus

Instructions For each of the clinical scenarios involving pregnancy, select the most likely diagnosis from the list of options.

79. Associated with the presence of lupus anticoagulant and/or antiphospholipid antibody and adverse pregnancy event (such as recurrent first-trimester miscarriage, abruption or early-onset pre-eclampsia).

80. Rare, but serious, systemic thrombo-haemorrhagic disorder that may be triggered by: amniotic fluid embolism, severe haemorrhage, stillbirth and placental abruption.

81. A genetically inherited condition associated with episodic attacks of pain and severe anaemia. The condition is associated with IUGR, perinatal mortality and vascular thrombosis.

82. Accounts for 70 % of cases of thrombocytopenia in pregnancy, occurs in the third trimester of pregnancy and characterised by the presence of normal platelet count first two trimesters, low platelets in third trimester, absence of any maternal bleeding complications or immunological/hypertensive disorders, absence of fetal thrombocytopenia and completely resolves in the postnatal period.

83. Rare life-threatening complication of third trimester of pregnancy associated with nausea, vomiting, jaundice, hypoglycaemia, elevated white cell count, deranged liver function and clotting profile

Options for Questions 84–88

Women's sexual and reproductive health: STIs

A. *Candida albicans*
B. *Gardnerella vaginalis*
C. *Chlamydia trachomatis*
D. Group B streptococcus
E. *Haemophilus ducreyi* (chancroid)
F. Hepatitis B
G. Herpes simplex virus
H. HIV
 I. Human papilloma virus
 J. Lymphogranuloma venereum
K. *Mycoplasma hominis*
 L. *Neisseria gonorrhoeae*
M. Syphilis
N. *Trichomonas vaginalis*

Instructions Listed are recognised infections of the female genital tract. Select the most single most likely infective organism responsible according to the clinical characteristics described.

84. Specifically targeted by national vaccination programme, with vaccine given to girls aged 12–13 years.

85. Vesicular lesions appear within 7 days and lead to painful shallow ulcers.
86. Associated with vaginal pH > 4.5, clue cells and fishy amine odour.
87. Associated with microscopic motile trophozoites and vaginal pH > 4.5.
88. Itchy white vaginal discharge with vaginal pH ≤ 4.5.

Options for Questions 89–93

Women's sexual and reproductive health: STIs

A. *Candida albicans*
B. *Gardnerella vaginalis*
C. *Chlamydia trachomatis*
D. Group B streptococcus
E. *Haemophilus ducreyi* (chancroid)
F. Hepatitis B
G. Herpes simplex virus
H. HIV
 I. Human papilloma virus
J. Lymphogranuloma venereum
K. *Mycoplasma hominis*
L. *Neisseria gonorrhoeae*
M. Syphilis
N. *Trichomonas vaginalis*

Instructions Listed are recognised infections of the female genital tract. Select the single most likely infective organism responsible according to the clinical characteristics described.

89. Associated with postabortal and postpartum fevers, but the organism lacks cell wall therefore unable to Gram stain
90. The common cause of painful genital ulceration and tender inguinal adenopathy in Africa and Asia
91. Associated with itchy vaginal discharge, sensitive to metronidazole and important to treat both woman and partner to prevent infective recurrence
92. Infection that is screened for as part of routine pregnancy booking (<13 weeks' gestation) serology and where mode of delivery can impact on the risk of vertical transmission
93. Asymptomatic vaginal carriage in 20 % of women and associated with stillbirth and newborn neonatal sepsis

Options for Questions 94–98

Women's sexual and reproductive health: contraception

A. Combined oral contraceptive pill (COC)
B. Combined oral contraceptive transdermal patch (Evra)
C. Combined oral contraceptive vaginal ring (NuvaRing)
D. Copper intrauterine device (Cu-IUD)
E. Progestogen-only injection (Depo-Provera)
F. Hysteroscopic sterilisation
G. Laparoscopic sterilisation
H. Levonelle
 I. Mirena (LNG-IUS)
 J. Natural family planning (Persona)
K. Progestogen-only pill (POP)
L. Progestogen-only implant (Nexplanon)
M. Ulipristal acetate
N. Vasectomy

Instructions Each clinical scenario refers to a woman seeking contraception given a particular set of medical circumstances and preferences. For each scenario, select the most appropriate contraceptive method from the options listed. The same contraceptive method may be valid in more than one clinical scenario.

94. 24 years old, strong FH of ovarian cancer with proven BRCA genetic mutation. Has had one child and is planning to have bilateral oophorectomy following birth of the second child. Seeks effective contraception that would be beneficial to her long-term health.

95. 30 years old, always forgetful with contraception. Wishes the longest possible interval between needing to renew contraception. In a stable relationship. Nulliparous. Not keen on having things inserted in her vagina or uterus.

96. 48 years old, infrequent-cycle heavy menstrual bleeding. Fed up with heavy periods and current contraception of POP. Stable relationship. Family complete. Considering starting oestrogen replacement therapy (HRT) when menopause occurs.

97. 40 years old, smoker, obese (BMI 40), 3 previous LSCSs, family complete, seeks permanent effective contraception. Partner refuses to take contraceptive precautions.

98. 18 years, painful periods, irregular menstrual cycles wishes contraception then can help normalise her periods. She is nulliparous. She does not like tablets, injections, implants or wishes to insert things in her vagina.

Options for Questions 99–103

Women's sexual and reproductive health: contraception

A. Combined oral contraceptive pill (COC)
B. Combined oral contraceptive transdermal patch (Evra)
C. Combined oral contraceptive vaginal ring (NuvaRing)
D. Copper intrauterine device (Cu-IUD)
E. Progestogen-only injection (Depo-Provera)
F. Hysteroscopic sterilisation
G. Laparoscopic sterilisation
H. Levonelle
 I. Mirena (LNG-IUS)
 J. Natural family planning (Persona; Clearblue)
K. Progestogen-only pill
L. Progestogen-only implant (Nexplanon)
M. Ulipristal acetate
N. Vasectomy

Each clinical scenario refers to a woman seeking contraception given a particular set of medical circumstances and preferences. For each scenario, select the most appropriate contraceptive method from the options listed. The same contraceptive method may be valid in more than one clinical scenario.

99. 20 years old, sickle cell disease, experiences painful sickle cell crises with menstruation. She is nulliparous. She has had some symptom alleviation when using POP, but she is occasionally forgetful with pill taking. She wants to start a family in 1 year.

100. 26 years old, infrequent periods, mild hirsutism, mild acne and polycystic ovaries on pelvic ultrasound. Wishes effective contraception that may also reduce her hirsutism and acne.

101. 24 years old, strong FH of ovarian cancer with proven BRCA genetic mutation. Has had one child and is planning to have bilateral oophorectomy following birth of the second child. Seeks effective contraception that would be beneficial to her long-term health.

102. 35 years old, trying to conceive by improving her understanding of when her fertile period is during her menstrual cycle to better time sexual intercourse. Has been told by a friend of a method that is obtainable over the counter without prescription.

103. 21 years old, unprotected sexual intercourse 4 days earlier. Currently she is day 18 of her 28-day menstrual cycle. Wishes the most effective method to avoid pregnancy. This is her third episode of requesting emergency contraception.

Options for Questions 104–108

A. IVF
B. Surgical treatment
C. Sperm washing
D. Laparoscopic ovarian drilling
E. Metformin
F. Reassurance/no treatment needed
G. Clomiphene citrate
H. Laparoscopic cystectomy
 I. IUI
J. Donor sperm

104. A 28-year-old known to have mild endometriosis which was treated by abla-
     tion has been trying to conceive for 18 months. There are no other factors
     affecting fertility.
105. A woman with unilateral 3 cm endometrioma.
106. A woman with hydrosalpinges needs IVF treatment.
107. A 36-year-old HIV-negative patient wishes to conceive with a man who is
     HIV positive. However, he is not compliant with HAART.
108. A 28-year-old has PCOS and a BMI of 33. She has a 2-year history of second-
     ary subfertility. There are no other factors affecting fertility.

Answers to EMQs

30

Answers with Explanation

1-C(CVS)—at 11 weeks gestation with a previous history of genetic syndrome, in this case beta-thalassemia, autosomal recessive with a 25 % chance of recurrence, a CVS would be ideal. CVS can be done at 11 weeks to obtain fetal DNA—allows for earlier diagnosis and, if results are unfavourable, gives the option of a first-trimester TOP.

2-A(Amniocentesis)—Amniocentesis is a method of obtaining fetal cells from the amniotic fluid which can then be cultured to obtain a fetal karyotype. It can be done after 15 weeks of gestation and in this scenario is the ideal option to confirm fetal karyotype as per the patient's wish.

3-H(Cervical length by TVS)—Women with a history of spontaneous second-trimester loss or preterm delivery who have not undergone a history-indicated cerclage may be offered serial sonographic surveillance, as there is evidence to suggest that those who experience cervical shortening are at an increased risk of subsequent second-trimester loss/preterm birth and may benefit from ultrasound-indicated cerclage, while those whose cervix remains long have a low risk of second-trimester loss/premature delivery.

References Cervical cerclage. RCOG Green-Top guideline No. 60. 2011. http://www.rcog.org.uk/files/rcog-corp/GTG60cervicalcerclage.pdf

4-I(Fetal ultrasound study)—Ultrasound scan assessment should be undertaken as part of the preliminary investigations of a woman presenting with RFM after 28+0 weeks of gestation if the perception of RFM persists despite a normal CTG or if there are any additional risk factors for FGR/stillbirth.

References Reduced fetal movements. RCOG Green-Top guideline No. 57. 2011. http://www.rcog.org.uk/files/rcog-corp/GTG57RFM25022011.pdf

© Springer India 2016
C. Ratha, J. Gupta, *SBAs and EMQs for MRCOG II*,
DOI 10.1007/978-81-322-2689-5_30

Answers with Explanation

5-G(Fetal blood transfusion)—Fetal parvovirus infection is known to cause fetal anaemia and hence hydrops. Intrauterine fetal blood transfusion will help correct the fetal anaemia and resolve the hydrops. As parvoviral infection is generally self-limiting, the overall results of fetal blood transfusion are very good.

References To M, Kidd M, Maxwell D. Prenatal diagnosis and management of fetal infections. Obstet Gynaecol. 2009;11:108–16.

6-D(Fetoscopic laser coagulation of placental anastomotic vessels)—This is a case of severe twin to twin transfusion in an MCDA twin pregnancy. The ideal treatment in this case is fetocopic LASER photocoagulation of the anastomotic vessels. Severe twin–twin transfusion syndrome presenting before 26 weeks of gestation should be treated by laser ablation rather than by amnioreduction or septostomy.

References Management of monochorionic twin pregnancy. RCOG Green-Top guideline No. 51. 2008. http://www.rcog.org.uk/files/rcog-corp/uploaded-files/T51ManagementMonochorionicTwinPregnancy2008a.pdf

7-C(Selective feticide)—Selective feticide is an invasive ultrasound-guided procedure. It is a reasonable alternative to expectant management or termination of the whole pregnancy in cases of twin pregnancy discordant for major fetal anomaly. Common indications are chromosomal anomalies, major structural anomalies and genetic disorders. The preferred route of fetal entry is transabdominal. Complications include pregnancy loss (6–12 %), preterm delivery (8 %), chorioamnionitis, placental abruption, bleeding, maternal coagulopathy, psychological stress and depression. The risk to the normal fetus is of extreme preterm delivery, neurodevelopment delay as a result of the death of its co-twin (much lower in dichorionic than monochorionic twins) and intrauterine death.
Termination may be granted if 'there is a substantial risk that if the child were born, it would suffer from such physical or mental abnormalities as to be seriously handicapped' (UK Abortion Act 1967, amended 1991, clause E). The risk of stillbirth after the procedure is 6–12 %, similar to the risk of stillbirth in multifetal gestation (12.3 %). The ongoing presence of the anomalous fetus potentially increases the complications in the antenatal period to those of a twin pregnancy, thereby putting the normal fetus at risk. Thus, selective feticide, by reducing the ongoing risks of the pregnancy, is beneficial to the mother in improving the chances of having at least one normal child.

References (a) National Collaborating Centre for Women's and Children's Health. Multiple pregnancy-the management of twin and triplet pregnancies in the antenatal period (NICE clinical guideline 129). National Institute for Health and Clinical Excellence. London; 2011.

(b) Selective termination in dichorionic twins discordant for congenital defect., Fetal Medicine Unit, Madrid, Spain. Eur J Obstet Gynaecol. 2012;161(1):8–11.

8-E-(Amniodrainage)—Therapeutic amniocentesis (amnioreduction/amniodrainage) has also been proposed in singleton pregnancies to reduce maternal symptoms, given by overdistension of the uterus in severe and acute hydramnios. The reduction in maternal distressing symptoms is significant.

References (a) Elliott JP, et al. Large volume therapeutic amniocentesis in the treatment of hydramnios. Obstet Gynecol. 1994;84:1025–7.
(b) Piantelli G, et al. Amnioreduction for treatment of severe polyhydramnios. Acta Biomed. 2004;75(1):56–8.

Answers

(9) A. Lichen sclerosus
Lichen sclerosus can occur in any age group. Skin in the whole genital region may be affected, including the perianal area and genitocrural folds. The skin has well-demarcated whitening that does not extend to the vaginal mucosa. Pruritus is a common associated symptom.
(10) A. Lichen sclerosus
The classical histological features are an atrophic epidermis with overlying hyperkeratosis, an effaced dermoepidermal junction, superficial dermal hyalinisation and lymphocytic infiltration.
(11) E. Psoriasis
Vulval psoriatic lesions are well defined, uniform and symmetrical. The appearance is that of a beefy-red area that may affect any part of the vulva, but not the vaginal mucosa. Characteristic lesions may be present in other locations. Histologically, there is papillomatosis, parakeratosis with neutrophil exocytosis and spongiform pustules.
(12) F. Herpes simplex
The lesions described are likely to represent herpes simplex. The differential diagnosis of genital ulcers also includes chancroid and syphilis.

Answers

(13) F–Power calculation
The power of a study is determined by the sample size and the difference between the magnitudes of difference between the outcomes. This needs to be determined so that sample size can be estimated.
(14) J—Systematic review

A comprehensive review of all the evidence, conducted with scientific methods, is
likely to give the most reliable evidence.

(15). C—Intention to treat analysis

A study that includes all the patients initially recruited in the final analysis is called
an intention to treat analysis.

Answers

(16) E—Nexplanon implant

Many of the options listed may be appropriate in such a scenario. However, one
must balance the risks with the failure rate. High-dose progesterone and oestrogens are absolute contraindications, but adequate contraception is essential as
pregnancy has a high risk of maternal mortality. In a 16 year old, Nexplanon is
more desirable than a levonorgestrel intrauterine system as the uterus may not
have fully developed. The patient must be counselled with regard to abnormal
vaginal bleeding that occurs with the use of Nexplanon.

(17) B—Copper IUCD

A previous failure, in consideration of her age and marital status and in the absence
of menorrhagia, the IUCD is the best choice.

(18) D—GyneFix IUD

The GyneFix IUCD is designed for the nulliparous patient. The use of condoms
should also be advised to avoid sexually transmitted infection.

Answers

(19) E—Endometrial outpatient biopsy

Endometrial biopsy is the most useful next step investigation as this is likely to give
a histological diagnosis. Hysteroscopy may also be useful but will not give a
histological diagnosis.

(20) F—Fsh, Lh and oestradiol

The only part missing in the history is 'hot flushes'. The single most useful diagnosis would be a hormonal profile. A hysteroscopy may be a useful investigation,
but alone may not give a diagnosis.

(21) B—Cervical smear

Women with HIV infection are more likely to develop cervical cancer, as the history
suggests here. A cervical smear should give a diagnosis. Any immunocompro-
mised woman should have annual smears.

Answers

(22) B—0.5 %

Bowel adhesions to the anterior abdominal wall are found in 0.5 % of patients without prior surgery, 20 % with a previous Pfannenstiel incision and 50 % with a previous midline incision.

(23) J—Reduces incidence of vascular trauma only

Open laparoscopy will reduce the incidence of vascular trauma and is advocated in patients with an anticipated complicated entry due to previous surgery. Current evidence suggests that bowel injury is not reduced, but is more readily identified.

References Preventing entry-related gynaecological laparoscopic injuries. RCOG Green-Top guideline No. 49. 2008. http://www.rcog.org.uk/files/rcog-corp/uploaded-files/GT49PreventingLaparoscopicInjury2008.pdf

(24) I

Explanation For women having continuous EFM, a documented systematic assessment based on these definitions and classifications should be undertaken every hour. During episodes of abnormal FHR patterns when the woman is lying supine, she should be advised to adopt the left-lateral position. Prolonged use of maternal facial oxygen therapy may be harmful to the baby and should be avoided. There is no research evidence evaluating the benefits or risks associated with the short-term use of maternal facial oxygen therapy in cases of suspected fetal compromise. In the presence of abnormal FHR patterns and uterine hypercontractility not secondary to oxytocin infusion, tocolysis should be considered. A suggested regimen is subcutaneous terbutaline 0.25 mg. In the event of abnormal CTG following epidural top up, it may be reasonable to infuse intravenous fluids to prevent hypotension.

References http://www.nice.org.uk/guidance/cg55/resources/guidance-intrapartum-care-pdf

(25) L

Explanation A diagnosis of delay in the established first stage of labour needs to take into consideration all aspects of progress in labour and should include:

- Cervical dilatation of less than 2 cm in 4 h for first labours.
- Cervical dilatation of less than 2 cm in 4 h or a slowing in the progress of labour for second or subsequent labours.
- Descent and rotation of the fetal head.
- Changes in the strength, duration and frequency of uterine contractions.

If slow progress is due to ineffective contractions, then oxytocin infusion should be started. Effective uterine contractions are defined as 3–5 contractions in ten minutes each lasting 45–55 s.

References http://www.nice.org.uk/guidance/cg55/resources/
guidance-intrapartum-care-pdf

(26) J

Explanation In view of the abnormal CTG and the vaginal exam findings fulfilling
criteria for safe instrumental delivery, it would be acceptable to resort to an instrumental delivery. The choice of instrument depends on the operator's experience.
    Classification for operative vaginal delivery:

Outlet.

– Fetal scalp visible without separating the labia.
– Fetal skull has reached the pelvic floor.
– Sagittal suture is in the anteroposterior diameter or right or left occiput anterior
  or posterior position (rotation does not exceed 45°).
– Fetal head is at or on the perineum.
– Low leading point of the skull (not caput) is at station plus 2 cm or more and not
  on the pelvic floor.

Two subdivisions:

• Rotation of 45° or less from the occipitoanterior position
• Rotation of more than 45° including the occipitoposterior position

Mid:

– Fetal head is no more than 1/5th palpable per abdomen.
– Leading point of the skull is above station plus 2 cm but not above the ischial
  spines.

Two subdivisions:

• Rotation of 45° or less from the occipitoanterior position
• Rotation of more than 45° including the occipitoposterior position

High:
Not included in the classification as operative vaginal delivery is not recommended
  in this situation where the head is 2/5th or more palpable abdominally and the
  presenting part is above the level of the ischial spines.

References Operative vaginal delivery. RCOG Green-Top guideline No. 26.

(27) D

Explanation Changing from intermittent auscultation to continuous EFM in low-
risk women should be advised for the following reasons:

– Significant meconium-stained liquor, and this change should also be considered
  for light meconium-stained liquor.

- Abnormal FHR detected by intermittent auscultation (less than 110 beats per minute [bpm], greater than 160 bpm, any decelerations after a contraction).
- Maternal pyrexia (defined as 38.0C once or 37.5C on two occasions 2 h apart).
- Fresh bleeding developing in labour.
- Oxytocin use for augmentation.
- The woman's request.

References http://www.nice.org.uk/guidance/cg55/resources/guidance-intrapartum-care-pdf

(28) M

Explanation Observations during the first stage of labour include:

- 4-hourly temperature and blood pressure
- Hourly pulse
- Half-hourly documentation of frequency of contractions
- Frequency of emptying the bladder
- Vaginal examination *offered 4-hourly*, or where there is concern about progress or in response to the woman's wishes (after abdominal palpation and assessment of vaginal loss)

In addition:

Intermittent auscultation of the fetal heart after a contraction should occur for at least 1 min, at least every 15 min, and the rate should be recorded as an average. The maternal pulse should be palpated if a FHR abnormality is detected to differentiate the two heart rates. Ongoing consideration should be given to the woman's emotional and psychological needs, including her desire for pain relief.

References http://www.nice.org.uk/guidance/cg55/resources/guidance-intrapartum-care-pdf

(29) B

Explanation Category 1 CS is when there is immediate threat to the life of the woman or fetus, and category 2 CS is when there is maternal or fetal compromise which is not immediately life threatening.

This patient requires a category 1 CS in the presence of fetal bradycardia.

References http://www.nice.org.uk/guidance/cg132/resources/guidance-caesarean-section-pdf

(30) G

Explanation Women with prelabour rupture of membranes at term (at or over 37 weeks) should be offered a choice of induction of labour with vaginal PGE2 or expectant management.

Induction of labour is appropriate approximately 24 h after prelabour rupture of the membranes at term. Vaginal PGE2 is the preferred method of induction unless there are contraindications. It should be used as a gel or tablets or a controlled release pessary. The recommended regimens are:

– One cycle of vaginal PGE2 tablets or gel: one dose, followed by a second dose after 6 h if labour is not established (up to a maximum of two doses)
– One cycle of vaginal PGE2 controlled release pessary: one dose over 24 h

References http://www.nice.org.uk/guidance/cg70/resources/guidance-induction-of-labour-pdf

(31) N

Explanation For women having continuous EFM, a documented systematic assessment based on these definitions and classifications should be undertaken every hour. During episodes of abnormal FHR patterns when the woman is lying supine, she should be advised to adopt the left-lateral position. Prolonged use of maternal facial oxygen therapy may be harmful to the baby and should be avoided. In the presence of abnormal FHR patterns and uterine hypercontractility not secondary to oxytocin infusion, tocolysis should be considered. A suggested regimen is subcutaneous terbutaline 0.25 mg.

References http://www.nice.org.uk/guidance/cg55/resources/guidance-intrapartum-care-pdf

(32) D

Explanation Changing from intermittent auscultation to continuous EFM in low-risk women should be advised for the following reasons:

– Significant meconium-stained liquor, and this change should also be considered for light meconium-stained liquor
– Abnormal FHR detected by intermittent auscultation (less than 110 beats per minute [bpm]; greater than 160 bpm; any decelerations after a contraction)
– Maternal pyrexia (defined as 38.0C once or 37.5C on two occasions 2 h apart)
– Fresh bleeding developing in labour
– Oxytocin use for augmentation
– The woman's request

References http://www.nice.org.uk/guidance/cg55/resources/guidance-intrapartum-care-pdf

(33) M

Explanation Observations during the first stage of labour include:

- 4-hourly temperature and blood pressure
- Hourly pulse
- Half-hourly documentation of frequency of contractions
- Frequency of emptying the bladder
- Vaginal examination *offered 4-hourly*, or where there is concern about progress or in response to the woman's wishes (after abdominal palpation and assessment of vaginal loss).

In addition:

Intermittent auscultation of the fetal heart after a contraction should occur for at least 1 min, at least every 15 min, and the rate should be recorded as an average. The maternal pulse should be palpated if a FHR abnormality is detected to differentiate the two heart rates. Ongoing consideration should be given to the woman's emotional and psychological needs, including her desire for pain relief.

References http://www.nice.org.uk/guidance/cg55/resources/guidance-intrapartum-care-pdf

(34) D

Explanation After delivery, the placental bed, caesarean section and episiotomy wounds, cervical and vaginal lacerations are all susceptible to bacterial infection. Prolonged rupture of membranes, prolonged labour, operative vaginal delivery, caesarean section, pre-existing vaginal infection or history of Group B streptococcal (GBS) infection, postpartum haemorrhage, wound haematoma, retained pieces of placenta, membranes or intrauterine clot, or retained swabs all increase the risk of postpartum infection. The condition presents with lower abdominal pain, fever and offensive vaginal discharge or secondary postpartum haemorrhage. Management consists of broad spectrum antibiotics with coverage for anaerobic organisms as well.

References Glackin K, Harper M. Postpartum pyrexia. Obstet Gynaecol Reprod Med. 22(11):327–31.

(35) H

Explanation Pregnancy itself affects the immune system, and conditions such as anaemia, impaired glucose tolerance or diabetes mellitus reduce resistance to infection. Obesity, an increasing problem in the developed world, is a risk factor for sepsis, as is multiparity. Antibiotic prophylaxis plays an important role in preventing surgical-site infection. Therapy should be directed towards likely offending organisms endogenous in the lower genital tract including: *Escherichia coli*, other Gram-negative rods, Streptococcus species, *Staphylococcus aureus*, coagulase-negative staphylococci, *Enterococcus faecalis*, *Gardnerella vaginalis* and anaerobes including Bacteroides species and Peptostreptococcus species. To optimise intraoperative tissue concentration, prophylactic antibiotics should be given at the time of induction. Repeated doses confer no further benefit and increase the risk of adverse effects and antibiotic resistance. The antibiotic of choice should be well tolerated, safe to use and will be determined by local microbial population and their known sensitivities.

References Glackin K, Harper M. Postpartum pyrexia. Obstet Gynaecol Reprod Med. 22(11):327–31.

(36) **J**

Explanation Caesarean section has become the most common obstetric surgery, with one in three of pregnant women having a caesarean delivery. The use of urinary catheters during and after CS is routinely used with caesarean delivery. Alleged benefits of using catheters include the following: it maintains bladder drainage that may improve visualisation during surgery and minimise bladder injury, and there is less retention of urine after operation, but it could be associated with an increased incidence of urinary tract infection, urethral pain, voiding difficulties after removal of the catheter, delayed ambulation and increased hospital stay. Prophylactic antibiotics reduce the rate of bacteriuria and other signs of infection, such as pyuria, febrile morbidity and Gram-negative isolates in patients' urine, in surgical patients who undergo bladder drainage for at least 24 h postoperatively.

References Abdel-Aleem H, Aboelnasr MF, Jayousi TM, Habib FA. Indwelling bladder catheterisation as part of intraoperative and postoperative care for caesarean section. Cochrane Database Syst Rev. 2014, Issue 4. Art. No.: CD010322.

Lusardi G, Lipp A, Shaw C. Antibiotic prophylaxis for short-term catheter bladder drainage in adults. Cochrane Database Syst Rev. 2013;7:CD005428.

(37) **B**

Explanation Aspiration pneumonitis is a syndrome resulting from the inhalation of gastric contents. The incidence in obstetric anaesthesia has fallen, largely due to improved anaesthetic techniques and the increased use of regional anaesthesia at caesarean section. However, aspiration pneumonitis is still a cause of maternal morbidity and mortality, and it is important to use effective prophylaxis. Antacids (like sodium citrate), H_2 receptor antagonists (like ranitidine) and proton pump antagonists (like omeprazole), all reduce the acidity of the stomach contents. An antacid plus an H_2 receptor antagonist also reduce acidity. In theory, a combination like this, where the antacid acts quickly and the H_2 receptor antagonists takes a little longer, should protect at periods of greatest risk, i.e. the beginning and end of the procedure (i.e. intubation and extubation).

References Paranjothy S, Griffiths JD, Broughton HK, Gyte GML, Brown HC, Thomas J. Interventions at caesarean section for reducing the risk of aspiration pneumonitis. Cochrane Database Syst Rev. 2014, Issue 2. Art. No: CD004943.

(38) A

Explanation The symptoms and signs of VTE include leg pain and swelling (usually unilateral), lower abdominal pain, low-grade pyrexia, dyspnoea, chest pain, haemoptysis and collapse. It is up to ten times more common in pregnant women than in nonpregnant women of the same age and can occur at any stage of pregnancy, but the puerperium is the time of highest risk. When suspected, objective testing should be performed expeditiously, and treatment with low molecular weight heparin (LMWH) started until the diagnosis is excluded by objective testing, unless treatment is strongly contraindicated. Where there is clinical suspicion of acute PTE, a chest X-ray should be performed. Compression duplex Doppler should be performed where this is normal. If both tests are negative with persistent clinical suspicion of acute PTE, a ventilation–perfusion (V/Q) lung scan or a computed tomography pulmonary angiogram (CTPA) should be performed.

References RCOG Green-Top guideline No. 37b. The acute management of thrombosis and embolism during pregnancy and the puerperium.

(39) J

Explanation Uterine rupture is a well-recognised complication of labour when a uterine scar exists. The risk is undoubtedly related to the site of the uterine scar and probably to the number of previous uterine surgeries. Rarely, rupture is recognised only after delivery of the baby and should be a differential diagnosis for postpartum collapse. If the rupture extends into the broad ligament, the woman can present with gradually increasing abdominal pain and a very tender abdominal mass. Diagnosis of uterine rupture warrants resuscitation and exploratory laparotomy. The importance of immediate senior involvement and teamwork cannot be overemphasised. Repair of the uterus is possible in the majority of women. In others, haemorrhage from extension of the rupture into the broad ligament or extensive damage to the uterus requires hysterectomy. Hysterectomy rates following uterine rupture have been quoted as 3.4/10 000 women choosing trial of labour following caesarean section.

References Manoharan M, Wuntakal R, Erskine K. Uterine rupture: A revisit. Obstet Gynaecol. 2010;12:223–30.

(40) E

Explanation After delivery, the placental bed, caesarean section and episiotomy wounds, cervical and vaginal lacerations are all susceptible to bacterial infection. Prolonged rupture of membranes, prolonged labour, operative vaginal delivery, caesarean section, pre-existing vaginal infection or history of Group B streptococcal (GBS) infection, postpartum haemorrhage, wound haematoma, retained pieces of placenta, membranes or intrauterine clot, or retained swabs all increase the risk of postpartum infection. The condition presents with lower abdominal pain, fever and offensive vaginal discharge or secondary postpartum haemorrhage. Management consists of broad spectrum antibiotics with coverage for anaerobic organisms as well.

References Glackin K, Harper M. Postpartum pyrexia. Obstet Gynaecol Reprod Med. 22(11):327–31.

(41) D

Explanation Disseminated intravascular coagulation (DIC) is a type of coagulopathy characterised by widespread intravascular activation of the coagulation system leading to vascular deposition of fibrin and a consumption of clotting factors. It is associated with certain obstetric complications including amniotic fluid embolisation, placental abruption and severe chorioamnionitis. It may also be triggered by massive blood loss. The management of a coagulopathy requires effective communication with the haematologist who will advise on the use of clotting factors. Ideally, coagulopathy should be prevented by anticipating depletion in clotting factors and transfusing appropriately. It is not necessary to wait for laboratory clotting results if a developing coagulopathy is suspected. A prothrombin time (PT) and APTT ratios of >1.5 are associated with an increased risk of a clinical coagulopathy; in the presence of ongoing bleeding, this requires correction with FFP.

References Moore J, Chandraharan E. Management of massive postpartum haemorrhage and coagulopathy. Obstet Gynaecol Reprod Med. 20(6):174–80.

(42) I

Explanation Uterine inversion, either partial or complete, is a rare but serious obstetric complication. It may present:

– Acutely—within 24 h of delivery
– Subacutely—over 24 h and up to the 30th postpartum day
– Chronic—more than 30 days after delivery

It presents most often with symptoms of a postpartum haemorrhage. The classic presentation is of:

- Postpartum haemorrhage
- Sudden appearance of a vaginal mass
- Cardiovascular collapse (varying degrees)
  Treatment should follow a logical progression.
  Hypotension and hypovolaemia require aggressive fluid and blood replacement.

Immediate uterine repositioning is essential for acute puerperal inversion. Measures may include:

- Preparing theatres for a possible laparotomy.
- Administering tocolytics to allow uterine relaxation. For example:
  - Nitroglycerin (0.25–0.5 mg) intravenously over 2 min
  - Terbutaline 0.1–0.25 mg slowly intravenously
  - Magnesium sulphate 4–6 g intravenously over 20 min
- Attempt prompt repositioning of the uterus. This is best done manually and quickly, as delay can render repositioning progressively more difficult. Reposition the uterus (with the placenta if still attached) by slowly and steadily pushing upwards.
- If this fails, then a general anaesthetic is usually required. The uterus may then be returned by placing a fist on the fundus and gradually pushing it back manually into the pelvis through the dilated cervix.
- Maintain bimanual uterine compression and massage until the uterus is well contracted and bleeding has stopped.
- If this is unsuccessful, a surgical approach is required. Laparotomy for surgical repositioning is more usual (find and apply traction to the round ligaments), but a vaginal or even laparoscopic approach can be used.
- General anaesthetic or uterine relaxant is then stopped and replaced with oxytocin, ergometrine or prostaglandins.
- Start antibiotics and continue the stimulant for at least 24 h. Monitor closely after repositioning, in order to avoid reinversion.

References Beringer RM, Patteril M. Puerperal uterine inversion and shock. Br J Anaesth. 2004;92(3):439–41.

(43) A

Explanation When uterine atony is perceived to be a cause of the bleeding, the following mechanical and pharmacological measures should be instituted, in turn, until the bleeding stops. These are done along with or following initial resuscitative efforts which include fluid replacement and continuous monitoring of maternal parameters.

- Bimanual uterine compression (rubbing up the fundus) to stimulate contractions.
- Ensure bladder is empty (Foley catheter, leave in place).
- Syntocinon 5 units by slow intravenous injection (may have repeat dose).

- Ergometrine 0.5 mg by slow intravenous or intramuscular injection (contraindicated in women with hypertension).
- Syntocinon infusion (40 units in 500 ml Hartmann's solution at 125 ml/h) unless fluid restriction is necessary.
- Carboprost 0.25 mg by intramuscular injection repeated at intervals of not less than 15 min to a maximum of 8 doses (contraindicated in women with asthma).
- Direct intramyometrial injection of carboprost 0.5 mg (contraindicated in women with asthma), with responsibility of the administering clinician as it is not recommended for intramyometrial use.
- Misoprostol 1000 micrograms rectally.

References http://www.rcog.org.uk/files/rcog-corp/GT52Postpartum Haemorrhage0411.pdf

(44) I

Explanation Rare meat should be avoided in pregnancy because of the risk of toxoplasmosis. The *Toxoplasma gondii* parasite can be found in meat, soil, cat faeces and untreated water. It is often asymptomatic in the mother, 10–15 % of people develop symptoms similar to mild flu or glandular fever. Infection in the early stages of pregnancy increases the risk of miscarriage and stillbirth. The symptoms of congenital toxoplasmosis in the baby tend to be more severe if the mother was infected at the time of conception or in the first or second trimester. Symptoms can include hydrocephalus, brain damage, epilepsy, jaundice, reduced vision, organomegaly (liver and spleen), growth problems and cerebral palsy. Retinochoroiditis is a common complication of congenital toxoplasmosis. In pregnancy, toxoplasmosis is treated with spiramycin.

References NHS choices. Toxoplasmosis. 2013. Available at http://www.nhs.uk/Conditions/Toxoplasmosis/Pages/Introduction.aspx

(45) C

Explanation Vertical transmission (mother to infant) of hepatitis B infection occurs in 90 % of pregnancies where the mother is hepatitis B e-antigen positive and in about 10 % of surface antigen-positive, e-antigen-negative mothers. Most (>90 %) of the infected infants become chronic carriers. Infants born to infectious mothers are vaccinated from birth, usually in combination with hepatitis B-specific immunoglobulin 200 i.u. i.m. This reduces vertical transmission by 90 %.

References British Association of Sexual Health and HIV. United Kingdom national guideline on the management of the viral hepatitides A, B & C. 2008. Available at http://www.bashh.org/documents/1927.pdf

(46) G

Explanation Mould ripened soft cheeses, and unpasteurised cheeses should be avoided in pregnancy. This is because they are less acidic than hard cheeses and contain more moisture, creating an ideal environment for bacteria such as Listeria to grow. A Listeria infection in pregnancy doesn't usually pose a serious threat to the mother's health. However, it can cause pregnancy and birth complications and can result in miscarriage. An estimated 22 % of pregnancy-related cases of listeriosis will result in the death of the baby.

References NHS choices. Listeriosis. 2013. Available at http://www.nhs.uk/conditions/Listeriosis/Pages/Introduction.aspx

(47) L

Explanation If a pregnant woman develops varicella or shows serological conversion in the first 28 weeks of pregnancy, she has a small risk of fetal varicella syndrome. Spontaneous miscarriage does not appear to be increased if chickenpox occurs in the first trimester. Fetal varicella syndrome is characterised by one or more of the following: skin scarring in a dermatomal distribution, eye defects (microphthalmia, chorioretinitis, cataracts), hypoplasia of the limbs and neurological abnormalities (microcephaly, cortical atrophy, mental restriction and dysfunction of bowel and bladder sphincters). It does not occur at the time of initial fetal infection but results from a subsequent herpes zoster reactivation in utero and only occurs in a minority of infected fetuses.

References Royal College of Obstetricians and Gynaecologists. Chickenpox in pregnancy. Green-Top guideline No. 13. London: RCOG Press; 2011. Available at http://www.rcog.org.uk/files/rcog-corp/uploaded-files/GT13Chickenpoxin Pregnancy2007.pdf

(48) A

Explanation Around 10 % of infants born with congenital CMV infection have symptomatic disease at birth. The remaining asymptomatic 90 % of infected children generally have a better prognosis but are at risk for hearing loss. Hepatomegaly and splenomegaly are the most common findings on physical examination in neonates with symptomatic congenital CMV. Cutaneous manifestations of congenital CMV infection include jaundice and a generalised petechial rash caused by thrombocytopenia. Mental function and/or hearing are impaired in almost 90 % of the children who survive with symptomatic congenital CMV infection. 70 % of children with symptomatic infection have psychomotor retardation, usually accompanied by neurological complications and microcephaly. Hearing loss occurs in 50 % of patients with symptomatic congenital CMV.

References Nassetta L, Kimberlin D, Whitley R. Treatment of congenital cyto-megalovirus infection: implications for future therapeutic strategies. J Antimicrob Chemother. 63(5):862–7. Oxford University Press; 2009. Available at http://jac.oxfordjournals.org/content/63/5/862.long

(49) B

Explanation Women with twin and triplet pregnancies should be offered a first-trimester ultrasound scan when crown-rump length measures from 45 mm to 84 mm (at approximately 11 weeks 0 days to 13 weeks 6 days) to estimate gestational age, determine chorionicity and screen for Down syndrome. Chorionicity should be determined at the time of detecting twin and triplet pregnancies by ultrasound using the number of placental masses, the lambda or T-sign and membrane thickness. Sensitivity and specificity for diagnosis of monochorionic placentas drops beyond 14 weeks of gestation.

References NICE. Multiple pregnancy: the management of twin and triplet pregnancies in the antenatal period. Cg 129 2011. Available at http://publications.nice.org.uk/multiple-pregnancy-cg129/guidance
    Royal College of Obstetricians and Gynaecologists. Management of monochorionic twin pregnancy. Green-Top guideline No. 51. London: RCOG Press; 2008. Available at h t t p : / / w w w . r c o g . o r g . u k / f i l e s / r c o g - c o r p / u p l o a d e d - f i l e s / T51ManagementMonochorionicTwinPregnancy2008a.pdf

(50) C

Explanation The quadruple test window starts from 14 weeks + 2 days to 20 weeks + 0 days. A maternal blood sample is required for the analysis of human chorionic gonadotrophin (hCG), alpha-fetoprotein (aFP), unconjugated oestriol (uE3) and inhibin-A. This test has been retained because there will always be women who book too late in pregnancy for combined testing (about 15 % of the pregnant population) and wish to have screening. It is therefore important that women are made aware of the lesser performance of the quadruple test and that commissioners have in place the offer of combined testing for those who book in the recommended time window (10 + 1 to 14 + 0).

References NHS Fetal Anomaly Screening Programme. Screening for Down's syndrome: UK NSC policy recommendations. 2011–2014 model of best practice. Exeter, NHS evidence: 2011. Available at http://anr-dpn.vjf.cnrs.fr/sites/default/files/NSCModel-of-Best-Practice-DS%20screening2011-2014Sept2011.pdf

(51) C

Explanation Women with a history of spontaneous second-trimester loss or pre-term delivery who have not undergone a history-indicated cerclage may be offered serial sonographic surveillance, as there is evidence to suggest that those who experience cervical shortening are at an increased risk of subsequent second-trimester loss/preterm birth and may benefit from ultrasound-indicated cerclage. Insertion of a cerclage as a therapeutic measure in cases of cervical length shortening can be seen on transvaginal ultrasound. Ultrasound-indicated cerclage is performed on asymptomatic women who do not have exposed fetal membranes in the vagina. Sonographic assessment of the cervix is usually performed between 14 and 24 weeks of gestation.

References http://www.rcog.org.uk/files/rcog-corp/GTG60cervicalcerclage.pdf

(52) A

Explanation Preimplantation genetic diagnosis (PGD) is a technique that enables people with a specific inherited condition in their family to avoid passing it on to their children. It involves checking the genes of embryos created through IVF for this genetic condition.

Before PGD clinics are permitted to test for a condition or combination of conditions, the HFEA must first agree that the condition they want to test for is sufficiently serious. This list of conditions is those that the HFEA has so far agreed that it is acceptable for clinics to use PGD to test for. The list is given in the following link:

References http://guide.hfea.gov.uk/pgd/

(53) E

Explanation Risk factors for gestational diabetes should be determined at the booking appointment (BMI > 30, previous macrosomia, previous gestational diabetes, first-degree relative with diabetes, family origin with a high prevalence of diabetes). Women with any one of these risk factors should be offered testing for gestational diabetes using the 2 h 75 g oral glucose tolerance test (OGTT). Women who have had gestational diabetes in a previous pregnancy should be offered early self-monitoring of blood glucose or OGTT at 16–18 weeks and a further OGTT at 28 weeks if the results are normal. Women with any of the other risk factors for gestational diabetes should be offered an OGTT at 24–28 weeks.

References NICE. Diabetes in pregnancy: management of diabetes and its complications from preconception to the postnatal period. Cg 63 2008. Available at http://www.nice.org.uk/nicemedia/live/11946/41320/41320.pdf

(54) D

Explanation Ultrasound screening for fetal anomalies should be routinely offered, normally between 18 weeks 0 days and 20 weeks 6 days. The 20-week anomaly scan is to reassure the woman that her baby appears to have no obvious structural abnormalities. About 50 % (detection rates vary according to individual units) of significant abnormalities will be identified by a screening scan. The value of identifying fetal abnormalities at this stage is that it offers parents options. Some, probably the majority, for serious lesions, will elect to terminate the pregnancy. Those couples who choose to continue the pregnancy have the opportunity to prepare themselves through discussions with healthcare personnel and self-help groups, while attendants can ensure appropriate care during pregnancy and following delivery.

References NICE. Antenatal care. Cg 62 2010. Available at http://www.nice.org. uk/nicemedia/live/11947/40115/40115.pdf

Royal College of Obstetricians and Gynaecologists. Ultrasound screening. Women's health article. London: RCOG Press; 2000. Available at http://www.rcog. org.uk/womens-health/clinical-guidance/ultrasound-screening

(55) C

Explanation The quadruple test window starts from 14 weeks + 2 days to 20 weeks + 0 days. A maternal blood sample is required for the analysis of human chorionic gonadotrophin (hCG), alpha-fetoprotein (aFP), unconjugated oestriol (uE3) and inhibin-A. This test has been retained because there will always be women who book too late in pregnancy for combined testing (about 15 % of the pregnant population) and wish to have screening. It is therefore important that women are made aware of the lesser performance of the quadruple test and that commissioners have in place the offer of combined testing for those who book in the recommended time window (10 + 1 to 14 + 0).

References NHS Fetal Anomaly Screening Programme. Screening for Down's syndrome: UK NSC policy recommendations. 2011–2014 model of best practice. Exeter, NHS evidence; 2011. Available at http://anr-dpn.vjf.cnrs.fr/sites/default/files/NSCModel-of-Best-Practice-DS%20screening2011-2014Sept2011.pdf

(56) C

Explanation Women with a history of spontaneous second-trimester loss or preterm delivery who have not undergone a history-indicated cerclage may be offered serial sonographic surveillance, as there is evidence to suggest that those who experience cervical shortening are at an increased risk of subsequent second-trimester loss/preterm birth and may benefit from ultrasound-indicated cerclage. Insertion of a cerclage as a therapeutic measure in cases of cervical length shortening can be seen on transvaginal ultrasound. Ultrasound-indicated cerclage is performed on asymptomatic women who do not have exposed fetal membranes in the vagina. Sonographic assessment of the cervix is usually performed between 14 and 24 weeks of gestation.

References http://www.rcog.org.uk/files/rcog-corp/GTG60cervicalcerclage.pdf

(57) A

Explanation Preimplantation genetic diagnosis (PGD) is a technique that enables people with a specific inherited condition in their family to avoid passing it on to their children. It involves checking the genes of embryos created through IVF for this genetic condition.

Before PGD clinics are permitted to test for a condition or combination of conditions, the HFEA must first agree that the condition they want to test for is sufficiently serious. This list of conditions are those that the HFEA has so far agreed that it is acceptable for clinics to use PGD to test for. The list is given in the following link:

References http://guide.hfea.gov.uk/pgd/

(58) G

Explanation All women require follow-up imaging if the placenta covers or overlaps the cervical os at 20 weeks of gestation. Asymptomatic women without a previous caesarean section whose placenta has just reached but not covered the cervical os at the 20-week scan and in whom pregnancy is progressing normally can be managed expectantly, with further imaging at 36 weeks of gestation. In cases with asymptomatic suspected major placenta praevia or a question of placenta accrete (e.g. previous caesarean section), imaging should be performed at around 32 weeks of gestation to clarify the diagnosis and allow planning for third-trimester management, further imaging and delivery.

References Royal College of Obstetricians and Gynaecologists. Placenta praevia, placenta praevia accreta and vasa praevia: diagnosis and management. Green-Top guideline No. 27. London: RCOG Press; 2011. Available at http://www.rcog.org. uk/files/rcog-corp/GTG27PlacentaPraeviaJanuary2011.pdf

(59) H

Explanation For patients < 25 years, a biopsy need not be performed if the following criteria are satisfied: ultrasound reveals a solid lesion which has benign ultrasound features (e.g. ellipsoid shape (wider than tall)), a well-defined outline with smooth edges or fewer than four gentle lobulations. If a biopsy has been performed and confirmed benign, then follow-up is advised.

References http://www.associationofbreastsurgery.org.uk/media/4585/best_practice_diagnostic_guidelines_for_patients_presenting_with_breast_symptoms.pdf

(60) A

Explanation Polymastia (supernumerary breasts) is a relatively common congenital condition in which abnormal accessory breast tissue is found in addition to normal breast tissue. However, it may not be evident until puberty. Although accessory breast tissue is usually found along the thoracoabdominal region of the milk line (67 %), which extends down to the groin, ectopic breast tissue may also be present in locations such as the face, back and thigh.

About 2–% of females and 1–3 % of males are affected by this condition, a third of whom have more than one area of supernumerary tissue growth. Occurrence rates vary widely on the basis of ethnicity and gender, ranging from as low as 0.6 % in Caucasians to as high as 5 % in Japanese females.

Symptoms include swelling and tenderness of the affected region, thickening of the axilla and limited range of shoulder motion, and irritation from clothing. These symptoms are usually worsened by the onset of puberty and pregnancy. Supernumerary breast tissue also develops during this period alongside normal breast tissue growth.

References Down S, Barr L, Baildam AD, Bundred N. Management of accessory breast tissue in the axilla. Br J Surg. 2003;90:1213–4.

(61) D

Explanation Most often, fibrocystic changes are diagnosed based on symptoms alone. These symptoms can include breast pain and tender lumps or thickened areas in the breasts. The symptoms may change as the woman moves through different stages of the menstrual cycle. Sometimes, one of the lumps might feel firmer or have other features that lead to a concern about cancer. When this happens, a biopsy may be needed to make sure that cancer is not present. Fibrosis and cysts can also be seen on a biopsy that is done for a lump that turns out to be something else.

Most women with fibrocystic changes and no bothersome symptoms do not need treatment, but closer follow-up may be advised. Women with mild discomfort may get relief from well-fitted, supportive bras, applying heat or using over-the-counter pain relievers. For a very small number of women with painful cysts, draining the fluid with a needle can help relieve symptoms.

It has been suggested that many vitamin supplements relieve symptoms, but so far none have been proven to be of any use, and some may have dangerous side effects if taken in large doses.

Some doctors prescribe hormones, such as oral contraceptives (birth control pills), tamoxifen or androgens. But these are usually given only to women with severe symptoms because they can have serious side effects.

References http://www.cancer.org/healthy/findcancerearly/womenshealth/non-cancerousbreastconditions/non-cancerous-breast-conditions-fibrocystic-changes

(62) J

Explanation Signs and symptoms of breast cancer may include:

- A breast lump or thickening that feels different from the surrounding tissue
- Bloody discharge from the nipple
- Change in the size or shape of a breast
- Changes to the skin over the breast, such as dimpling
- Inverted nipple
- Peeling, scaling or flaking of the nipple or breast skin
- Redness or pitting of the skin over your breast, like the skin of an orange

For most patients, whether they are referred following breast screening or after presentation to a GP, diagnosis in the breast clinic is made by triple assessment (clinical assessment, mammography and/or ultrasound imaging, and core biopsy and/or fine needle aspiration cytology). It is best practice to carry out these assessments at the same visit.

Pretreatment ultrasound evaluation of the axilla should be performed for all patients being investigated for early invasive breast cancer, and, if morphologically abnormal lymph nodes are identified, ultrasound-guided needle sampling should be offered.

The routine use of magnetic resonance imaging (MRI) of the breast is not recommended in the preoperative assessment of patients with biopsy-proven invasive breast cancer or ductal carcinoma in situ.

References http://www.nice.org.uk/guidance/cg80/resources/guidance-early-and-locally-advanced-breast-cancer-pdf

(63) C

Explanation As far as hormone replacement therapy (HRT) is concerned, some studies have shown an increased incidence of benign breast disease in long-term HRT users, whereas other investigations have found either no effect or a protective effect. The use of HRT does not appear to influence the clinical pattern of benign breast disease in postmenopausal women, although enlargement of pre-existing cysts or fibroadenomas has been sometimes reported. The limited available data failed to detect a deleterious effect of HRT use in women with benign breast disease, even in those with increased breast cancer risk due to a family history or high-risk benign breast conditions.

References Gadducci A, Guerrieri ME, Genazzani AR. Benign breast diseases, contraception and hormone replacement therapy. Minerva Ginecol. 2012;64(1):67–74.

(64) J

Explanation Speculum examination will allow inspection of the vulva, vagina and cervix (ectropion, cervical polyps, discharge), for local causes of bleeding. A cervical screen for sexually transmitted infections can be done at the same time. However, cervical screening is not recommended if prior routine screen was found negative.

References Rao S. Intermenstrual and post coital bleeding. Obstet Gynaecol Reprod Med. 21(10):288–93.

(65) I

Explanation Retained products of conception following a medical abortion may be picked up ultrasound scan. However, decision to evacuate the uterus should be based on clinical findings rather than on the ultrasound features.

References http://www.rcog.org.uk/files/rcog-corp/Abortion_Guideline_ Summary.pdf

(66) L

Explanation Complete molar pregnancies are not associated with fetal parts, so suction evacuation is the method of choice for uterine evacuation. Medical evacuation of complete molar pregnancies should be avoided if possible. There is theoretical concern over the routine use of potent oxytocic agents because of the potential to embolise and disseminate trophoblastic tissue through the venous system. In addition, women with complete molar pregnancies may be at an increased risk for requiring treatment for persistent trophoblastic disease, although the risk for women with partial molar pregnancies needing chemotherapy is low (0.5 %).

References http://www.rcog.org.uk/files/rcog-corp/GT38Management Gestational0210.pdf

(67) D

Explanation In this woman, the diagnosis of ruptured ectopic pregnancy should be considered unless proven otherwise. However, the patient must be appropriately and rapidly resuscitated. This requires the insertion of two large-bore cannulae and the infusion of crystalloid or blood if significant haemorrhage is thought to have occurred. Resuscitation can take place while the patient is being prepared for theatre and should not delay surgical intervention, although this cannot and must not go ahead until the patient is stable and the anaesthetic team is happy.

References Raine-Fenning N, Hopkisson J. Management of ectopic pregnancy: a clinical approach. Obstet Gynaecol Reprod Med. 19(1):19–24.

(68) C

Explanation NICE guideline recommends offering systemic methotrexate as a first-line treatment to women who are able to return for follow-up and who have all of the following:

- No significant pain
- An unruptured ectopic pregnancy with an adnexal mass smaller than 35 mm with no visible heartbeat
- A serum hCG level less than 1500 IU/l
- No intrauterine pregnancy (as confirmed on an ultrasound scan)

References http://www.nice.org.uk/nicemedia/live/14000/61854/61854.pdf

(69) C

Explanation 'Pregnancy of uncertain viability' is defined as presence of an intra-uterine sac <25 mm mean diameter with no obvious yolk sac or fetus, or fetal echo >7 mm crown-rump length with no obvious fetal heart activity. In these circumstances, a repeat scan at a minimum interval of 1 week is necessary.

References Sagili H, Divers M. Modern management of miscarriage. Obstet Gynaecol. 2007;9:102–8.

(70) B

Explanation Also known previously as missed abortion, delayed miscarriage, silent miscarriage or anembryonic pregnancy. These reflect different stages in the same process. It is diagnosed when ultrasound detects fetal pole >7 mm with no fetal heart or gestation sac >25 mm with no fetal pole or yolk sac. Patient usually presents with minimal vaginal bleeding or pain and loss of pregnancy symptoms, but with a closed cervix.

References Sagili H, Divers M. Modern management of miscarriage. Obstet Gynaecol. 2007;9:102–8.

(71) H

Explanation Pregnancy of unknown location, defined as 'no signs of either intra- or extrauterine pregnancy or retained products of conception in a woman with a positive pregnancy test', occurs in approximately 8–31 % of pregnancies. Rates are lower, around 10 %, in departments with a specialised scanning service or if the patient is assessed by an expert and can be kept to a minimum by the critical application of transvaginal ultrasound and strict diagnostic criteria.

References Raine-Fenning N, Hopkisson J. Management of ectopic pregnancy: a clinical approach. Obstet Gynaecol Reprod Med. 19(1):19–24.

(72) D

Explanation Defined as bleeding without passage of tissue but with an open cervix. The patient may be managed by expectant, medical or surgical management. Surgical evacuation remains the treatment of choice if bleeding is excessive, vital signs are unstable or infected tissue is present in the uterine cavity (in which case surgery must be done under antibiotic cover). Fewer than 10 % of women who miscarry fall into these categories. Expectant management can be continued as long as the woman is willing and provided there are no signs of infection. For medical management, a variety of equally effective prostaglandin regimens have been described, including gemeprost 0.5–1 mg, vaginal misoprostol and oral misoprostol. However, vaginal misoprostol is as effective as oral misoprostol, with a significant reduction in the incidence of diarrhoea. Success rates varied from 61 to 95 %, mild–moderate bleeding lasted 4–6 days, side effects were tolerable in 96 % and satisfaction rates were 95 %.

References Sagili H, Divers M. Modern management of miscarriage. Obstet Gynaecol. 2007;9:102–8.

(73) J

Explanation In a case of ruptured ectopic pregnancy, the aim should be to prevent further blood loss as quickly as possible. Obviously there is no role for methotrexate. Once the abdomen has been opened, or a laparoscope safely inserted, the pelvis needs to be carefully inspected before proceeding. If this cannot be performed quickly or safely endoscopically, the abdomen must be opened to ensure further bleeding is stopped. The consultant gynaecologist on call must be informed and involved in the care of the patient. A team leader should be identified to ensure good communication. The timing of events must be noted and recorded and the whole event documented in detail, although this is often done in retrospect due to the urgency of the situation.

References Raine-Fenning N, Hopkisson J. Management of ectopic pregnancy: a clinical approach. Obstet Gynaecol Reprod Med. 19(1):19–24.

(74) G

Explanation As many women of reproductive age only present for the first time when pregnant, chronic hypertension is often revealed in the first half of pregnancy.

Approximately 90–95 % of cases of chronic hypertension are considered to be essential. Secondary causes account for approximately 5–10 %.

Causes of secondary chronic hypertension:

- Idiopathic (essential hypertension)
- Vascular disorders
Renovascular hypertension
Aortic coarctation
- Endocrine disorders
Diabetes mellitus
Hyperthyroidism
Hypothyroidism
Phaeochromocytoma
Acromegaly
Cushing's syndrome
Conn's syndrome
- Renal disorders
Renal failure resulting from:
Diabetic nephropathy
Reflux nephropathy
Chronic glomerulonephritis
Nephritic and nephrotic syndrome
Polycystic kidney
- Connective tissue disorders
Systemic lupus erythematosus
Systemic sclerosis
Polyarteritis nodosa
Rheumatoid disease

References McCarthy FP, Kenny LC. Hypertension in pregnancy. Obstet Gynaecol Reprod Med;22(6):141–6.

(75) C

Explanation The outcome of pregnancy in women with chronic renal disease depends on the following factors: the degree of renal impairment, the presence of chronic hypertension, the presence of proteinuria and the underlying renal pathology. These women should be cared for by a multidisciplinary team that includes midwives, specialists in maternal medicine and nephrologists, ideally in a tertiary centre. A baseline renal profile, including serum urea, creatinine, electrolytes, albumin and full blood count; urinalysis; and urine culture, should be performed. In addition, an assessment of proteinuria is necessary. These tests should be repeated every 4 weeks or more frequently, depending on the clinical situation.

They may need more frequent hospital visits, depending on the clinical situation. Regular scans are recommended every 4 weeks from 28 weeks of gestation onwards to check growth as well as liquor volume. Blood pressure monitoring and adequate control are important determinants of outcome. Preterm labour is common. In the absence of maternal or fetal deterioration, delivery should be planned at or near term. Early delivery is usually necessary for obstetric indications such as pre-eclampsia and fetal growth restriction or for rapidly deteriorating maternal renal function. Obstetric considerations should be the main determinant for caesarean section outcome.

References Kapoor N, Makanjuola D, Shehata H. Management of women with chronic renal disease in pregnancy. Obstet Gynaecol. 2009;11:185–91.

(76) E

Explanation Gestational hypertension is defined as a rise in the blood pressure in the absence of proteinuria after 20 weeks' gestation. True non-proteinuric pregnancy-induced hypertension does not appear to be associated with an increase in maternal or fetal morbidity. However, the risk of progression from pregnancy-induced hypertension to pre-eclampsia is approximately 20–30 %, and therefore vigilance is required. This increases to approximately 50 % when pregnancy-induced hypertension develops before 32 weeks' gestation. As a result of this risk of progression to pre-eclampsia, weekly urinalysis and BP checks are generally recommended in women with pregnancy-induced hypertension.

References McCarthy FP, Kenny LC. Hypertension in pregnancy. Obstet Gynaecol Reprod Med;22(6):141–6.

(77) H

Explanation Pre-eclampsia is defined by the International Society for the Study of Hypertension in Pregnancy as gestational hypertension of at least 140/90 mmHg on two separate occasions measured at least 4 h apart accompanied by significant proteinuria of at least 300 mg in a 24 h collection of urine, arising de novo after the 20th week of gestation in a previously normotensive woman and resolving completely by the 6th postpartum week. It usually occurs during the second half of pregnancy and complicates 2–8 % of pregnancies, depending on population studied.

Pre-eclampsia is twice as common in primigravid women as in women having second or later pregnancies. It is a potentially life-threatening hypertensive disorder of pregnancy characterised by vascular dysfunction and systemic inflammation involving the brain, liver and kidneys of the mother.

Pre-eclampsia also carries implications in adult life, with offspring of affected pre-eclamptic pregnancies demonstrating poor growth in childhood and an increased risk of hypertension, heart disease and diabetes.

References McCarthy FP, Kenny LC. Hypertension in pregnancy. Obstet Gynaecol Reprod Med;22(6):141–6.

(78) B

Explanation Chronic hypertension is defined as hypertension preceding pregnancy. Women with high blood pressure before the 20th week of pregnancy are assumed to have pre-existing or essential hypertension. As many women of reproductive age only present for the first time when pregnant, chronic hypertension is often revealed in the first half of pregnancy. Approximately 90–95 % of cases of chronic hypertension are considered to be essential. With superimposed pre-eclampsia, the principles of management include control of hypertension, prevention of seizures and optimising maternal and fetal outcome by appropriately timed delivery.

References McCarthy FP, Kenny LC. Hypertension in pregnancy. Obstet Gynaecol Reprod Med. 22(6):141–6.

(79) B

Explanation Antiphospholipid syndrome (APS) is an established cause of fetal loss. Explanations for the pathophysiology of APS-associated pregnancy loss include defective placentation due to a direct effect of anticardiolipin antibodies on trophoblast, activation of the complement system or thrombosis of the placental vasculature.

APS is defined by at least one clinical and one laboratory criterion. The clinical criteria include three or more spontaneous miscarriages or one fetal loss after 10 weeks' gestation. The laboratory criteria include persistent abnormality of one of the following tests measured at least twice and more than 6 weeks apart, a raised titre of IgG or IgM antibodies to cardiolipin (ACA) and B2 glycoprotein 1 antibodies or presence of lupus anticoagulant.

Two tests are necessary as mild viral infections can cause falsely positive results. The testing for lupus coagulant can be done using a number of coagulation-based assays, such as the dilute Russell viper venom test. Testing for ACA is done using the enzyme-linked immunosorbent assay technique. Patients with APS should be offered low-dose aspirin and heparin during pregnancy as this has shown to be effective in randomised controlled trials. Most units use low molecular weight heparin as this only has to be administered once a day.

References Quenby S. Recurrent miscarriage. Obstet Gynaecol Reprod Med. 20(10):305–10.

(80) D

Explanation   Disseminated intravascular coagulation (DIC) is a type of coagulopathy characterised by widespread intravascular activation of the coagulation system leading to vascular deposition of fibrin and a consumption of clotting factors. It is associated with certain obstetric complications including amniotic fluid embolisation, placental abruption and severe chorioamnionitis. It may also be triggered by massive blood loss. The management of a coagulopathy requires effective communication with the haematologist who will advise on the use of clotting factors. Ideally, coagulopathy should be prevented by anticipating depletion in clotting factors and transfusing appropriately. It is not necessary to wait for laboratory clotting results if a developing coagulopathy is suspected. A prothrombin time (PT) and APTT ratios of >1.5 are associated with an increased risk of a clinical coagulopathy; in the presence of ongoing bleeding, this requires correction with FFP.

References   Moore J, Chandraharan E. Management of massive postpartum haemorrhage and coagulopathy. Obstet Gynaecol Reprod Med. 20(6):174–80.

(81) I

Explanation   Sickle cell disease (SCD) is an autosomal recessive condition, which leads to lifelong haemolytic anaemia. Clinical features are intermittent episodes of severe pain and chronic complications including a high risk of stroke, renal dysfunction, retinopathy and cardiopulmonary disease. Advances in treatment have enabled affected women to live to childbearing age. Pregnancy and childbirth with SCD are considered high risk and are associated with increased maternal and fetal morbidity and mortality. A universal newborn screening programme provides for early identification of all affected newborns. The antenatal screening programme identifies women with haemoglobinopathies and offers them the option of fetal screening. Management of women with SCD begins with preconceptual care, which involves counselling, screening for end organ damage and a review of their medications. Multidisciplinary antenatal care is desirable. Contraception should be discussed post pregnancy.

References   Oteng-Ntim E, Nazir S, Singhal T, Howard J. Sickle cell disease in pregnancy. Obstet Gynaecol Reprod Med. 22(9):254–60.

(82) E

Explanation   This is the most common cause of thrombocytopenia in pregnancy, occurring in approximately 75 % of cases of thrombocytopenia and 8 % of all pregnancies. It is a benign condition usually found incidentally later in pregnancy, and there is no bleeding risk to mother or fetus. Counts are typically >70 and usually >100. Many of the features are similar to mild immune thrombocytopenia, and it can be difficult to distinguish between the two disorders. There are no specific diagnostic tests for either, and both conditions are diagnoses of exclusion. Rarely, cases of gestational thrombocytopenia with platelet counts as low as 50 have been described. Again, the outcome appears good.

References Myers B. Thrombocytopenia in pregnancy. Obstet Gynaecol. 2009;11:177–83.

(83) A

Explanation This rare disorder is associated with abnormalities in mitochondrial b oxidation and LCHAD deficiency. There is considerable overlap of the symptoms and signs with pre-eclampsia and HELLP syndrome. It is more common in multiple pregnancies, primis, obese women and with a male fetus. For features and investigations, the presentation is similar to that in HELLP syndrome with nausea, vomiting and abdominal pain, although the rise in serum transaminases, creatinine and leucocytosis tends to be more marked. Other discriminating features are hypoglycaemia and coagulopathy which are much more evident in AFLP. It may present postpartum with severe haemorrhage.

AFLP carries a high maternal and fetal mortality of between 2–18 % and 7–58 % respectively. Maternal complications include disseminated intravascular coagulation, renal failure, pancreatitis and (transient) diabetes insipidus. There is also a risk of progression to hepatic encephalopathy and fulminant liver failure.

If AFLP presents antenatally, then coagulopathy and hypoglycaemia should be treated aggressively, and delivery expedited. HDU and/or ITU involvement are/is usually required and early liaison with a specialist liver unit in case of progression to liver failure.

Postdelivery most women recover quickly, and management is conservative and supportive. Liver function may take up to 4 weeks to recover, and liver transplantation should be considered in those with liver rupture, severe encephalopathy or failure of liver recovery. The recurrence rate for AFLP is around 25 %.

References Cuckson C, Germain S. Hyperemesis, gastro-intestinal and liver disorders in pregnancy. Obstet Gynaecol Reprod Med 21(3):80–6.

(84) I

Explanation Vaccines are available to protect against the two most common HPV types (16 and 18) that cause cervical cancer and the two most common HPV types that cause genital warts (6 and 11). The national immunisation programme began in 2008 using a vaccine (Cervarix) against HPV 16 and 18. In 2012, the programme changed to use a vaccine (Gardasil) against HPV 6, 11, 16 and 18. Both HPV vaccines are over 99 % effective in preventing cervical abnormalities associated with HPV types 16 and 18 in women who have not already been infected by these types (Lu et al., 2011). The vaccines have not been shown to protect against disease if a woman has an active HPV infection. However, they may protect a woman who has already been exposed to HPV infections and is no longer infected. The vaccines will protect individuals against infection by the HPV vaccine types they have not already contracted. These vaccines do not protect against all HPV types that cause cervical cancer.

References https://www.gov.uk/government/uploads/system/uploads/attachment_data/file/207669/dh_133346.pdf

(85) G

Explanation Herpes simplex virus (HSV) is the most common cause of genital ulceration in the UK Symptomatic, primary infections are equally likely to be caused by type 1 or type 2 HSV, but recurrence is more likely with HSV type 2. Incidence rates of primary genital herpes simplex infection are highest in the 20- to 24-year age group (3/1000).

Most of those infected have subclinical or latent infection. Severity of symptoms is determined by prior immunity to HSV. The incubation period is 2–20 days. Most patients with primary infection have a 'flu-like' illness with fever and myalgia. Meningitis is possible. Genital lesions are vesicles, which rapidly ulcerate and remain painful for 10–12 days.

The urethra is often involved and dysuria might progress to urinary retention. HSV can also cause an autonomic neuropathy resulting in urinary retention. Vaginal discharge might reflect vaginal ulcers or cervicitis. Perianal involvement is common and does not necessarily result from anal intercourse. Proctitis symptoms might ensue. Inguinal lymphadenopathy is also common. Extragenital lesions might occur on the buttocks or thighs.

References Kieran E, Hay DP. Sexually transmitted infections. Curr Obstet Gynaecol. 2006;16:218–25.

(86) B

Explanation Up to 50 % of women with a clinical diagnosis of BV are asymptomatic. When present, however, the symptoms include a profuse, malodorous vaginal discharge. The offensive smell is due to the production of amines by anaerobic bacteria and is often worse after sex and during menses, when the higher pH causes further release of the amines. The discharge itself is usually white, thin and homogenous and not associated with any inflammation of the vulva or vagina.

References McCathie R. Vaginal discharge: common causes and management. Curr Obstet Gynaecol. 2006;16:211–7.

(87) N

Explanation Women infected with *T. vaginalis* might be asymptomatic at the time of diagnosis; however, if left untreated, they often develop symptoms. The most common complaint is vaginal discharge, classically described as green and frothy, although—practically speaking—it can be any colour. About 50 % of women find the discharge to be malodorous, and it often has a pH of >4.5. Other signs and symptoms of infection with *T. vaginalis* include vulval or vaginal itching, evidence of a vaginitis or a cervicitis on speculum examination and, very rarely, punctuate haemorrhages of the cervix (so-called strawberry cervix). Symptoms might be worse during or just after the menses.

References McCathie R. Vaginal discharge: common causes and management. Curr Obstet Gynaecol. 2006;16:211–7.

(88) A

Explanation The diagnosis of a candida infection can be made entirely clinically, based on the symptoms and signs. They include vulval itching or soreness, curdy white vaginal discharge without a smell, dysuria or superficial dyspareunia. Vulval itching is the most common symptom, and the discharge might be absent in 50 % of cases. The clinical signs include erythema of the vulva or vagina, vulval fissuring and oedema, and satellite lesions.

References McCathie R. Vaginal discharge: common causes and management. Curr Obstet Gynaecol. 2006;16:211–7.

(89) K

Explanation Mycoplasma hominis and ureaplasma spp. organisms (ureaplasmas) are those isolated most frequently from the human GU tract. Both mycoplasmas and ureaplasmas have a trilayered external membrane, rather than a rigid cell wall, rendering them resistant to b-lactam antibiotics. They are found to be associated with pregnancy-related complication—namely, preterm labour, PPROM, low birth weight as well as neonatal conjunctivitis and respiratory disease.

References Taylor-Robinson D, Lamont R. Mycoplasmas in pregnancy. BJOG. 2011;118:164–74.

(90) E

Explanation Chancroid is caused by a type of bacteria called *Haemophilus ducreyi*. The infection is found mainly in developing and third-world countries. Within 1 day–2 weeks after getting chancroid, the infected person develops a painful ulcer, with sharply defined borders and a grey base which bleeds easily when scraped. About half of infected men have only a single ulcer. Women often have four or more ulcers. In women the most common location for ulcers is the labia majora. 'Kissing ulcers' may develop. Other areas, such as the labia minora, perineum and the inner thighs, may also be involved. The most common symptoms in women are pain with urination and intercourse. The ulcer may look like a chancre, the typical sore of primary syphilis. About half of the people who are infected with a chancroid will develop enlarged inguinal lymph nodes. These nodes may l break through the skin and cause draining abscesses, also called buboes.

References   http://www.nlm.nih.gov/medlineplus/ency/article/000635.htm

(91) N

Explanation The most common complaint is vaginal discharge, classically described as green and frothy, although—practically speaking—it can be any colour. About 50 % of women find the discharge to be malodorous, and it often has a pH of >4.5. Other signs and symptoms of infection with *T. vaginalis* include vulval or vaginal itching, evidence of a vaginitis or a cervicitis on speculum examination and, very rarely, punctuate haemorrhages of the cervix (so-called strawberry cervix). Symptoms might be worse during or just after the menses. First-line treatment of infection with *T. vaginalis* requires systemic rather than topical treatment because the infection is not always confined to the vagina but may involve other parts of the urogenital tract. Recommended treatment regimens for *T. vaginalis*:

– Metronidazole 2 g orally in a single dose
   or
– Metronidazole 400 mg orally twice daily for 5 days

Both treatment regimens result in cure rates of 95 % in combination with partner notification and treatment. Providing the patient is compliant and the symptoms settle (if symptomatic), a repeat test following treatment is not necessary.

References   McCathie R. Vaginal discharge: common causes and management. Curr Obstet Gynaecol. 2006;16:211–7.

(92) H

Explanation The rate of mother-to-child transmission (MTCT) is almost 25 % without any interventions. But with uptake of interventions, especially HAART (highly active retroviral therapy), the MTCT is reduced to <1 %. For women taking HAART, a decision regarding recommended mode of delivery should be made after review of plasma viral load results at 36 weeks.

Vaginal delivery is recommended for women on HAART with an HIV viral load <50 HIV RNA copies/mL plasma. For women with a plasma VL of >50 HIV RNA copies/mL at 36 weeks, prelabour CS (PLCS) should be considered. In women in whom a vaginal delivery has been recommended and labour has commenced, obstetric management should follow the same guidelines as for the uninfected population.

References http://www.bhiva.org/documents/Guidelines/Pregnancy/2012/hiv1030_6.pdf

(93) D

Explanation Group B streptococcus (*Streptococcus agalactiae*) is recognised as the most frequent cause of severe early-onset (at less than 7 days of age) infection in newborn infants. However, there is still controversy about its prevention. The current US guidelines advise that all women colonised with GBS at 35–37 weeks of gestation (or labouring before this time) should be offered IAP, usually in the form of high-dose intravenous benzylpenicillin or ampicillin. IAP has been shown to significantly reduce the risk of culture-positive early onset but not late-onset disease (occurring 7 or more days after birth). According to RCOG guidelines, IAP is offered when women are found to have GBS bacteriuria or GBS positive on vaginal swabs (not offered routinely though) during pregnancy. Women presenting in established preterm labour with intact membranes with no other risk factors for GBS should not routinely be offered IAP unless they are known to be colonised with GBS. Immediate induction of labour and IAP should be offered to all women colonised with GBS and with prelabour rupture of membranes at 37 + 0 weeks of gestation or more. IAP should be offered to women with a previous baby with neonatal GBS disease.

References http://www.rcog.org.uk/files/rcog-corp/GTG36_GBS.pdf

(94) A

Explanation A collaborative reanalysis of 45 epidemiological studies demonstrated that with every 5 years of use, there is approximately a 20 % reduction in the risk of ovarian cancer. A woman's risk after 15 years of use was around half of those who had never used COC. The protective effect increases with increasing duration of use, and while it decreases over time after stopping, it has been shown to last up to several decades after use.

Among BRCA mutation carriers too, COC use has been shown to provide a protective effect against ovarian cancer. It is strongly recommended that COC be offered to women desirous of contraception until more definitive interventions can be planned.

References http://www.fsrh.org/pdfs/CEUGuidanceCombinedHormonalContraception.pdf

(95) L

Explanation Nexplanon® is a progestogen-only subdermal implant that has now replaced the contraceptive implant, Implanon. Nexplanon and Implanon are bio-equivalent (i.e. they both contain 68 mg etonogestrel and they have the same release rate and 3-year duration of action). The progestogen-only implant is a long-acting reversible method of contraception (LARC). The primary mode of action is to prevent ovulation. Implants also prevent sperm penetration by altering the cervical mucus and possibly prevent implantation by thinning the endometrium.

References http://www.fsrh.org/pdfs/CEUGuidanceProgestogenOnlyImplants.pdf

(96) I

Explanation Most of the contraceptive effect of the LNG-IUS is mediated via its progestogenic effect on the endometrium which prevents implantation. Within 1 month of insertion, high intrauterine concentrations of levonorgestrel induce endometrial atrophy. In addition, changes in the endometrial stroma, an increase in endometrial phagocytic cells and a reduction in sperm penetration through cervical mucus contribute to the contraceptive effect. Apart from contraceptive efficacy, it is also useful in the treatment of heavy menstrual bleeding and in women on ERT.

References http://www.fsrh.org/pdfs/CEUGuidanceIntrauterine ContraceptionNov07.pdf

(97) F

Explanation Hysteroscopic sterilisation by tubal cannulation and placement of intrafallopian implants is usually performed with the patient under local anaesthesia and/or intravenous sedation. A hysteroscope is inserted through the vagina and cervix. A flexible microinsert is passed through the hysteroscope using a guidewire and placed into each of the fallopian tubes. The microinserts induce scar tissue formation, which occludes the fallopian tubes and prevents conception. An additional form of contraception should be used until imaging has confirmed satisfactory placement of the microinserts. Imaging may be by X-ray or ultrasound scanning initially, followed by hysterosalpingogram (HSG) in selected patients or by HSG as a routine test to ensure that the fallopian tubes have been occluded.

References Hysteroscopic sterilisation by tubal cannulation and placement of intrafallopian implants. NICE interventional procedures guidance [IPG315].

(98) B

Explanation Combined vaginal ring (CVR) releases EE and etonogestrel at daily rates of 15 µg and 120 µg, respectively. A ring is inserted into the vagina and left in continuously for 21 days. After a ring-free interval of 7 days to induce a withdrawal bleed, a new ring should be inserted. It works primarily by inhibiting ovulation via action on the hypothalamo–pituitary–ovarian axis to reduce luteinising hormone and follicle-stimulating hormone. Alterations to cervical mucus and the endometrium may also contribute to the efficacy.

References http://www.fsrh.org/pdfs/CEUGuidanceCombinedHormonal Contraception.pdf

(99) E

Explanation DMPA is a 3 monthly injectable contraception that acts primarily by inhibiting ovulation. There is thickening of cervical mucus, inhibiting sperm penetration into the upper reproductive tract. In addition, changes to the endometrium make it an unfavourable environment for implantation. In addition, it has been shown that it can reduce sickling crises in women with sickle cell anaemia.

References http://www.fsrh.org/pdfs/CEUGuidanceProgestogenOnly Injectables09.pdf

(100) A

Explanation COCs are a reasonable treatment for acne in women who also desire contraception. A systematic review of 25 randomised controlled trials concluded that COCs reduced acne severity and lesion counts compared with placebo. This review was unable to show that one type of COC was clearly superior to another in the treatment of acne. Therefore, any COC is likely to be effective in the treatment of acne. COC treatment for hirsutism has not been as well studied as for acne. Nevertheless, physiologically, it makes sense that COCs should also improve hirsutism and COCs are used clinically for that purpose. While COCs can prevent an increase in hirsutism, any existing hair will need to be treated cosmetically. Two small trials have shown that drospirenone-, levonorgestrel- and desogestrel-containing COCs are effective in improving hirsutism.

References Carey MS, Allen RH. Non-contraceptive uses and benefits of combined oral contraception. Obstet Gynaecol. 2012;14:223–8.

(101) A

Explanation A collaborative reanalysis of 45 epidemiological studies demonstrated that with every 5 years of use, there is approximately a 20 % reduction in the risk of ovarian cancer. A woman's risk after 15 years of use was around half of those who had never used COC. The protective effect increases with increasing duration of use, and while it decreases over time after stopping, it has been shown to last up to several decades after use.

Among BRCA mutation carriers too, COC use has been shown to provide a protective effect against ovarian cancer. It is strongly recommended that COC be offered to women desirous of contraception until more definitive interventions can be planned.

References http://www.fsrh.org/pdfs/CEUGuidanceCombinedHormonal Contraception.pdf

(102) J

Explanation Persona works by monitoring the changes in hormones (luteinising hormone and oestrogen) which control the cycle and identifies the days when one is at significant risk of becoming pregnant. PERSONA consists of Test Sticks and a hand-held Monitor. The Test Sticks collect hormones from the first urine of the day and process them into information that the Monitor can read. The Monitor reads, stores and uses the information from the Test Sticks to let you know whether you are at risk of becoming pregnant ('Red' Day) or not ('Green' Day).

References http://www.persona.info/uk/

(103) D

Explanation All eligible women presenting between 0 and 120 h of UPSI or within 5 days of expected ovulation should be offered a Cu-IUD because of the low documented failure rate. This may also provide the advantage of ongoing contraceptive use in a person not on regular use of any particular method. The other options are oral ulipristal acetate and LNG.

The efficacy of ulipristal acetate (UPA) has been demonstrated up to 120 h and can be offered to all eligible women requesting EC during this time period. It is the only oral EC licensed for use between 72 and 120 h. The efficacy of levonorgestrel (LNG) has been demonstrated up to 96 h; between 96 and 120 h efficacy is unknown. Use of LNG beyond 72 h is outside the product licence.

References http://www.fsrh.org/pdfs/CEUguidanceEmergencyContraception11. pdf

(104) F – *Reassurance/No treatment needed*

Explanation Advise them to try to conceive for a total of 2 years before IVF will be considered.

References NICE guideline –Fertility.

(105) H Explanation: *Laparoscopic cystectomy* Women with ovarian endometriomas should be offered laparoscopic cystectomy because this improves the chance of pregnancy.

References NICE guideline –Fertility.

(106) B Explanation: *Surgical treatment* Women with hydrosalpinges should be offered salpingectomy, preferably by laparoscopy, before IVF treatment because this improves the chance of a live birth.

References NICE guideline –Fertility.

(107) C Explanation: *Sperm washing* If the man is HIV positive but he is not compliant with HAART or the viral load is greater than 50 copies/ml, sperm washing should be offered. It reduces, but does not eliminate, the risk of HIV transmission.

References NICE guideline –Fertility.

(108) E Explanation: *Metformin* The treatment options in any order are clomiphene citrate or metformin or a combination of both. Women with a BMI of 30 or over should be encouraged to lose weight. Metformin may be more successful in ovulation induction in women with raised BMI.

References NICE guideline –Fertility.